Human Virology

Human Virology

A text for students of medicine, dentistry, and microbiology

Third edition

Leslie Collier

Emeritus Professor of Virology
University of London

and

John Oxford

Professor of Virology
Scientific Director of Retroscreen Virology Ltd
Professor of Virology at St Bartholomew's and The
Royal London Hospital, Queen Mary's School
of Medicine and Dentistry

With illustrations by

Jim Pipkin

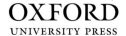

OXFORD
UNIVERSITY PRESS

OXFORD

UNIVERSITY PRESS

Great Clarendon Street, Oxford OX2 6DP

Oxford University Press is a department of the University of Oxford.
It furthers the University's objective of excellence in research, scholarship,
and education by publishing worldwide in

Oxford New York

Auckland Cape Town Dar es Salaam Hong Kong Karachi
Kuala Lumpur Madrid Melbourne Mexico City Nairobi
New Delhi Shanghai Taipei Toronto

With offices in

Argentina Austria Brazil Chile Czech Republic France Greece
Guatemala Hungary Italy Japan South Korea Poland Portugal
Singapore South Korea Switzerland Thailand Turkey Ukraine Vietnam

Oxford is a registered trade mark of Oxford University Press
in the UK and in certain other countries

Published in the United States
by Oxford University Press Inc., New York

British Library Cataloguing in Publication Data
Data available

Library of Congress Cataloging in Publication Data
Data available

Typeset by
Expo Holdings Sdn Bhd, Malaysia

Printed in Italy by Lito Terrazzi s.r.l.

ISBN 0-19-856660-3 (Pbk.) 978-0-19-856660-1 (Pbk.)

10 9 8 7 6 5 4 3 2 1

Preface to the second edition

We planned the first edition of this book on a 'need to know' basis, its primary object being to provide students and medical and dental practitioners with the knowledge essential for an informed approach to the prevention and treatment of viral infections. We aimed also at supplying just enough basic virology to underpin the more practical aspects—clinical manifestations, epidemiology, pathogenesis, immune responses, and so forth. And not least, we tried our best to make the text as readable as is possible, given the highly technical nature of some of the material.

The success of *Human Virology* prompted us to produce a second edition, which, in view of the accelerating pace of advance in this field, is already overdue. The general arrangement of the book in four parts is the same: General principles, Specific infections, Special syndromes, and Practical aspects. There are, however, some important changes and additions:

- Every chapter has been revised and updated.

- There are more diagrams than previously, and those being reused have been improved to aid clarity.

- Both of the large and unwieldy chapters on herpesviruses and hepatitis viruses have been broken down into an introductory section followed by three chapters, each dealing with a specific group of viruses, including the more recently discovered agents in both families.

- As might be expected, the chapter on prion diseases has been considerably amplified.

- There are two new mini-chapters summarizing respiratory and sexually transmitted infections.

- Looking to the future, there is a new chapter on emerging infections.

However, those already familiar with the first edition of *Human Virology* will immediately recognize a more fundamental alteration in its scope. Since its first appearance in 1993, the expansion of molecular biology in the world of microbes has been immense, and nowadays even the medical weeklies contain articles that quite recently would have been relegated to the more abstruse specialist journals. In recognizing this trend, we have supplied considerably more details of genome structure and replication than hitherto. At the same time, we do not wish to overburden those with little interest in these aspects, which are identified by the use of italics; the more clinically oriented can skip these sections without feeling unduly guilty.

That said, there is an irreducible minimum of molecular biology that must be assimilated, and here we have done our best to make life easier by improving diagrams and simplifying explanations. Representative genome maps are provided for some of the viruses described.

In matters of nomenclature and classification we continue to follow the Reports of the International Committee on Taxonomy of Viruses (ICTV), the sixth and latest available of which appeared in 1995; it recommended a number of changes, which we have adopted.

This new edition appears at a time when our understanding of microbes and their diseases is increasing exponentially. Virology is at the leading edge of these advances; and we hope that this book will provide both a helpful guide to current knowledge and a glimpse of the exciting possibilities to come as we enter the new Millennium.

London
2000

L.H.C.
J.S.O.

Preface to the third edition

The appearance of this, the third edition of *Human Virology* confirms its acceptance as a valuable teaching aid and as a source of information on virology in general and its clinical aspects in particular. Its popularity has been confirmed with its publication in Italian, French, and Polish editions.

The aim of the book and the approaches adopted were set out in the prefaces to the previous two editions and we strongly recommend reading them as a prelude to the main body of the work. Readers of the previous editions will recognize the format, in which the text is divided into four main parts: General principles, Specific infections, Special syndromes, and Practical aspects. As previously, these are supplemented by appendices dealing respectively with safety precautions, notifiable infections, and recommendations for further reading. Readers of past editions will thus often recognize familiar territory, which may, however, have undergone substantial modification during extensive revision and updating since the last edition.

It has always been our aim to produce a text that is clear, concise, and readable. We hope our readers will agree that the third edition of *Human Virology* meets these criteria.

London L.H.C.
2006 J.S.O.

Contents

Abbreviations

Although abbreviations are defined in the text at first mention, a complete list is given here for ease of reference.

ACV	aciclovir
AIDS	acquired immunodeficiency syndrome
APC	antigen-presenting cell
ARC	AIDS-related complex
AZT	azidothymidine
bDNA	branched DNA
BL	Burkitt's lymphoma
BMT	bone-marrow transplant
BSE	bovine spongiform encephalopathy
CD	cluster of differentiation
CDC	Centers for Disease Control (USA)
cDNA	complementary DNA
CELO	chick embryo lethal orphan virus
CIN	cervical intraepithelial neoplasia
CIS	Commonwealth of Independent States (formerly USSR)
CJD	Creutzfeldt–Jakob disease
CJD^{nv}	new variant Creutzfeldt–Jakob disease
CMI	cell-mediated immunity
CMV	cytomegalovirus
CNS	central nervous system
CPE	cytopathic effect
CSF	cerebrospinal fluid
D&V	diarrhoea and vomiting
ddI	didanosine
DHSS	dengue haemorrhagic shock syndrome
DNA	deoxyribonucleic acid
ds	double-stranded (nucleic acid)
EA	early antigen (of EBV)
EBNA	Epstein–Barr (virus) nuclear antigen
EBV	Epstein–Barr virus
ELISA	enzyme-linked immunosorbent assay
EM	electron microscope, microscopy

FITC	fluorescein isothiocyanate
GSSD	Gerstmann–Sträussler–Scheinker disease
HA	haemagglutinin
HAART	highly active antiretroviral therapy
HAM	HTLV-I-associated myelopathy
HAV	hepatitis A virus
HBcAg	hepatitis B core antigen
HBeAg	hepatitis B e antigen
HBsAg	hepatitis B surface antigen
HBV	hepatitis B virus
HCC	hepatocellular carcinoma
HCV	hepatitis C virus
HDCS	human diploid cell strain virus (of rabies virus)
HDV	deltavirus (hepatitis D virus)
HEV	hepatitis E virus
HFRS	haemorrhagic fever with renal syndrome
HGV	hepatitis G virus
HHV	human herpesvirus
HI	haemagglutination inhibition
HIV	human immunodeficiency virus
HLA	human leucocyte antigen
HNIG	human normal immunoglobulin
HPS	hantavirus pulmonary syndrome
HPV	human papillomavirus
HRIG	human rabies immunoglobulin
HSV	herpes simplex virus
HTLV	human T-cell leukaemia virus
HuCV	human calicivirus
ICAM	intercellular adhesion molecule
ICTV	International Committee on Taxonomy of Viruses
IDDM	insulin-dependent diabetes mellitus
IEM	immunoelectron microscopy
IFN	interferon
IL	interleukin

IPV	inactivated poliomyelitis vaccine	RNA	ribonucleic acid
kb	kilobase	RNase	ribonuclease
kbp	kilobase pairs	RNP	ribonucleoprotein
kDa	kilodalton	RSV	respiratory syncytial virus
LCM	lymphocytic choriomeningitis virus	RT	reverse transcriptase
LTR	long terminal repeat	SARS	severe acute respiratory syndrome
LYDMA	lymphocyte-detected membrane antigen (of EBV)	snRNPs	small nuclear ribonucleoprotein particles
MBM	meat and bonemeal (cattle dietary supplement)	SRSV	small round structured virus
ME	myalgic encephalomyelitis	ss	single-stranded (nucleic acid)
MHC	major histocompatibility complex	STD	sexually transmitted disease
MMR	measles–mumps–rubella (vaccine)	SV	simian vacuolating (virus)
MP	mononuclear phagocytic cell	Taq	Thermophilus aquaticus (polymerase)
MRC	Medical Research Council (UK)	Tc	cytotoxic T cell
mRNA	messenger RNA	Tdh	delayed hypersensitivity cell
NA	neuraminidase	Th	T-helper cell
NANB	non-A, non-B hepatitis	TK	thymidine kinase
NK	natural killer (cell)	TNF	tumour necrosis factor
NPC	nasopharyngeal carcinoma	ts	temperature-sensitive (mutants)
NS	non-structural	Ts	T-suppressor cell
NS1	non-structural protein 1	TSE	transmissible spongiform encephalopathy
ntr	non-translated regions	TSP	tropical spastic paraparesis
OPV	oral (attenuated) polio vaccine	VAIN	vaginal intraepithelial neoplasia
ORF	open reading frame	VCA	viral capsid antigen (of EBV)
PCR	polymerase chain reaction	VEE	Venezuelan equine encephalitis
PHLS	Public Health Laboratory Service (UK)	VIN	vulvar intraepithelial neoplasia
PML	progressive multifocal leucoencephalopathy	VSV	vesicular stomatitis virus
PrP	proteinaceous infectious particle (prion)	VZV	varicella-zoster virus
PrPC	normal cellular PrP	WHO	World Health Organization
PrPSc	scrapie-type PrP	YF	yellow fever
RIA	radioimmunoassay	ZIG	zoster immune globulin

Part 1

General principles

Virology: how it all began

History is more or less bunk
Henry Ford (1863–1947)

1 Introduction

Although not many would agree entirely with the great industrialist's dismissal of the past, there is certainly a tendency for today's students of science to regard the history of their subjects as a waste of time. Given the sheer volume of material that has to be absorbed, digested, and regurgitated in the examinations, this feeling is understandable; but it is a pity, because history, especially that of virology, provides not only a fascinating account of technological developments in microbiology, but also the intellectual challenge of thinking about how life began.

Viruses do not leave fossils, and our views on their origin must be based on the most slender of clues; the rest is at present speculation, based mostly on our knowledge of the behaviour of today's viruses, bacteria, and cells, but influenced sometimes by individual ideas of religion and even cosmology. For example, some believe that viruses, like all other life forms, were divinely created, and others that they originated in comets or elsewhere in outer space. However, most people would probably take the intuitive approach that simple organisms preceded more complicated ones, and that bacteria evolved from what were once free-living, self-replicating molecules that resemble today's viruses. However, this superficially attractive argument ignores the fact that modern viruses have an absolute requirement for living cells in which to multiply, and that—as far as we know—no such organic, self-replicating molecules exist nowadays. An alternative notion is that viruses evolved from cellular components—nucleic acids and proteins—as semi-independent agents able to replicate only by exploiting the energy and reproductive machinery of the cells of higher organisms.

Scientists can speculate endlessly about such theories, and some have been stimulated to test them in the laboratory; others again are searching for clues in meteorites, and in samples taken from Mars by space probes. All findings are as yet inconclusive, so we must leave this fascinating topic and take a look at the more down to earth story of how virology, rather than the viruses themselves, evolved. Many of the points in this introductory chapter are dealt with in more detail later in the book.

2 How viruses were discovered

As a science, virology evolved later than bacteriology; this is not surprising, because the comparatively large size of bacteria made them visible even with the simple microscope invented by Antonie van Leeuwenhoek, a Dutch optician, who in 1673 first described their appearances. However, it was not until the nineteenth century that Louis Pasteur, Robert Koch, and others established the biological properties of bacteria and yeasts, first as the causes of fermentation and putrefaction, then as causes of disease. But, although the physical nature of viruses was not fully revealed until the invention of the electron microscope (EM), the infections they caused have been known and feared since the dawn of history. Two examples from ancient Egypt are shown in Chapters 14 (Fig. 14.2) and 16 (Fig. 16.1).

The Latin word *virus* means 'poisonous fluid', and this is just what they seemed to the first virologists. In the latter part of the nineteenth century, huge strides were being made in the study of microbes. In Pasteur's laboratory, Charles Chamberland devised a filter that would hold back even the smallest bacteria; next, Iwanowski in Russia and Beijerinck in Holland both showed that a plant infection, tobacco mosaic, could be transmitted by extracts that had been passed through a Chamberland filter, and hence could not contain bacteria. Soon afterwards, foot-and-mouth disease of cattle was also transmitted by bacteria-free filtrates, and it came to be realized that living agents, smaller than any known bacteria but capable of multiplying, could cause a wide range of diseases in plants and animals.

3 How they were grown in the laboratory

Very quickly, Beijerinck realized that whatever it was that caused tobacco mosaic would grow only in living cells and could not be cultivated in the media used for bacteria. At that time, there was no way of growing cells in the laboratory, and so it was that all the early work on virus infections had to be done with intact plants or animals. Thus Pasteur used dogs and rabbits in the development of a rabies vaccine, and rabbits, calves, and sheep were used for work on smallpox vaccine. But, in addition to humanitarian considerations, for much experimental work the use of animals is unsatisfactory on grounds of expense and reproducibility, and biologists have always sought to replace them by tests *in vitro* (i.e. in the test tube). This goal was achieved in 1928, when a virus was first grown in suspensions of minced kidney tissue. During the following decade, a great advance was made with the propagation of many viruses in developing chick embryos, but the really big breakthrough came with the discovery of antibiotics in the 1940s and 1950s. Until then, it was very difficult to keep cell and tissue cultures free from contamination with airborne bacteria and moulds, but the addition of antibiotics to the culture medium inhibited these unwanted contaminants and permitted the handling of cultures on the open bench.

The new millennium is witnessing a great expansion of molecular techniques for studying micro-organisms. In particular, the ability to identify, isolate, clone, and express specific nucleotide sequences has led to the identification of hitherto unknown viruses that cannot be propagated in the laboratory by conventional methods. Polio virus has been synthesized as an infectious entity in the laboratory. The polio virus genome can now be manipulated at will. Undoubtedly we are on the edge of new discoveries. However, the latest virus to be discovered (SARS) was first identified not by molecular biology but by more traditional cell culture and EM.

4 Sizes and shapes

Light microscopes were well advanced by the end of the nineteenth century and the appearances of many bacteria—cocci, rods, spirals, and so forth—were already familiar. Furthermore, the vast majority proved larger than 0.25 µm, which is about the limit of resolution of the light microscope, and so were easy to see. The reverse is true of viruses, which are smaller than this limit (Fig. 1.1). Poxviruses are an exception, and it is a scientific oddity that, as long ago as 1886, one of them was actually seen and measured accurately by John Buist, a Scottish microscopist. However, study of the shapes and sizes—the **morphology** of viruses—had to await the coming of the EM in 1939. Whereas the resolving power of the conventional microscope is limited by the wavelength of light, the EM is under no such constraint, functioning as it does with a beam of electrons focused by electromagnets. It is interesting that the first virus to be identified—

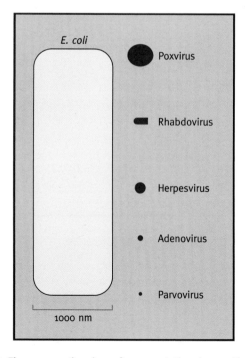

Fig. 1.1 The comparative sizes of representative viruses. The viruses are compared with a typical bacterium (*Escherichia coli*).

tobacco mosaic— was also the first to be seen under the EM, appearing as regular rod-shaped particles measuring about 25 × 300 nanometres. (A nanometre (nm) is the unit used for expressing the sizes of viruses. It is 1/1000 of the micrometre unit (μm) used for bacteria.) At about the time that the EM started to come into its own, other methods of measuring viruses were developed. One involved the passing of suspensions through a series of filters with accurately graded pore diameters; the size of the virus was determined from the smallest pore diameter through which it could be filtered; another was high-speed centrifugation, whereby the sizes of viruses could be estimated from their sedimentation characteristics. These were quite good methods, but were eventually replaced by the less cumbersome and more precise EM technique, which had the great additional advantage of revealing the shapes of viruses; it was soon found that the morphology of nearly all of them conforms to one of two basic patterns, spherical or helical; these terms will be explained more fully in Chapter 2.

5 Replication

To reproduce, bacterial cells and all higher life forms must undergo some form of fission, a complex process involving many synthetic and other biochemical activities mediated by a battery of enzymes, terminating in division of the genetic material between two or more daughter cells. Viruses, with their minute size and simple structure, could not possibly replicate in this way. But, if not, how? The answer to this question was to prove crucial in defining the fundamental difference between viruses and all other life forms.

Yet again, it was the tobacco mosaic virus that yielded the first clue. In 1937, it was shown that this virus consisted not just of protein, as was first thought, but also contained ribonucleic acid (RNA). Other viruses were then found to contain deoxyribonucleic acid (DNA) rather than RNA, and in 1944, Avery and his colleagues showed that the genetic information of a bacterium, the pneumococcus, was stored in its DNA. We now know that this is true of all organisms from the bacteria upwards: viruses are unique in that their genetic material may be either DNA or RNA; in fact, the RNA viruses well outnumber those with DNA. In all viruses, the nucleic acid core is surrounded by an outer shell of protein that functions as a protective coat during their journeys from one cell to another.

The next major event, which laid the foundation of the whole field of molecular biology, was the description by Watson and Crick in 1953 of the structure of DNA and of the way in which genetic information is encoded within it. Even this discovery did not answer the central question of how viruses replicate and thus pass their genetic information to subsequent generations. The main elements of this complicated puzzle were solved in the 1940s and 1950s, largely as a result of work on viruses

that infect bacteria (bacteriophages). Chapter 3 describes the process in more detail, but in brief, it was found that, within the cell, viruses use enzymes, either encoded in their own nucleic acid or provided by the host cell, to transcribe and replicate their genetic information; they also make use of the host cell's synthetic machinery (e.g. ribosomes) to produce the protein components of the progeny virus. Some even carry the enzyme into the cell.

Modern molecular virology techniques allowing dissection and indeed reconstruction of viral genomes can also lead to the development of rapid diagnostic tests. The genome of the new SARS virus was sequenced in a few weeks and a polymerase chain reaction (PCR) test developed for rapid diagnosis.

6 The control of viral diseases

The understanding of viral replication brought immediate practical benefits in the form of antiviral drugs. The earliest of these were discovered by random screening of compounds likely to inhibit nucleic acid synthesis, some of which proved remarkably successful (e.g. aciclovir (ACV), which acts against certain herpesviruses, and a range of drugs against human immunodeficiency virus (HIV)). With more complete understanding of how viruses replicate, this approach is giving way to the synthesis of drugs 'tailor-made' to attack various specific points in the replication cycle. In parallel, advances in the immunology of virus infections are leading to the development of ever more safe and effective vaccines (see Chapter 37).

Some viruses such as adenovirus vaccine and Venezuelan equine encephalitis (VEE) are being used as vectors to carry into the cell genes for virus vaccines or to correct host genetic faults. However, the most potent way of controlling viruses is our own immune system, and recent discoveries of RNA interference within cells to block messenger RNAs (mRNAs) have reminded us of the power of our own bodies.

7 Conclusions

In conclusion, virological history is being made as we write, probably faster than in most other biological subjects. In addition to propagation in cell cultures and EM, many highly sensitive techniques, involving the detection and analysis of nucleic acids and proteins, are being brought to bear on the characterization of viruses, not least for diagnostic purposes. Not only are new viruses constantly coming to light, but strange infective proteins with some virus-like properties, the prions (proteinaceous infective particle, PrP), are, by adding to our understanding of the world of infective agents, exploding previous notions that genetic information can be transferred only via nucleic acids. These topics, and other important aspects of virology, will be explored in the following chapters.

General properties of viruses

1 Introduction

Viruses have the following characteristics:

- They are small, retaining infectivity after passage through filters small enough to hold back bacteria (Fig. 1.1). Bacteria are measured in terms of the micrometre (μm), which is 10^{-6} of a metre. For viruses, we use the nanometre (nm) as the unit, which is a thousand times smaller (i.e. 10^{-9} of a metre). Viruses range from about 20 nm to 150 nm in diameter.

- They are totally dependent on living cells, either eukaryotic or prokaryotic, for replication and existence. Some viruses do possess enzymes of their own, such as RNA-dependent RNA polymerase or reverse transcriptase (RT), but they cannot reproduce and amplify and translate into proteins the information in their genomes without the assistance of the cellular scaffolding and machinery.

- They possess only one species of nucleic acid, either DNA or RNA.

- They have a component—a receptor-binding protein—for attaching or 'docking' to cells so that they can commandeer them as virus production factories.

Within the past few years, the possibility of a novel class of infective agents that possess no nucleic acid has been investigated intensively, notably by Stanley Prusiner, who was awarded a Nobel Prize for his work. These agents, which he terms **prions** (proteinaceous infectious particles), appear to cause Creutzfeldt–Jakob disease (CJD) and other spongiform encephalopathies affecting both humans and animals. They are described in Chapter 29.

Viruses are both subversive and subtle in their operations; in a way, they are the ultimate evolutionary end-point. They have colonized most living beings on this planet, whether plant, animal, insect, or bacterium. Their small size and total dependence on a host cell for replication delayed studies of viruses to the twentieth century. Only the techniques of EM, cell culture, high-speed centrifugation, and electrophoresis of RNA or DNA genomes, and now nucleotide sequencing, allowed their detailed characterization. Surprisingly, a major step forward in the techniques of virology was the discovery of penicillin and other antibiotics in the 1940s and 1950s; as these compounds inhibit bacteria but not viruses; their addition to cell cultures minimized the risk of bacterial contamination and thus greatly facilitated the propagation of viruses in the laboratory. This advance was brilliantly exploited by the Nobel prize winners, Enders, Weller, and Robbins, who first grew and studied poliomyelitis, mumps, and measles viruses in cell cultures; their researches opened the gate to a flood of discoveries about these and other viruses, which is still gathering momentum. During the 1980s the acquired immunodeficiency syndrome (AIDS) viruses and new hepatitis and herpesviruses came to light; it is certain that other viruses remain to be discovered. In 2003 two new human coronaviruses were discovered, one of them the cause of SARS. Nowadays they are often first encountered by molecular biologists as novel nucleotide sequences in diseased tissues, rather than being detected by EM or growth in the laboratory but SARS was the exception to the rule. Last year a virus, polio, was constructed in a laboratory from common chemicals, and this year the dreaded Spanish influenza virus was reconstructed by reverse operatics.

2 The architecture of viruses

Knowledge of the structure of viruses is, of course, important in their identification; it also helps us to deduce many potentially important properties of a particular virus. As an example, the processes of attachment and penetration of cells and, later, maturation and release differ greatly according to whether the virus possesses a lipid-containing outer envelope. Such enveloped viruses tend to cause fusion of host cells at some stage during their entry. Viruses without this envelope tend to be more resistant to heat and detergents. There are thus important practical consequences of knowledge about virus structure.

2.1 Basic components of viruses

The proteins that make up the virus particle are termed **structural proteins**. The viral genome also codes for very important enzymes that are needed for viral replication but that do not become incorporated in the virion: these are the non-structural or **NS proteins**.

The protein coat of a virus is termed a **capsid** and is itself made up of numerous **capsomeres** (Fig. 2.1(a,b)), visualized by EM as spherical proteins, although X-ray crystallography reveals that they are in fact long polypeptide strands woven into complex structural patterns, much like a ball of wool. The functions of the capsid are to facilitate entry into the host cell and to protect the delicate viral nucleic acid. The complex of protective protein and viral nucleic acid is the **nucleocapsid**.

Some viruses possess an outer envelope containing lipid, derived from the plasma membrane of the host cell during their release by budding from the cell surface. In these, the capsomeres take the form of 'spikes' protruding through a lipid bilayer. There may be a stabilizing protein membrane beneath the lipid bilayer, called the membrane protein, and a further core structure consisting of protein and the viral genome. The whole virus particle, that is the nucleocapsid with its outer envelope (if present), is called the **virion**.

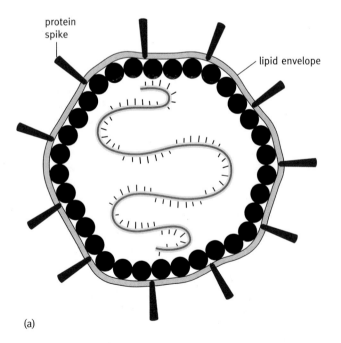

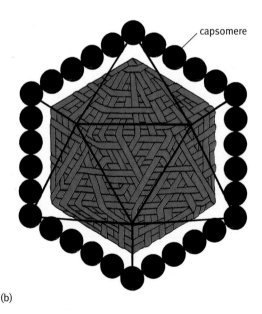

(a)   (b)

Fig. 2.1 Stylized structures of helical and icosahedral viruses. **(a)** A helical virus. The nucleocapsid is in the form of a spiral staircase, the viral nucleoproteins forming the 'steps' surrounding the nucleic acid. These viruses are often pleomorphic, with a lipid envelope, through which protrude protein spikes. **(b)** An icosahedral virus. The 20-sided protein shell (capsid) encloses the nucleic acid, which is in a non-helical configuration and may be packaged as a condensed or crystal structure. Little is known about the exact packaging of nucleic acids in virus particles.

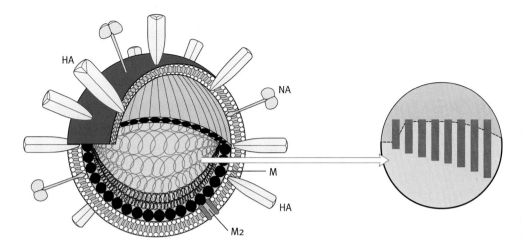

Fig. 2.2 Structural features of influenza virus. The spikes of HA and NA protrude from the lipid bilayer; beneath this is a layer of M protein, which in turn encloses the segmented RNA genome, each segment of which is covered with the nucleocapsid protein and has attached additional structural proteins PB1, PB2, and PA, which are involved in genome replication. 'Pores' of M2 penetrate through the lipid and function as ion channels.

Most of this knowledge of basic virion structure has come from EM studies, and there is still much to be learned. In recent years X-ray crystallographers have probed many viral capsomeres and we now know the precise three-dimensional configuration of the polypeptides of capsomeres of most animal viruses.

Perhaps the most investigated virus spike protein is the haemagglutinin (HA) of influenza and we will digress a little to use this virus as an example of modern molecular studies of a virus structural protein. The influenza HA spike protein is shaped like a 'Toblerone' chocolate bar and protrudes from the virus surface, there being about 500 spikes on each virion (Fig. 2.2). Biochemical studies and X-ray crystallography show each spike to be composed of three identical subunits with a bulb-shaped hydrophilic portion furthest from the viral membrane, while a narrower hydrophobic stalk attaches the spike to the viral lipid and protrudes through it to anchor the spike to the underlying membrane of matrix protein. The most exposed and distant region of the HA contains the antigenic sites, which often protrude from the HA, and a receptor-binding site, a saucer-shaped depression near the HA tip. Two polypeptides (HA1 and HA2), joined together by disulphide bonds, constitute the HA. These two polypeptides originate from a complete HA molecule, which during synthesis in the cell is cleaved into the two pieces by a protease. An influenza virion with a cleaved HA is more infectious than one in which the HA remains as a single protein.

*It had been appreciated that the low pH environment of cytoplasmic endosomes—where the influenza virus finds itself soon after infecting an epithelial cell in the nose or pharynx—must 'do' something to the virus. In fact, it triggers a massive movement of the chain of amino acids in HA1/HA2 and the whole HA molecule becomes contorted. The central junction of HA1 and HA2 mentioned above, normally buried deep in the molecule near the proximal (lipid membrane) end, suddenly finds itself where, in reality, it needs to be, i.e. nearer the far or distal end, which naturally comes into contact with the lipid membrane of the endosome. The HA2 has a particular sequence of amino acids called a **fusion motif** at one end. The contortion triggered by low pH places the motif in the correct position to carry out its fusion function. Fusion of viral and endosome lipids enables the viral RNA to be released and infect the nucleus of the cell, where it will replicate.*

The second spike protein of influenza, the mushroom-shaped neuraminidase (NA), has also been crystallized and studied by X-ray crystallographers. Antigenic sites were identified around the periphery of the enzyme active site on the mushroom head, and the enzyme site itself was located. This knowledge has led directly to a series of anti-influenza drugs, designed to sit precisely in the NA active site and so block enzyme action. NA is essential for release of virus from infected cells, so that these NA inhibitors may provide an important advance in the chemotherapy of influenza. Apart from its intrinsic scientific interest, knowledge of the structure of viral capsids and capsomeres is thus leading to new therapies.

2.2 Virus symmetry

The vast majority of viruses are divided into two groups, according to whether their nucleocapsids have helical or icosahedral (cubic) symmetry. These terms need some explanation. A staircase is a good example of helical symmetry. If one were to look directly down the centre of a spiral staircase, and if it were possible to rotate it around its central axis, the staircase would continue to have the same appearance; it would be symmetrical about the central axis. In viruses with helical symmetry, the protein molecules of the nucleocapsid are arranged like the steps of the spiral staircase and the nucleic acid fills the central core.

Cubic symmetry is more complicated, but we do not wish to delve too far into three-dimensional geometry! It is enough to say that several solids with regular sides, among them the cube and the icosahedron, share certain features of rotational symmetry, a term referring to the fact that they can be rotated about various axes and still look the same. With few exceptions, all viruses that are not helical are icosahedral, that is, they have 20 equal triangular sides. Because they belong to the same geometric group as the cube, they are often referred to as having cubic symmetry, but we shall use the term 'icosahedral symmetry'. The icosahedral formation is the one that permits the greatest number of capsomeres to be packed in a regular fashion to form the capsid.

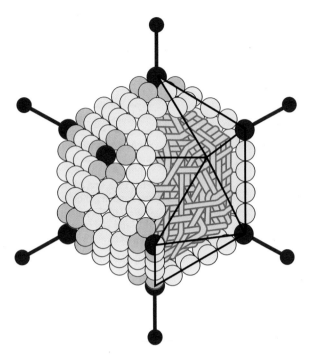

Fig. 2.3 Structural features of adenovirus. Long thin fibres extend from the 12 points, or vertices, of the icosahedral protein coat. The DNA is represented here as a ribbon-like molecule, although its precise physical structure is unknown.

Icosahedral symmetry

These viruses have a highly structured capsid with 20 triangular facets and 12 corners or apices (Fig. 2.3). The individual capsomeres may be made up of several polypeptides, as in the case of poliovirus, in which three proteins constitute the capsomeres. The capsomeres have a dual function, contributing both to the rigidity of the capsid and to the protection of nucleic acid. Except for the complex poxviruses, all DNA containing animal viruses have these icosahedron-shaped capsids, as do certain RNA viruses (see Table 2.1). The DNA-containing herpesviruses have icosahedral symmetry but, in addition, the virion is surrounded by a lipid envelope.

Helical symmetry

Examples of these viruses are the ssRNA viruses such as influenza (Fig. 2.2), the parainfluenza viruses, and rabies. The flexuous helical nucleocapsid is always contained inside a lipoprotein envelope, itself lined internally with a matrix protein. The lipid of the envelope is derived from the cellular membranes through which the virus matures by budding. Viral glycoprotein spikes project from the lipid bilayer envelope and often extend internally through the lipid bilayer to contact the underlying protein shell, referred to as the membrane or matrix (M) protein. This M protein may be rather rigid, as in the case of the bullet-shaped rhabdoviruses, or readily distorted, as in influenza and measles viruses. More recently it has been realized that with influenza virus, ion channels also penetrate through the lipid and allow entry of ions into the virion

interior. In the influenza virus these ions are often protons and cause a change of pH, which can trigger vital structural alterations between the four internal proteins surrounding the RNA genome and so 'activate' its infectiousness (see Section 2.1).

Complex symmetry

Perhaps not unexpectedly, viruses with large genomes have a correspondingly complicated architecture. Such an example is the poxvirus, which has lipids in both the envelope and the outer membranes of the virus; these viruses are neither icosahedral nor helical, and are referred to by the rather unsatisfactory designation of '**complex**' viruses.

Figure 2.4 shows the appearance of typical icosahedral, helical, and complex viruses under the EM.

2.3 Virus genomes

The hereditary information of the virus is encoded in the sequence of nucleotides in the RNA or DNA. This information has to be passed on to new viruses through replication of the viral nucleic acid. Furthermore, this genetic information directs the synthesis of viral proteins. The nucleic acid of DNA viruses does not direct protein synthesis itself. RNA copies of the appropriate segments (genes) of DNA are used as templates to direct the synthesis of the protein. Some RNA viruses contain a positive-strand (or positive-sense) RNA genome that acts directly as mRNA. By contrast, negative-strand RNA viruses possess an enzyme that copies the viral negative-sense RNA genome into a positive-stranded copy, which is then used as an mRNA to direct protein synthesis.

In bacteria most proteins are encoded by an uninterrupted stretch of DNA that is transcribed into an mRNA. By contrast, mammalian genes have their coding sequences (**exons**) interrupted by non-coding sequences (**introns**). The introns have to be removed by **RNA splicing**, which in essence involves a complex series of cuts followed by a 'stitching' together of the exons to form a true mRNA transcript. Splicing of precursor mRNAs can allow different proteins to be produced by the same gene and is particularly important for viruses with small genomes.

Conformation of genomes

Viral genomes can have a number of conformations. The molecules may be double stranded, as in higher life forms, but uniquely they may also be single stranded; they may be linear, circular, continuous, or segmented. Furthermore, as we have already noted, many viruses have genetic information stored in RNA, which is quite unlike the system in bacteria or mammalian cells. Table 2.1 lists the characteristics of the genes of all the virus families and Figs 2.5 and 2.6 show representative DNA and RNA genomes. Quite often the viral DNA or RNA, when carefully solubilized from the virus, may be infectious, but this depends on the precise nature of the genome. Certainly the infectivity of viral nucleic acids, either DNA or RNA, is considerably less than that of the corresponding intact virions.

Table 2.1 Characteristics of viral nucleic acids and properties related to classification

Family name	Page	Positive- or negative-stranded genome[†]	Genome*	Infectivity of isolated nucleic acid	Approximate genome size[‡]
DNA viruses					
Parvoviridae	107	ss	±	+	5
Papovaviridae	119	ds	±	+	8
Adenoviridae	71, 100	ds	±	+	36
Herpesviridae	137	ds	±	+	150
Poxviridae	111	ds	±	+	200
Hepadnaviridae	160–163	ds	±	?	3
RNA viruses					
Astroviridae	101	ss	+	+	v8
Picornaviridae	127	ss	+	+	8
Flaviviridae	175, 198	ss	+	+	10
Togaviridae	103	ss	+	+	12
Coronaviridae	73	ss	+	+	30
Bunyaviridae	198	ss	–	0	16
Orthomyxoviridae	87	ss	–	0	13
Paramyxoviridae	79	ss	–	0	15
Rhabdoviridae	189	ss	–	0	15
Arenaviridae	208	ss	±	?	12
Retroviridae	179	ss	+	?	10
Reoviridae	97	ds	–	0	20
Filoviridae	206	ss	+	0	19
Caliciviridae	100	ss	+	?	8

* ss, single stranded; ds, double stranded.

[†] ±, strands of both polarities present (ambisense).

[‡] kilobases (kb) for single-stranded genomes, kilobase pairs (kbp) for double-stranded genomes.

We do not want students to memorize all these details of viral genes, but rather to appreciate the general principles of how viruses encode the information for manufacture of their proteins, which also enables them to commandeer a host cell and take over its machinery to manufacture virus rather than cellular proteins.

Genome size

The sizes of viral genomes vary greatly but there is considerable pressure to minimize them because of the difficulty of packaging the genes into the small space within in the virion. Human cells have more than 60 000 genes and the bacterium, *Escherichia coli*, has 4000 genes. Even the largest viruses (e.g. poxviruses) may contain only 200 or fewer genes.

The smallest virus may have the equivalent of only three or four genes. In general, RNA viruses have smaller genomes and code for fewer proteins than DNA viruses. RNA genomes are more fragile than DNA and this feature limits their size.

It is usual to measure viral genomes in terms of the number of bases (or nucleotides) in their nucleic acid. As they are quite large, these numbers are often expressed as thousands of bases (kilobases, or kb). For **single-stranded genomes**, the notation **kb** is used. For **double-stranded genomes**, numbers are expressed as kilobase pairs (**kbp**). Thus the single-stranded measles virus genome is 16 000 bp (16 kb) in length, and the double-stranded adenovirus genome contains about 36 000 bp (36 kbp).

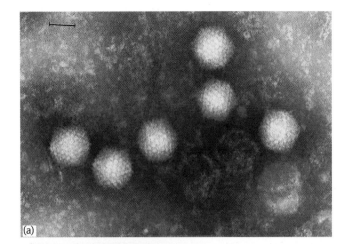

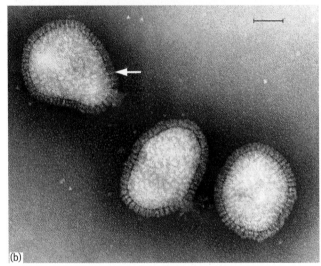

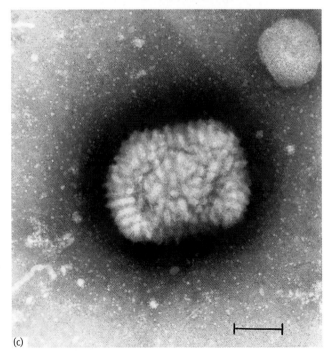

Fig. 2.4 Electron micrographs of typical icosahedral, helical, and complex viruses. **(a)** Adenovirus (icosahedral); **(b)** influenza virus (helical); and **(c)** poxvirus (complex). Scale bar = 100 nm.

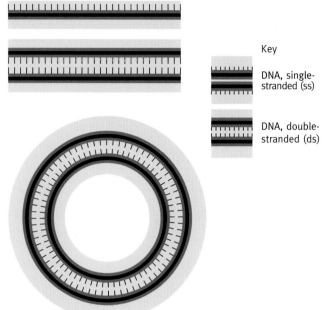

Fig. 2.5 DNA virus genomes.

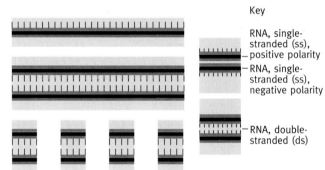

Fig. 2.6 RNA virus genomes.

2.4 Virus genome and transcription maps

Figure 2.7 illustrates genome maps of two RNA viruses. Further details of particular viruses are presented in the relevant chapters. It is virtually impossible to illustrate a 'typical' viral genome or a typical transcription strategy.

DNA viruses

Adenoviruses have a more orthodox genome of linear dsDNA of 36 kbp, containing 30 genes. There is a terminal protein attached to the 5′ end of each DNA strand, which acts as a primer during genome replication and initiates synthesis of new DNA strands. Groups of genes are expressed from a limited number of shared promoters; to extend the genetic information, viral-spliced mRNAs are utilized to produce a variety of polypeptides from each promoter.

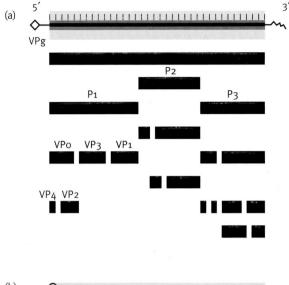

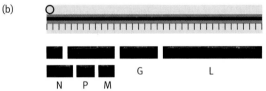

Fig. 2.7 **(a)** Poliovirus, a positive-strand RNA virus. The virion RNA molecule is polyadenylated (⌇) at the 3′ end and a small virus-coded protein (VPg) is present at the 5′ end. The genome has a single open reading frame whose primary translation product is a polyprotein, which is cleaved to produce viral capsid proteins (VP1, VP2, VP3, and VP4), the RNA polymerase, two proteases, and some minor products (unlabelled). Non-translated regions (ntr) at each end of the genome are not translated into proteins. The 5′ end non-coding region has an important function in the initiation of protein synthesis. **(b)** Rabies, a negative-strand RNA virus. A virion-associated polymerase transcribes the five genes, which are arranged sequentially on the ssRNA genome into 5′ capped, methylated, and polyadenylated mRNAs (not shown); these are translated into the nucleocapsid (N), core phosphoprotein (P), matrix (M), glycosylated membrane spike (G), and polymerase (L) polypeptides.

Herpes and **poxviruses** have large DNA genomes with over 150 genes. Gene splicing is not used with either of these viruses and, in particular, not with poxviruses, which replicate in the cytoplasm. There is precisely regulated transcription with early and late switches, which ensure that gene products involved in DNA replication are synthesized early in the cycle and viral structural proteins much later. Both these viruses, and particularly poxviruses, have a range of unique enzymes that are carried by the viruses themselves.

The DNA **hepatitis B virus** has a very unusual circular genome, consisting of two strands of DNA, which is described in Chapter 22.

The smallest in terms of genome size and complexity are the **parvoviruses**, in which ssDNA replication and gene expression depend on cellular functions. Not unexpectedly with such a small genome, the coding regions overlap and there is splicing to produce a variety of subgenomic mRNAs.

Positive-strand RNA viruses

Poliovirus is a typical positive-strand RNA virus. Its RNA is polyadenylated at the 3′ end and a small virus-coded protein (VPg) is present at the 5′ end; the viral RNA is used directly as mRNA. The genome has a single open reading frame (ORF) whose primary translation product is a single polyprotein. This is cleaved to produce viral capsid proteins (VP1, VP2, VP3, and VP4), the RNA polymerases, two viral proteases, and some minor viral protein products. There are non-translated regions (ntr) at each end of the genome that have important functions. The 5′ ntr (600 nucleotides) has a significant role in the initiation of viral protein synthesis, virulence, and encapsidation, whereas the 3′ ntr is necessary for synthesis of negative-strand RNA.

By contrast, **coronaviruses** utilize subgenomic RNA molecules in the form of a nested set of six overlapping RNAs with common 3′ ends. Each viral mRNA is capped and polyadenylated and only the 5′ ends are translated.

Negative-strand RNA viruses

These genomes are more diverse than their positive-stranded RNA counterparts. They are not infective for cells. Furthermore, some of the viruses in this group have ambisense genomes with both negative- and positive-stranded regions.

Characteristically of this group of viruses, **rabies** carries the RNA transcriptase in the virus itself. This virion-associated polymerase transcribes the single virus RNA strand by a start/stop mechanism followed by reinitiation. The five viral genes are arranged sequentially on the ssRNA genome as the nucleocapsid (N), core phosphoprotein (P), matrix (M), glycosylated membrane spike (G), and polymerase (L).

Influenza has an RNA composed of eight ssRNA segments, each encoding at least one protein. Using a splicing mechanism, genes 7 and 8 code for two proteins so that one protein is translated from an unspliced mRNA, whereas a smaller protein is translated from a spliced mRNA; both, however, share the same AUG initiation codon and nine subsequent amino acids. Oddities among DNA and RNA viruses may occur, in the sense that one often sees by EM 'empty' particles that contain no nucleic acid at all. These virus particles cannot, of course, replicate. Other virions may look normal by EM yet have a defective genome, lacking part of the nucleic acid needed to infect a cell; these are termed **defective interfering** virus particles, because although defective for their own replication, they interfere with the replication of normal viruses. This property could conceivably be harnessed to prevent virus infections.

It is useful to remember that:

- **the nucleic acid of all DNA viruses except parvoviruses is double stranded** (but note that hepadnavirus DNA is partly single stranded when not replicating);

- the nucleic acid of all RNA viruses except reoviruses is single stranded.

The evolution of viruses

In the absence of fossil remains of viruses, calculations of rates of change of viral genes must remain as estimates. Viruses evolve rapidly because they undergo many genome duplications in a short time. Adenovirus, for example, may produce 250 000 DNA molecules in an infected cell. The host cell has evolved an editing system to test for mismatched base pairs during DNA synthesis but RNA viruses may be unable to perform this function. With RNA viruses the rate of divergence of RNA genomes at the nucleotide level can be as high as 2 per cent per year. This is a million times the rate for eukaryotic DNA genomes. Both viral RNA polymerases and viral RT have a very high frequency of transcription error and this, together with a lack of editing, explains why some RNA viruses, such as influenza and HIV, are so heterogeneous. By mutation of genes coding for target proteins, these formidable RNA viral pathogens are able to evade vaccine-induced immunity and the effects of antibody or antiviral drugs. It is a sobering thought that, because of this extraordinary genetic diversity, mutants of HIV and influenza already exist that will be resistant to antiviral drugs not as yet discovered.

3 Classification of viruses

The precise pigeon-holing of a virus in a classification system is not only scientifically satisfying, but also of practical consequence. Two examples illustrate this assertion. For example, the AIDS virus (HIV-1) was at first thought to belong to the tumour virus group of the family *Retroviridae* (Chapter 6). When, by examination of its detailed morphology and establishment of its genome structure, HIV-1 was shown to be more related to the lentivirus group (Chapter 25), certain features of its biology (e.g. a long latency period and absence of oncogenicity) could be filled in by reference to other viruses of the same group. The identification of the virus causing severe acute respiratory syn-

Table 2.2 Important structural characteristics of the families of viruses of medical importance

Family name	Representative viruses	Approximate diameter of virion (nm)	Symmetry of nucleocapsid*
DNA viruses			
Parvoviridae	Human parvovirus	20	I
Papovaviridae	Wart viruses	50	I
Adenoviridae	Adenoviruses	80	I
	Herpes simplex virus	180	I
Poxviridae	Vaccinia virus	250	C
Hepadnaviridae	Hepatitis B virus	40	I
RNA viruses			
Astroviridae	Astroviruses	30	I
Picornaviridae	Polioviruses	25	I
Flaviviridae	Yellow fever virus	30	I
Togaviridae	Rubella virus	80	I
Coronaviridae	Infectious bronchitis virus	100	H
Bunyaviridae	California encephalitis virus	100	H
Orthomyxoviridae	Influenza viruses	100	H
Paramyxoviridae	Measles virus	150	H
Rhabdoviridae	Rabies virus	150	H
Arenaviridae	Lassa fever virus	100	H
Retroviridae	HIV-1	100	I
Reoviridae	Rotaviruses	70	I
Flaviviridae	Marburg virus	Variable	H
Caliciviridae	Calicivirus	35	I

* H, helical; I, icosahedral; C, complex.

drome (SARS) in Southeast Asia in 2003 as a member of a previously known family of the human coronavirus brought rapid dividends, e.g. enabling diagnostic kits to be made and also giving the first intimation, compared with other members of the family that a successful vaccine could be made.

The following are the main criteria used for the classification of viruses:

- the type of nucleic acid (DNA or RNA);
- the number of strands of nucleic acid and their physical construction (single- or double-stranded, linear, circular, circular with breaks, segmented);
- polarity of the viral genome-RNA viruses in which the viral genome can be used directly as mRNA are by convention termed 'positive-stranded' and those for which a transcript has first to be made are termed 'negative-stranded';
- the symmetry of the nucleocapsid;
- the presence or absence of a lipid envelope.

On these criteria, viruses are grouped into families, subfamilies, genera, and species. Further subdivision is based on the degree of antigenic similarity. Classification lacks precision beyond this point, but antigenically identical viruses can sometimes be further categorized by differences in biological characteristics, such as virulence or cellular receptors; or in terms of molecular structure, for example their nucleotide sequences. Statistical comparison of the number of nucleotide sequence changes between individual members of a family enables a pictorial representative of similarity or diversity to be made, called a phylogenetic tree. The tree trunk represents the main evolutionary thrust, whereas various mutant viruses occupy branches of the tree. Viruses in the same or adjacent branches are more related to each other than those on more distant branches. An example of the usefulness of this system is shown in the case of SARS virus. Phylogenetic analysis of four principal genes of the newly discovered virus showed that it was indeed new and had not simply emerged from an existing grouping. Tables 2.1 and 2.2 summarize the genetic, biological, and structural characteristics of the families of viruses known to cause disease in humans.

4 The nomenclature of viruses

This topic has been in a state of flux for many years, and the names now in general use are based on characteristics that vary from family to family. Some viruses are named according to the type of disease they cause (e.g. poxviruses and herpesviruses); other familial names are based on acronyms, for example papovaviruses (*papilloma–polyoma–va*cuolating agent) and picornaviruses (*pico*, small; *rna*, ribonucleic acid); others again are based on morphological features of the virion, (e.g. coronaviruses, which have a halo or corona of spikes). Some individual viruses are named after the place where they were first isolated (e.g. Coxsackie, Marburg). More recently, in the

case of hantavirus outbreaks in the USA, residents strongly objected to a newly discovered strain being named after their locality. Occasionally, viruses have been named after their discoverers (e.g. Epstein–Barr virus (EBV)).

The descriptions, classification, and nomenclature of viruses are specified by the International Committee on Classification of Viruses (ICTV), which issues a report every few years. In this book we have followed the recommendations in the latest of these, the Seventh Report published in 2000. The complexity and expansion of the subject may be judged by the fact that it is twice the size of its predecessor, weighing in at nearly 3 kg. We shall not burden you with much detail, but you should know that the approved names of the various taxa (classes) of viruses (orders, families, subfamilies, genera, and species) are printed in italics with upper case initial letters, e.g. 'Rubella is caused by a member of the '*Togaviridae*', whereas names that have not yet been approved are printed in roman (standard) type. Names used colloquially, as in '*adenoviruses* cause some respiratory infections' are also printed in roman.

5 The range of diseases caused by viruses

We have so far dealt with viruses only as micro-organisms; we shall now start to look at them in relation to the diseases that they cause in humans and, where relevant, in animals. Viruses vary greatly not only in their host range, but also in their affinity for various tissues within a given host (**tissue tropism**) and the mechanisms by which they cause disease (**pathogenesis**). Some viruses are predominantly neurotropic, others replicate only in the liver or skin, and others again can infect many of the body systems. These variables are reflected in the ranges of diseases caused by viruses of different families. Despite their similarity in properties such as size, structure, and genome, the members of some families cause a wide variety of **syndromes** (sets of symptoms and physical signs occurring together); by contrast, the range of syndromes caused by other families is much more restricted. There may be considerable overlap between the syndromes caused by very different viruses. Respiratory symptoms are an excellent example. Members of five families of viruses cause cough, sore throat, and runny nose. As may be imagined, this can create problems in diagnosis, most of which can, however, be solved by studying the clinical picture as a whole and enlisting the aid of the virology laboratory as early in the illness as possible.

5.1 A little 'non-human' virology

So far, in line with the intention of this book, we have considered only viruses that infect humans or other mammalian or avian species that interact with them. For the sake of completeness, however, we should mention that there are many other viruses that affect most—possibly all—of the diverse life-forms on our planet. They include vertebrates, insects, plants, algae, fungi, and bacteria. Fortunately, we need concern ourselves briefly with only two of these groups.

It seems extraordinary that some of the smallest life-forms on our planet should harbour even smaller living entities: but they do. As Swift (1713) wrote:

> So, naturalists observe, a flea
> Hath smaller fleas that on him prey;
> And these have smaller fleas to bite 'em,
> And so proceed *ad infinitum*.

Bacteriophages ('phage' for short) as their name suggests, are viruses that infect bacteria. They have been isolated from many species, including chlamydias, and fall into two main categories: *virulent* phages that lyse their host bacteria, and *temperate* phages that set up a non-lytic (lysogenic) cycle of replication. Their nucleic acid may be either DNA or RNA. The host range, morphology, sizes (roughly 20–2000 nm) and replication strategies of these agents vary greatly and we shall not deal with them at any length. That is not to say that they are of no importance. The following points are worth noting.

- Phages have proved invaluable as tools for studying the genetics of bacteria and for demonstrating that their nucleic acid is physically separable from their protein coats.

- Species and subspecies of various bacteria, e.g. *Staphylococcus aureus* and various salmonellas can be identified by their patterns of susceptibility to a range of phages. Rapid phage typing is particularly useful for studying outbreaks of infection with these and some other bacteria.

- Attempts have been made, notably in eastern Europe and the former Soviet Union, to exploit the lytic properties of bacteriophages for treating enteric infections, e.g. cholera, but such measures were not very successful and have been largely superseded by the use of antibiotics. Nevertheless, in the face of widespread resistance to antibiotics, there has been a revival of interest in the possibility of using phages for therapeutic purposes.

- The presence of a phage in its lysogenic state (prophase) may give rise to phenotypic changes in the bacterial host.

- Some bacterial toxins, e.g. those of cholera and diphtheria are encoded by prophages.

- Contamination with phages may interfere with certain industrial processes, e.g. manufacture of dairy products and antibiotics.

5.2 Viroids

These very small circular ssRNA molecules are hardly worthy of being regarded as true viruses, hence their name. They affect plants only and are responsible for some commercially important diseases; but their main interest lies in how they manage to replicate with such a tiny genome (approximately 300 nucleotides). They are too small to encode proteins, and thus must rely on the host-cell enzymes for replication. They have rather jolly names, such as *coconut cadang–cadang viroid* and *tomato 'planta macho' viroid*.

6 Reminders

- Viruses are characterized by their small size, obligate intracellular parasitism, possession of either an RNA or a DNA genome, and of a receptor-binding protein.

- Viral genomes vary in size from three to 150 genes but most commonly have 10–15 genes. Such compression of genetic information forces viruses into strategies to extend the genetic information by **splicing** or **utilizing different reading frames**.

- The genome is protected by a coat or **capsid** consisting of protein subunits (**capsomeres**). Each capsomere is made of one to three polypeptides. Some viruses also have a lipid envelope. The nucleic acid is often complexed with a protein. The nucleic acid core and the capsid are together known as the **nucleocapsid**. The complete virus particle (nucleocapsid with envelope, if present) is termed the **virion**.

- The tertiary structure of many capsid proteins has been established by X-ray crystallography. This knowledge, together with nucleotide sequence of the corresponding gene, now gives chemotherapists a good start in designing inhibitors that will bind to these proteins.

- The nucleocapsids of most viruses are built either like **helices**, with the capsids arranged like the steps in a spiral staircase around the central genome core, or like **icosahedra**, in which the capsids are arranged to form a solid with 20 equal triangular sides, again enclosing the genome. These forms are referred to, respectively, as having helical or icosahedral (cubic) symmetry. The large poxviruses have complex structures not falling into either category.

- Viruses are classified into families according to the characteristics of their nucleic acid, whether **DNA** or **RNA**, the **number of strands**, and their **polarity**. Positive-stranded viruses use the viral genome as mRNA. Negative-stranded viruses must first make a transcript of the genome RNA to be used as a message and carry an RNA transcriptase in the virus particle to perform this function.

- Some families are divided into subfamilies on the basis of gene structure. Further subdivisions into genera depend on antigenic and other biological properties. Phylogenetic trees can be constructed, which outline relatedness between members of a family and give indications of evolution and change.

- There is a single order of *Mononegavirales*, which contains four families with similar genomes and mode of replication (*Paramyxoviridae*, *Rhabdoviridae*, and *Filoviridae*).

- Viruses vary widely in the range of hosts and tissues that they can infect; members of some families cause a wide range of syndromes, whereas the illnesses due to others are much more limited in number.

- **Bacteriophages** are very small viruses that infect most, perhaps all, bacteria. They have been very useful in the study of molecular biology and for typing certain strains of bacteria. **Viroids** are also very small, containing a circular ssRNA molecule. They infect plants only, in which they may cause commercially important diseases.

Chapter 3

Viral replication and genetics

1 Introduction

In the task of reproducing themselves, viruses are at a major disadvantage compared with higher forms of life. The latter all multiply by some form of fission, so that the daughter cells start their existence with a full complement of genetic information and with the enzymes necessary to replicate it and to catalyse the synthesis of new proteins. A virus, on the other hand, enters the cell with nothing but its own puny molecule of nucleic acid, which may have only 20 or so genes compared with 100 000 genes for a mammalian cell, and sometimes without even a single enzyme to start the process of replication. This is why it must rely so heavily on the host cell for the materials it needs for reproduction and why the replication of viruses is more complicated in some respects than that of other microorganisms. Although we now have a fairly detailed picture of the main steps, we still do not know everything about the strategies that viruses have developed over the millennia to continue their existence. In fact, detailed investigations of viral replication continue to uncover major facts about control mechanisms and genetic strategies in our own cells.

As the replication of viruses is so intimately related to cellular activities, it may be helpful to provide an outline of the molecular biology of the host cell, with which you are probably already familiar, and will serve as a basis of comparison between these very different life forms.

2 The molecular biology of the mammalian cell

There are over 100 types of cell in the human body and these are mostly assembled into tissues. A typical animal cell is 20 μm in diameter. The most prominent organelle is the **nucleus**, which is enclosed by two concentric membranes that form the **nuclear envelope**. The nucleus contains dsDNA, which encodes the genetic specification of the cell. The nuclear pores allow certain molecules to enter and exit from the nucleus, but this procedure is strictly controlled. The cell interior is composed of transparent cytoplasm that is full of organelles and in which extensive traffic takes place, involving proteins and various chemical messengers, all of which may be important during viral replication. All the cell organelles are enclosed by membranes, thus enabling the cell to carry out many different processes at the same time. An important organelle is the **endoplasmic reticulum**, an irregular structure enclosed by lipid membranes. Also present is the Golgi organelle, which has the appearance of a stack of empty sacks. **Lysosomes** are balloon-like structures in which intracellular digestion occurs. Many viruses uncoat and initiate infection in this organelle. Ribosomes are the framework upon which new proteins are made, under the direction of mRNAs. Continual exchange of material takes place between these organelles and the outside of the cell, itself surrounded by a lipid bilayer **plasma membrane**. Underlying this is a **cytoskeleton** of filaments, such as actin, that strengthen the cell and give it a particular shape. The plasma membrane is packed with receptors for different molecules, many essential for the functioning of the cells. Viruses may use some of these receptors to enter and infect cells.

2.1   DNA as the carrier of genetic information

The life of the cell depends on its ability to store, retrieve, and translate genetic instructions, which are stored as **genes**. In the 1940s, DNA was identified as the carrier of genetic information. A DNA molecule consists of two strands of nucleotides held together by hydrogen bonds—a DNA double helix. The two strands of the helix each have a sequence of nucleotides that is complementary to that of the partner strand. DNA is an example of a **linear message**, encoded in the sequence of nucleotides along each strand. The DNA of a human cell is composed of 3×10^9 nucleotides and has a four-letter nucleotide 'alphabet' (A, C, T, and G). During replication this information must be copied faithfully.

2.2   Replication of cellular dsDNA

At replication, each DNA strand acts as a **template**, or mould, for the synthesis of a new **complementary strand**. DNA replication produces two complete double helices from the original DNA molecule. An enzyme, **DNA polymerase**, is central to this process. It catalyses addition of nucleotides to the 3′ end of a growing DNA strand by the formation of a phosphodiester bond between this end and the 5′-phosphate group of the incoming nucleotide. Virus DNA or RNAs are replicated in a similar manner.

2.3   Transcription of DNA to form mRNAs

When a particular protein is required by the cell, the correct small portion of this immense DNA molecule is copied into RNA. In turn these RNA copies (**mRNAs**) are used as templates to direct the synthesis of the protein. Many thousands of these **transcription** events occur each minute in mammalian cells. The information in the mRNA is used to make a protein, a process called **translation**. The virus can utilize this system with high efficiency. The virus can subvert the system or completely blockade translation of host-cell proteins.

2.4   Processing of primary RNA transcripts

The mRNA produced must be processed in the nucleus from a **primary transcript** to the final mRNA. First, the RNA is **capped** at the 5′ end by addition of a guanine nucleotide with a methyl group attached. Then a **poly(A) tail** is added at the 3′ end.

Mammalian cell genes (and many viral genes) have their coding sequences interrupted by non-coding sequences (**introns**) perhaps as long as 10 000 nucleotides. These introns are removed by **RNA splicing**. At each intron a group of small nuclear ribonucleoprotein particles (snRNPs) assembles in the nucleus, cuts out the intron, and rejoins the RNA chain. In fact, this splicing was first discovered in cells infected with viruses.

2.5   Translation of mRNAs into proteins

After migrating from the nucleus to the cytoplasm, the mRNAs are translated into proteins. Each group of three consecutive nucleotides in mRNA is called a **codon** and each specifies one amino acid. It follows therefore that an RNA sequence can be translated in three different **reading frames** (Fig. 3.9). Particular codons in the mRNA signal the sites where protein synthesis starts and stops. **Initiation factors** and the mRNA interact with a small ribosomal subunit which moves forward (5′–3′) along the mRNA, searching for the first **start codon**, namely AUG. The end of the protein-coding message is signalled by UAA, UAG, or UGA, termed **stop codons**. Viral mRNAs are translated in a similar manner but may have to compete with cellular mRNAs.

Note that genes are indicated by italics (e.g. *tax*) and their products by roman script (e.g. tax).

2.6   Control of gene expression

Gene expression must be controlled and a particularly important stage is at initiation of transcription. The **promoter region** of a gene attracts RNA polymerase: it has an **initiation site** and an associated 'upstream' region. Most genes also have **regulatory DNA sequences** that are required to switch genes on; they are recognized by regulatory proteins that bind to the DNA and act as activators or repressors. The process also requires the co-operation of a large set of proteins called **general transcription factors**. Some viruses code for their own transcription factors, which thereby interrupt the normal gene expression in the cells. The most recent discovery is RNA interference, the 'silencing' of gene expression by dsRNA molecules. RNA interference has evolved to silence viruses and rogue genetic elements that make dsRNA intermediates, types of RNA not usually produced by cells.

3   Virus infection and replication in a host cell

The initial infection of a cell is a rather hit or miss process, depending upon chance contact, but is greatly helped if a virus enters the body at a suitable site and in large numbers. Often

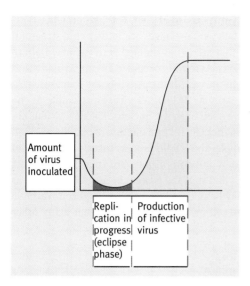
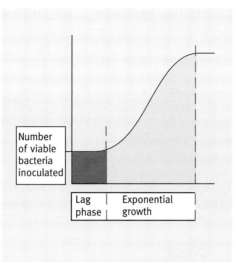

Fig. 3.1 Typical growth curve of a virus compared with that of a bacterium.

thousands of viruses may enter the body and yet only two or three actually establish an infection. The remainder are destroyed by the general defences before they have a chance to infect. There follows a period of a few hours during which nothing seems to be happening. This appearance is, however, deceptive because much is going on inside the cell at the molecular level, such as **transcription** of the 'incoming' viral genes to form viral mRNAs, and their translation to produce early viral proteins, including the enzymes necessary to replicate viral DNA or viral RNA. Thus although there are no visible signs in the cell, at the molecular level sensitive probes for viral genes indicate subtle but definite changes. Figure 3.1 illustrates a fundamental difference between the replication of viruses and bacteria; the latter retain their structure and infectivity throughout the growth cycle, whereas viruses lose their physical identity and most or all of their infectivity during the initial stage of replication, which for this reason has been termed the **eclipse phase**. The next stage, the **productive phase**, is even more full of action as new virus particles are produced and released from the cell.

3.1 General plan of viral replication

We shall look first at the main steps in the replication of a DNA virus (steps numbered as in Fig. 3.2). There is an approximate indication of the time scale. You will appreciate that no single virus is typical of them all. We have chosen a DNA poxvirus because the sequential steps in its replication are comparatively easy to follow. It should, however, be mentioned that this example is not typical of DNA viruses in that it replicates entirely in the cytoplasm, carries many of the enzymes needed for viral transcription and replication and sets up small virus 'factories'.

(1) Penetrating any mucus or other physical barriers, the virus adsorbs to a host cell using a specific receptor on the cell membrane. (2) A few minutes later it has entered the cytoplasm of the cell, after which (3) it 'uncoats' (i.e. sheds its pro-

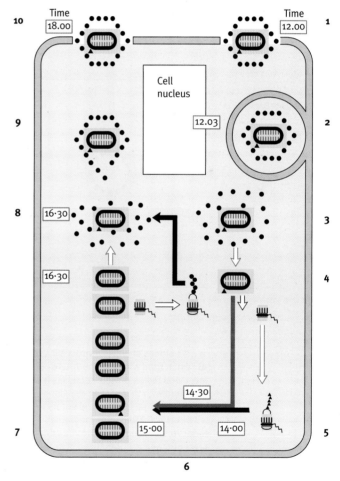

Fig. 3.2 Life cycle of vaccinia, a DNA virus. Adsorption and penetration occur rapidly. Unlike other DNA viruses, vaccinia replicates exclusively in the cytoplasm. Initial transcription takes place in the core of the virion. The genomic DNA strands are covalently linked at their ends. Early mRNAs, coding for enzymes that have an early function, such as replication of input DNA, are transcribed from input DNA. Late mRNAs coding for viral structural proteins are transcribed from newly synthesized DNA. See text for further details.

tective protein shell). In the case of poxvirus this uncoating is only partial. In other viruses the uncoating is more complete and the viral nucleic acid completely frees itself. (4) The poxvirus input DNA is transcribed to produce various viral mRNAs, which code for (5) 'early' viral proteins. Viral proteins are produced by the ribosomes of the host cell. There are as many as 100 **early genes** distributed throughout the poxvirus genome. Other viruses have only a handful of genes. The early viral proteins may have various functions; for example, some are **DNA-dependent DNA polymerases** that catalyse and direct the synthesis of new viral DNA molecules (7) and others are **transcriptional activators** that speed up the viral transcription process. In contrast, the **late viral mRNAs** are transcribed

only from newly synthesized viral DNA. The 'late' proteins translated from these late viral messages are mostly viral structural polypeptides (8) that are (9) assembled with the new DNA to form progeny virions. **Assembly** occurs in circumscribed areas of the cytoplasm in the case of the poxvirus and immature virions can be seen easily by EM. Other viruses assemble at the plasma membrane itself or in the nucleus. The new virions are then released from the cell (10) by a mixture of budding and cell lysis; in this example, the whole process takes a minimum of 6–8 hours. The new infective virions are then free to infect neighbouring cells and start the process over again. As many as 10 000 virions may be released from an infected cell. Vaccinia virus may kill the cell in which it replicates, but many other

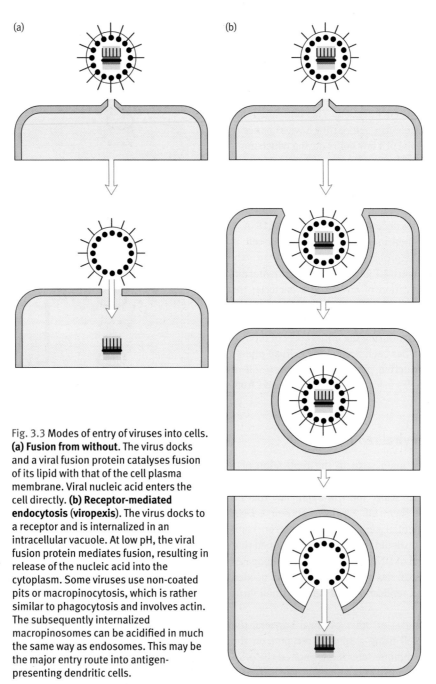

(a)

(b)

Fig. 3.3 Modes of entry of viruses into cells. **(a) Fusion from without.** The virus docks and a viral fusion protein catalyses fusion of its lipid with that of the cell plasma membrane. Viral nucleic acid enters the cell directly. **(b) Receptor-mediated endocytosis (viropexis).** The virus docks to a receptor and is internalized in an intracellular vacuole. At low pH, the viral fusion protein mediates fusion, resulting in release of the nucleic acid into the cytoplasm. Some viruses use non-coated pits or macropinocytosis, which is rather similar to phagocytosis and involves actin. The subsequently internalized macropinosomes can be acidified in much the same way as endosomes. This may be the major entry route into antigen-presenting dendritic cells.

viruses, particularly enveloped viruses, bud from the cell surface while the cell maintains its normal structure and produces wave upon wave of new virions.

We shall now describe these steps in viral replication in more detail, and explore the important variations adopted by both RNA and DNA viruses.

3.2 Recognition of a 'target' host cell

All viruses have on their outside a receptor-binding protein, which often has a saucer-shaped pocket that reacts specifically with a corresponding **receptor** on a cell surface. These receptors usually have other functions and viruses simply use them for attachment. The virus receptors on cells are often glycoproteins or glycolipids. Once attached, which may be a more or less instantaneous process, viruses are almost impossible to dislodge. This precise key-and-lock interaction explains why many viruses are restricted to a given host and, within that host, to particular cells and tissues.

*For example, the AIDS virus, HIV-1, recognizes and reacts specifically with two receptors on certain T lymphocytes and other cells, and can thus attach to and infect only these cells. The **primary receptor** is the CD4 molecule found on immune T cells and a **secondary receptor** is a chemokine receptor molecule, CXCR-4, or a β-chemokine receptor molecule, CCR-5. (CD = 'cluster of differentiation'.)*

3.3 Internalization of the virus

Having attached to the viral host cell, the virus must penetrate the external plasma membrane of the cell rapidly and release its genome into the cellular milieu for subsequent replication. This **internalization** is accomplished in one of three ways.

Fusion from without

Fusion at the cellular external plasma membrane, namely 'fusion from without', is the strategy of entry of paramyxoviruses such as measles and mumps viruses, and also HIV (Fig. 3.3(a)). Such viruses have a '**fusion protein**', with a short stretch of catalytic hydrophobic amino acids, which mediates fusion between the lipids of the virus and the lipids of the cell membrane.

Receptor-mediated endocytosis (viropexis)

Viropexis is the most common cellular entry technique for viruses (Fig. 3.3(b)). Mammalian cells have had to develop methods of attachment and entry of a range of essential molecules, such as nutrients and hormones. Viruses can exploit these existing avenues of entry. Viruses attach at special virus receptor areas on the cell membrane. The cellular protein, clathrin, which underlies the membrane, forms a so-called **coated pit** and, once the virus has attached, inversion of the cellular membrane and associated virus occurs. The virus is now in the cytoplasm but is still bounded by the cell membrane, through which it has to negotiate a route to the true internal environment and often to the nucleus of the cell. It is a

mystery how the viral nucleic acid, particularly ssRNA, protects itself from destruction by the many nucleases present in the cytoplasmic vacuole, but presumably the tightly bound viral nucleoproteins provide protection. These endosomes offer a convenient and rapid transit system across the plasma membrane and also through the cytoplasm to the nuclear pore.

Some viruses, such as influenza, achieve release from the internal endosomal vacuole by internal fusion ('fusion from within') mediated by the viral HA protein. A further requirement of internal fusion with influenza is a low pH in the cytoplasmic vacuole; this triggers a movement of the three-dimensional structure of the HA protein, so allowing juxtaposition of the HA fusion sequence, normally buried deep in the HA spike protein, with both viral and cellular lipid membranes.

Non-clathrin-mediated endocytosis

A few viruses may enter by a third technique known as non-clathrin-mediated endocytosis or via a caveolae assisted entry. In all cases quite extensive internal trafficking occurs before the virus RNA is released from the internalized virus and enters the nucleus via the nuclear pore.

3.4 Formation of viral mRNAs: a vital step in replication

When viruses infect cells, two important and separate events must be orchestrated, namely production of **virus structural proteins and enzymes**, and **replication of the viral genome**. Viruses have various methods of ensuring that their mRNAs are produced and then translated into viral proteins, often in preference to normal cellular mRNAs.

In the **Baltimore classification scheme** RNA viruses are categorized by their three strategies of forming viral mRNA, which depend upon the sense of their genome RNA. In this context, 'sense' refers to whether the genome is homologous with the viral mRNA ('positive-sense' or 'positive-stranded') or complementary to it ('negative-sense' or 'negative-stranded').

Positive-stranded RNA viruses

The **positive-stranded parental viral RNA** (Figs 3.4 and 3.5), with the addition of a poly(A) (AAA) tract at the 3′ end of the molecule and a cap at the 5′ end, is used directly as viral mRNA, from which 'early' and 'late' viral proteins (see Section 3.1) are translated directly.

Polio and flaviviruses are good examples of positive-stranded RNA viruses. Another feature of these viruses is that the viral genome is itself infectious for cells, but much less so than the complete virus.

Negative-stranded RNA viruses

In the case of the **negative-stranded RNA viruses**, for example influenza (Fig. 3.6) or rabies (Fig. 3.7), a virus-associated RNA polymerase (transcriptase), which is carried into the cell by the virus, must first make mirror-image copies of the original nega-

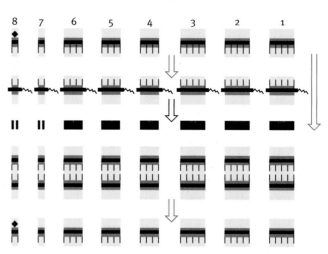

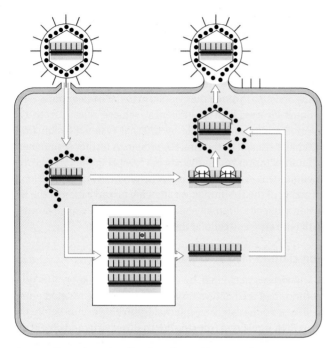

Fig. 3.4 Life cycle and replication of a positive-stranded RNA virus.

Fig. 3.6 Replication strategy of influenza, a negative-stranded RNA virus. The viral genome is in the form of eight loosely linked single-stranded RNA segments. Most transcribed mRNAs are monocistronic, i.e. they code for a single protein. However, the mRNAs of genes 7 and 8 have undergone splicing and each now codes for two viral proteins. The mode of transcription and replication of influenza virus is unique as it requires co-operation with cellular RNA polymerase II ('cap snatching'). ∿, poly(A) tail; ◆, RNA-dependent RNA polymerase.

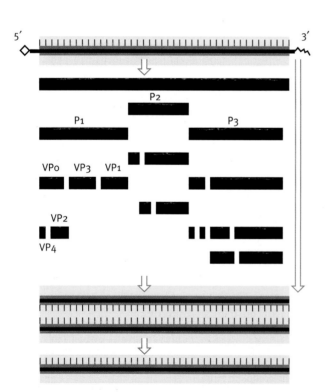

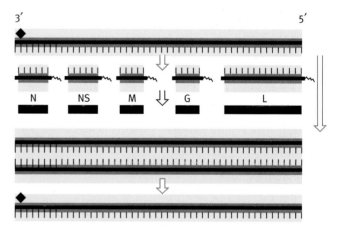

Fig. 3.7 Replication strategy of rabies, a negative-stranded RNA virus. The viral genome is in the form of a single complete strand of RNA. The five genes are positioned in a linear manner. There is an intergenic sequence, a translation start signal and a poly(A) signal at the end of each gene. Five mRNAs are transcribed by a start-and-stop mechanism and each is translated into a viral protein. ∿, poly(A) tail; ◆, RNA-dependent RNA polymerase.

Fig. 3.5 Replication strategy of polio, a positive-stranded RNA virus. The genomic RNA acts directly as mRNA and is translated to give a polyprotein, which is rapidly cleaved by virus-coded proteases into 12 or more smaller proteins (not all illustrated). At a later stage during replication the number of positive RNA strands increases and these are used either as mRNAs or are packaged into virions. ∿ poly(A) tail; ◇ 5′ cap.

tive-strand viral RNA segments. These copies, now positive-stranded and termed **antigenome** are exact complements of the genome, are capped at the 5′ end, polyadenylated at the 3′ end, and then function as viral mRNAs, which, in turn, are translated to give viral proteins.

Retroviruses

The third group of RNA viruses—the **retroviruses**—have a more complex strategy of producing viral mRNAs. The essentials of replication and integration are illustrated in Chapter

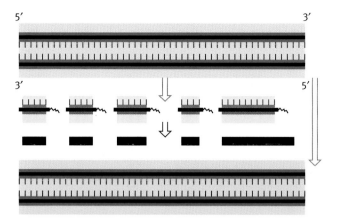

Fig. 3.8 Replication strategy of adenovirus, a DNA virus. The adenovirus genome is transcribed and replicated in the cell nucleus. Replication is mediated by a protein (P) at the 5' end of each DNA strand. Multiple mRNAs (not all shown) are transcribed from both DNA strands. Early mRNAs are encoded by input parental DNA. Later mRNAs are encoded on both DNA strands. Splicing is extensively utilized and can provide control of different regions of the genome, as well as a means of changing the reading frame. ∿, poly(A) tail.

25 (Fig. 25.4). As soon as the virus infects a cell the parental viral RNA is transcribed by a virus-associated **RT** (RNA-dependent DNA polymerase), which converts the viral RNA genome to a DNA–RNA hybrid. The RNA strand is digested away from the hybrid and replaced by a DNA copy to give a dsDNA molecule. This is **integrated** into the chromosomal DNA of the host cell by a virally encoded integrase, and is now termed **proviral DNA**. Viral mRNAs are transcribed from the proviral DNA in much the same way as host-cellular mRNAs are transcribed from host-cell chromosomal DNA. The viral messages are translated and viral proteins are synthesized.

DNA viruses

Obviously, DNA viruses must also produce viral mRNA transcripts soon after the infection of a cell (Fig. 3.8). This is usually achieved by a host-cell enzyme, **DNA-dependent RNA polymerase II,** although we have seen with poxviruses that, exceptionally, a DNA virus may carry the appropriate enzyme into the cell. **Early** and **late viral mRNAs** are transcribed from either DNA strand in the case of dsDNA viruses, and are translated to give 'early' and 'late' viral proteins, respectively. Early mRNAs are transcribed from input parental virus DNA, whereas late mRNAs are transcribed from newly replicated viral DNA (see Fig. 3.2).

3.5 Replication of viral genomes

RNA viruses

In contrast to the host genetic information, which is encoded in dsDNA, many viruses have an **RNA genome**. With the positive-stranded RNA viruses, a virus-coded RNA polymerase ('**replicase**') is translated directly from the viral genome,

whereas the replicase of negative-stranded RNA viruses is carried by the virus itself. In general RNA viral genes are transcribed from the 3' end. Either way, the RNA replicase synthesizes a complementary RNA strand that serves as a template for new rounds of viral RNA synthesis. These RNA duplexes are unstable and occur only as transient '**replicative intermediates**'.

In this manner the RNA virus faithfully—or sometimes, as the transcription process is error-prone, unfaithfully—copies its own genome into offspring genomes. The process is rapid, with production of tens of thousands of new viral genomes in a matter of a few hours after the cell has been infected.

DNA viruses

All DNA viruses except poxviruses replicate their genomes in the cell nucleus. Various methods are used, depending on the configuration of the DNA, which may be linear and single-stranded (parvovirus), circular (papillomavirus), or linear and double-stranded (poxvirus). Replication of ssDNA involves the formation of a **double-stranded intermediate**, which serves as a template for the synthesis of single-stranded progeny DNA. Replication of dsDNA molecules uses a **replication fork**. At these forks the DNA polymerase moves along the DNA, opening up the two strands of the double helix and using each strand as a template to make a new daughter strand. The forks move rapidly at 100 nucleotide pairs per second.

3.6 The intracellular location of viral genome replication

A positive-stranded RNA virus, whose genome can act as the mRNA, may not need to enter the nucleus of the cell. This is also true of the DNA poxviruses, which carry all the necessary DNA polymerases with them. Other DNA viruses replicate in the nucleus alongside host-cell DNA, although not necessarily by the same mechanisms.

3.7 Control of viral replication

As viruses depend totally on the apparatus and mechanisms of the cell for replication, it is essential that the viral genome exerts control of these processes and so must use its genetic information to the maximum. Perhaps the most important mechanism for achieving this control is a viral code for strong positive signals to promote viral gene expression and other signals to repress expression of cellular genes. Virus transcription itself may have to be blocked and some viruses use their M protein to carry this out. Other strategies for enhancing access to this information by the small viral genomes are **primary RNA transcript splicing, overlapping reading frames**, or other methods of encoding multiple proteins in single mRNAs.

Viral protein synthesis is completely dependent on the translation machine in the cell and so mechanisms have developed for reducing their dependence at this critical stage. Most eukaryotic mRNAs depend for initiation of translation on a 5′ terminal cap structure. Some viruses mediate initiation of translation through the internal binding of ribosomes on to mRNA at an internal ribosome entry site (IRES), a method used by hepatitis C, polio, and hepatitis A. This removes competition from host-cell caps giving advantage for the virus. For example, two NS proteins of hepatitis C enhance IRES directed translation.

Further control is exerted by the various properties of the viral mRNA, including its half-life and the actual flow of RNA from the nucleus to the cytoplasm. Control of viral gene replication may thus be exerted at the levels of transcription, post-transcription, or translation.

The expression of groups of virus genes is often carried out in critically timed phases. Thus **immediate early viral genes** of a virus such as herpes or adenovirus may code for activation proteins and **early viral genes** for other regulatory proteins, whereas **late viral genes** code for structural proteins.

3.8 Synthesis of viral proteins

All viruses use the cellular ribosomes to translate viral mRNAs. The viral messages are translated into the **structural proteins** that constitute the virus particle itself, or **NS proteins**, which are enzymes or transcription factors for virus replication, but not incorporated in the virus.

The message is read continuously from the start codon AUG (Fig. 3.9), but this continuity may be interrupted by the insertion or deletion of a base that causes a **frame shift**. In other words, from the point of such a mutation the message

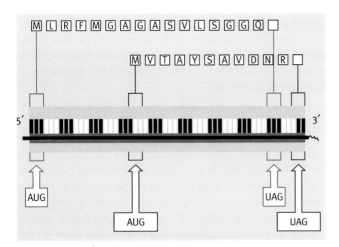

Fig. 3.9 Overlapping reading frames. The diagram shows how two or more polypeptides can be coded in a single length of nucleic acid. Starting at an initiation codon AUG, the nucleotide sequence is read to give a protein MLRFMG...., etc. An alternative start codon situated farther down the nucleic acid molecule allows a different protein, MVTAYS...., etc. to be translated from the same gene, as the nucleotide triplets are now read in a different sequence. The boxed letters are the conventional codes for the various amino acids: M, methionine; V, valine; L, leucine, etc. For clarity, the base triplets are represented alternatively as open and solid bars: the shading has no other significance. ∿, poly(A) tail.

is read as a different set of triplets and thus the viral protein will have a completely different amino acid sequence from that specified in the original message. It can even be a very shortened protein if the frame shift produces a **stop codon**. In this manner, the number of proteins that can be engendered from a small viral genome is increased. Several viruses use this strategy, including HIV and paramyxoviruses. Retroviruses have a special signal on the mRNA that triggers the ribosome to 'jump' and begin reading the triplet code in a different frame.

3.9 Post-translation modification of viral proteins

Even after synthesis of viral proteins our biochemical story is far from complete, as the viral protein must fold correctly into a precise three-dimensional structure. Important post-translation events must occur as a preparation for this folding. The initiator amino acid is removed while the polypeptide is still attached to the ribosome. Other important events may be **glycosylation** (attachment of carbohydrate), covalent attachment of lipoic acid, and addition of phosphate, sulphate, and acyl groups.

Some viruses, particularly positive-strand RNA viruses such as polio, rhinoviruses, and flaviviruses, have a strategy whereby a very large viral polyprotein is translated initially from a single viral messenger mRNA. This **polyprotein** is then cleaved at specific sites by viral or cellular proteolytic enzymes to give a series of smaller viral proteins, some of which are incorporated into the virus.

4 Virus assembly, release from the host cell, and maturation

4.1 Virus assembly and release

The virus is now nearing the time of release and maturation. Its structural proteins have been synthesized by a host cell that appears relatively normal, or that may be irretrievably damaged. Some viruses (e.g. poliovirus) assemble completely in the cytoplasm, whereas others (e.g. adenoviruses) are predominantly nuclear in location. Most enveloped viruses bud through the plasma membrane, but a few, such as rotavirus, exploit the endoplasmic reticulum membrane. Some viruses have signals on their glycoprotein spikes for specific targeting or retention. For negative-stranded RNA viruses the nucleocapsid has to be inactivated before packaging. The viral M protein acts as a blocker.

Lytic viruses, for example polio, are released on lysis and death of the cell. Others (e.g. influenza, HIV, and measles) escape by **budding** from the cell surface. Viral proteins are transported by the existing cell machinery and are, in the case of 'budding' viruses, inserted in the external plasma membrane of the cell; other virus structural proteins migrate to the inside of the plasma membrane. The proteins and nucleic acids self-assemble, and viral RNA or DNA is packaged as the completed virion buds by protrusion through the cellular plasma membrane. The bud is pinched off and a new virus is born. Some viruses, such as HIV and herpes, do not emerge from the cell, but may spread to contiguous cells via connecting pores or by inducing fusion of their membranes.

4.2 Viral maturation

For some viruses, such as HIV and influenza, there is a further stage in the replication cycle, termed **post-release maturation**. Certain capsid proteins in HIV have to be cleaved by a viral protease, which leads to changes in morphology of the new virion, quite easily detected by EM. In the case of the influenza virus, cellular proteases are needed to cleave the viral HA spike protein. Some cells do not have the correct protease and so the virus does not normally initiate a successful multicycle infection in that organ: virus replication is restricted. The cleavage often occurs before the HA reaches the plasma membrane and before budding, but may take place at or after budding, particularly if a protease is supplied exogenously. An example is co-infection of the lung with influenza virus and staphylococcus or streptococcus, which provide the protease and hence enhance the infectivity of the virus itself. The resulting pneumonia can be catastrophic.

5 Genetic variation of viruses

5.1 Low fidelity of reverse transcriptases and RNA replicases

Mutations such as removal or insertion of a nucleotide or a group of nucleotides (**deletion** or **insertion mutants**) are not uncommon during viral replication. Such mutations are more frequent in RNA than in DNA viruses because of the low fidelity of transcription of RT and RNA transcriptase, and absence of proof-reading and correction ability, compared with DNA polymerase. In fact, all RNA viruses are thought to exist as mixtures of countless genetic variants with slightly different genetic and antigenic compositions: so-called quasi-species. These mixtures of virions exist as a dynamic equilibrium within the host, so that under a particular set of conditions one virus in the mixture is dominant but others are still present, albeit in much lower numbers. Development of specific immunity to a particular variant or use of an antiviral drug provides the pressure to force viral evolution.

5.2 Recombination

An important way in which viruses may vary their genomic structure is by **recombination**. This is brought about in DNA viruses by DNA strand breakage and covalent linkage of genome DNA fragments, either from a single gene or from two infecting viruses of the same kind. It is thought to occur in RNA viruses when the virus polymerase switches template strands during genome synthesis. Fortunately, such genetic interactions do not occur among unrelated viruses (such as polio and influenza),

otherwise our problems would be greatly compounded. Nevertheless, this type of genetic interaction may give rise to a virus with hitherto unknown characteristics and may also give the mutant a selective advantage over its relatives. More often though, the new recombinant virus has properties incompatible with survival.

5.3 Gene reassortment

With certain RNA viruses, such as influenza and rotaviruses, in which the genome exists as separate fragments, simple exchange of genes may occur, a process known as **gene reassortment**. Such reassortant progeny viruses have characteristics that differ from those of the parental viruses. The frequency of such gene exchanges may be very high, much higher, for example, than that of true recombination. Such genetic reassortment can extend the gene pool of the virus and allow the emergence of new and successful variants. An example is the infrequent appearance of pandemics of influenza (in 1918, 1957, and 1968), caused by reassortment of genes between human, avian, and pig influenza A viruses. A novel mutant may be created that can cross the species barrier and infect humans.

6 Reminders

- The stages of viral infection of cells are **cellular recognition** and attachment to a cell receptor, **internalization**, **genome transcription** to form viral mRNA, **mRNA translation**, **genome replication**, **encapsidation**, and release of new virions from the cell. The complete viral life cycle characteristically takes 6–8 h and as many as 10 000 new viruses are released from each infected cell.

- Some RNA-containing viruses such as polio are **positive stranded** and the genome acts directly as mRNA. **Negative-stranded** RNA viruses, such as influenza, possess a virion-associated **RNA transcriptase** that produces a positive-stranded mRNA transcript from the genome RNA upon infection of the cell.

- Transcription of DNA viruses, with the exception of pox viruses, is carried out by cellular **DNA-dependent RNA polymerases**.

- The **Baltimore scheme** designates seven viral genome coding strategies: dsDNA; ssDNA; dsRNA; ss positive-sense RNA; ss negative-sense RNA; ss positive-sense RNA with DNA intermediate, and dsDNA with RNA intermediate.

- Primary RNA transcripts may be **spliced**, thus allowing several mRNAs to be coded in a single piece of viral genome. Viral messages may also be read in different **reading frames** at the translation stage, again allowing more extensive use of viral genetic information.

- **Control of viral gene expression** occurs at four levels:
  - configuration of viral DNA or RNA,

- at transcription itself (rate of initiation, utilization of upstream transcription factors);
- mRNA half-life, splicing of mRNA precursors, and flow of mRNA from the nucleus; and
- at translation.

- Viruses may **bud** in many waves from infected cells (which continue to be viable) or may be released instantaneously by **cell lysis**.

- The replication of RNA viral genomes is error prone; this generates **genomic diversity**. In contrast, replication of DNA viruses is extremely faithful, as the viral DNA polymerase has proof-reading and correction functions.
- Genetic recombination and gene reassortment may both lead to **genetic diversity**.

How viruses cause disease

1 Introduction

Figure 4.1 shows a child with measles, an elderly patient with severe herpes zoster ('shingles'), and another child with a malignant tumour of the jaw known as Burkitt's lymphoma (BL). Each of these people is under attack by a virus; however, the manifestations differ greatly, not only in appearance but also in the way in which the viruses concerned caused these unpleasant effects. This chapter is concerned with the complex interactions between viruses and hosts that result in disease, in other words, with the **pathogenesis** of viral infection. It is written primarily from the point of view of the virus; the next chapter describes the defences put up by the host.

2 Viral factors: pathogenicity and virulence

The terms **pathogenicity** and **virulence** are often used interchangeably, but this is not strictly correct. 'Pathogenicity' compares the severity of disease caused by **different micro-organisms**: rabies virus is more pathogenic than measles. 'Virulence', on the other hand, compares the severity of the disease caused by **different strains of the same micro-organism**. In practice, this may be related to the numbers of organisms needed to produce a given effect (e.g. the death of a mouse). For example, two strains of herpes simplex virus (HSV) inoculated into the skin may cause vesicular lesions, and are thus both pathogenic; but as few as 10 virions of strain A may kill the mouse, whereas 10 000 virions of strain B are needed to do so. Strain A is thus a thousand times more virulent than strain B.

What is it that makes one strain of virus more virulent than another? The development of rapid methods for determining nucleotide sequences within DNA and RNA is helping virologists to answer this intriguing question, which is important both from the points of view of preparing attenuated viruses for vaccines and of trying to predict whether viruses of enhanced virulence, for example, AIDS, could suddenly be created as the result of a small mutational change.

In at least some RNA viruses only very few nucleotide substitutions in the viral genome are needed to control a switch from virulence to avirulence. Poliomyelitis and influenza viruses provide two excellent examples. The complete genomes of a virulent type 3 poliovirus and an attenuated strain derived from it have been sequenced and compared. Only 10 **point**

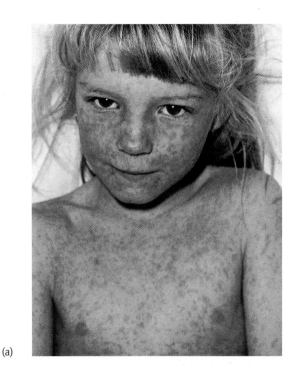

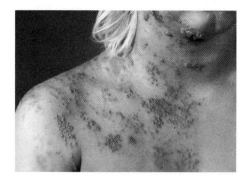

(b)

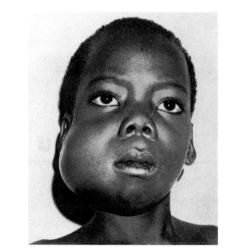

(a)

(c)

Fig. 4.1 Differing manifestations of viral infections. **(a)** Child with measles). **(b)** Elderly patient with herpes zoster. **(c)** Seven-year-old boy with Burkitt's lymphoma involving the right mandible (by courtesy of Dr Joan Edwards).

mutations (i.e. changes in single nucleotides) out of a total of about 7430 bases were detected in the attenuated strain; it now appears that only three of them give rise to amino acid substitutions and, of these, only one point mutation may be responsible for attenuation of virulence. Likewise, a single change in amino acid sequence near the receptor-binding site on the HA molecule had a decisive influence on the virulence of influenza B for volunteers (Fig. 4.2). Changes at this position may also allow influenza viruses to emerge from an avian reservoir to cause a global pandemic in humans, as mutation in the receptor binding site could allow the virus to bind on to both avian and mammalian cells.

The finding that virulence, or lack of it, depends upon such small molecular changes in the genome was unexpected and opens up new vistas both for vaccine development and for epidemiology.

3 Interactions between viruses and host cells

The interactions between the virus and the cells within which it replicates are of decisive importance in determining whether infection takes place at all, the type of infection that is established, and the final outcome for the host.

3.1 Cellular factors

The presence of appropriate receptors on the surface of the cell determines whether virus can adsorb to it (Chapter 3). Once

this takes place and the virus gets into the cell it must replicate in order to establish infection, which may take several forms. These are described in Sections 4 and 5 below, but the general

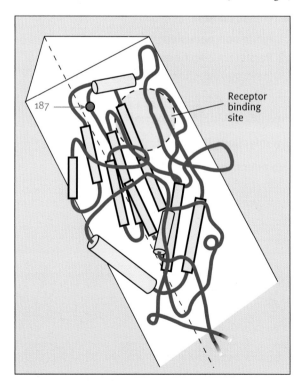

Fig. 4.2 X-ray crystallographic structure of influenza HA. The arrow indicates where substitution of a single amino acid (no. 187) causes a change in virulence.

point to be made here is that none of these outcomes are possible unless the internal, physical, and molecular environment of the host cell is suitable for the initial replication cycle. The temperature of the cell is important. For example, respiratory viruses that replicate well at 33°C are limited to the upper respiratory tract where this is the prevailing temperature, whereas those that replicate well at 37°C but not at 33°C predominantly infect the warmer environment of the lower respiratory tract.

3.2 Cytopathic effects

Many viruses kill the cells in which they replicate, sometimes with characteristic appearances or cytopathic effect (CPEs). These effects occur in the intact host as well as in cell cultures, and are often distinctive enough to give an idea of the virus concerned, a property that is occasionally useful in the diagnostic laboratory (Chapter 36). Furthermore, the type of CPE may give clues as to the sort of immune response to be expected.

Cell lysis

The 'early' virus-coded proteins (Chapter 3) may **shut down synthesis of macromolecules**, particularly polypeptides, by the host cell. Later in the multiplication cycle of some viruses (e.g. adenoviruses) accumulation of large amounts of capsid protein may cause a general inhibition of both host cell and viral synthetic activities. Death of the cell is followed by lysis and release of large numbers of virions. We can think of these viruses as 'bursters'.

Cell fusion

We saw in Chapter 3 that virus-specified **fusion proteins** mediate the entry of certain viruses through the plasma membrane of the cell; they also cause the formation of multinucleated giant cells (**syncytia**, Fig. 4.3) by **paramyxoviruses**, such as respiratory syncytial virus (RSV), parainfluenza viruses, and measles. **Herpesviruses** and some **retroviruses** also give rise to

syncytia. Viruses that behave in this way tend to **pass from cell to cell** rather than to be liberated in bursts by lysis. These are the 'creepers'.

Inclusion bodies

Inclusion bodies are eosinophilic or basophilic bodies that appear within cells as a result of infection with some—but not all—viruses and with certain bacteria (notably *Chlamydia*). Viral inclusions may be **intracytoplasmic**, **intranuclear**, or **both**. Some examples are given in Fig. 4.3.

The nature of the inclusions varies with the virus concerned. They may represent aggregations of mature virions (papovaviruses, reoviruses), but are more often areas of altered staining at sites of viral synthesis, or simply degenerative changes. The finding of characteristic inclusions in exfoliated cells or tissue sections stained by conventional methods was formerly much used in diagnosis, but has been superseded by the more reliable methods of molecular biology.

3.3 New cell-surface antigens

Another major consequence of many virus infections is the induction of **new antigens** on the cell surface. This is particularly important in the case of enveloped viruses that bud from the cell surface (e.g. herpes-, myxo-, paramyxo-, and retroviruses). As they are specified by the virus rather than the host cell, these antigens mark the infected cells as being in a sense 'foreign', so that they are susceptible to attack by cytotoxic T cells, an important element in the immune response. The surface antigens induced by viruses can be made visible by immunofluorescence staining.

Some viruses induce malignant changes in cells; the important topic of the relationship between viruses and cancer will be dealt with in Chapter 6.

4 The spread of viruses in the host

We must now move from events in individual cells to consider how viruses cause disease in the intact host.

4.1 Important events in pathogenesis

To cause disease, a virus has to clear a number of hurdles, that vary somewhat in type and number according both to the virus concerned and its host. The following sequence of events is typical. The virus must, sequentially:

1. **invade** the host;

2. **establish a bridgehead** by replicating in susceptible cells at the site of inoculation;

3. **overcome the local defences**, for example lymphocytes, macrophages, and interferon (IFN);

4. **spread from the site of inoculation** to other areas, often via the bloodstream;

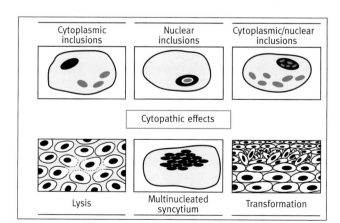

Fig. 4.3 Cytopathic effects of viral infection. *(top)* Inclusion bodies: intracytoplasmic, e.g. rabies; intranuclear, e.g. herpesviruses; or both, e.g. measles virus. *(bottom)* The three main types of cytopathic effect: lysis, syncytium formation, and transformation.

Table 4.1 Examples of viruses entering through the skin

Virus	Disease
Entry via abrasions	
Papillomaviruses	Warts
Poxviruses (cowpox, orf)	Vesicular or nodular lesions on milkers' fingers
Herpes simplex viruses	Herpetic lesions on face, fingers, genitalia
Entry via abrasions or inoculation with contaminated needle	
Hepadnavirus	Hepatitis B
Lentiviruses (HIV)	AIDS
Entry via insect or animal bites	
Arboviruses	Various tropical fevers
Lyssavirus	Rabies

Table 4.2 Examples of viruses entering through mucous membranes

Virus	Disease
Entry via respiratory tract	
Orthomyxoviruses	Influenza
Paramyxoviruses	Measles, mumps, parainfluenza, respiratory syncytial disease
Rhinoviruses	Common cold
Varicella-zoster	Chickenpox
Entry via gastrointestinal tract	
Poliovirus	Poliomyelitis
Other enteroviruses	Febrile illnesses affecting muscles or CNS
Rotavirus	Gastroenteritis
Entry via conjunctiva	
Enterovirus type 70	Conjunctivitis
Adenovirus type 8	Keratoconjunctivitis
Entry via genital tract	
Lentivirus (HIV)	AIDS
Hepadnavirus	Hepatitis B
Herpes simplex	Herpetic lesions of cervix, urethra
Papillomavirus	Genital warts, cancer

5. **undergo further replication** in its target area, whether this be localized (e.g. adenovirus conjunctivitis) or generalized (e.g. measles);

6. **exit from the host** in numbers large enough to infect other susceptible hosts and thus ensure its own survival.

Some of these activities relate to specific properties of the virus itself and others to interactions between virus and host, both within individual cells and with the body as a whole and its array of immune defences.

4.2 Invasion routes

Viruses gain access to the host either through the skin or mucous membranes. Examples are given in Tables 4.1 and 4.2. Please note that these lists are not exhaustive, since routes of infection will be given in more detail in the chapters dealing with individual viruses. They show:

- the diversity of routes adopted;
- the ability of some viruses to infect by more than one route.

The stratified squamous epithelium of the **skin** is a formidable barrier to microbes and some degree of trauma is necessary before infection can take place. Table 4.1 shows that some viruses (e.g. papilloma and some pox- and herpesviruses) cause more or less localized lesions at the site of implantation, whereas others go on to produce generalized infections involving a variety of body systems.

By contrast, many viruses entering through **mucous membranes** (Table 4.2) need little or no trauma, as they adsorb directly to the epithelial cells, in which they undergo an initial cycle of replication. The infections caused by some of these viruses, notably those affecting primarily the conjunctiva, are localized. Most, however, are more general; and here it is important to appreciate that the body system by which a virus enters is not necessarily the one that will ultimately be mainly affected. Thus, although varicella virus enters by the respiratory tract, its main target organ is the skin; likewise enteroviruses, which, as their name suggests, do indeed invade and multiply within the enteric canal, cause disease of the CNS or muscles rather than enteritis.

In temperate climates the most common infections are those acquired by the **respiratory route.** An unstifled sneeze results in an aerosol, an ideal medium for carrying microbes into someone else's respiratory tract. The smaller the droplets, the more widely they will be disseminated and the further down the bronchial tree they will penetrate. Especially in wintertime, crowded stores, buses, and trains are ideal places in which to exchange viruses transmitted by the respiratory route.

Respiratory infections are also very prevalent in the tropics; and because standards of hygiene are poor in many developing countries, these areas also bear the brunt of infections acquired via the **gastrointestinal tract**. This mode of infection is known as the **faecal–oral** route, which sounds revolting and is, as it means that viruses shed in faeces have got into someone else's mouth. Figure 4.4 shows a number of ways in which this can happen. Such infections are by no means confined to Third World countries; they are prevalent wherever sanitary conditions are indifferent, for example in some mental institutions.

Not surprisingly, viruses that infect via the alimentary tract, such as the enteroviruses, are resistant to the acid environment

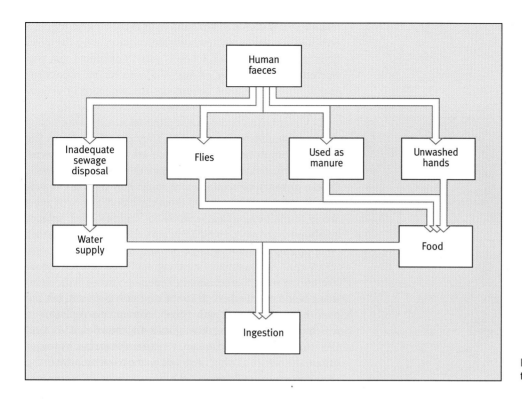

Fig. 4.4 The faecal–oral route of transmission of viruses.

of the stomach, whereas those with other portals of entry (e.g. the respiratory viruses) are not.

The incidence of **sexually transmitted diseases** (STDs) has increased enormously since the end of the Second World War in 1945 and has risen still further in the first years of the new millennium. Much of the increase is due to viruses and chlamydia: but the 'classical' venereal infections, gonorrhoea and syphilis, have also increased in prevalence. Although some syndromes such as AIDS and hepatitis B are, in Western countries, particularly associated with promiscuous male homosexuals, all the STDs mentioned in Table 4.2 can also be spread by heterosexual intercourse (see also Chapter 34).

The third and increasingly frequent, way of acquiring infection is from **transplants**, particularly of bone marrow and kidneys. Two herpesviruses—cytomegalovirus (CMV) and EBV— are notorious in this respect. Both cause persistent but asymptomatic infections in a substantial proportion of the general population; if an organ donor is infected in this way, the recipient is liable to suffer, particularly if he or she has no pre-existing immunity, or if the immune responses have been impaired by immunosuppressive treatment (Chapter 32). **Blood transfusions** and **blood products** such as Factor VIII are also a potential source of infection with certain viruses, such as the hepatitis viruses B and C and possibly vCJD. However, rigorous screening and the exclusion of high-risk donors such as drug addicts has greatly reduced, but not eliminated, the number of infections from such sources.

Other infections resulting from **surgical treatment** have been described, but are rare. More than one person has died from rabies after receiving a corneal transplant from a donor who was incubating the disease—surely the ultimate in bad luck stories! Others again have acquired CJD, another fatal infection of the CNS, from surgical instruments contaminated with the causal agent, which is unusually resistant to sterilization (Appendix A).

Spread of infection from mother to fetus is a special form of transmission from one person to another and is described in Chapter 31.

Like bacterial and fungal infections, those caused by viruses can be classified under two main headings:

- those localized to tissues at or contiguous with the site of entry; and
- those that spread to one or more organs remote from this area.

4.3 Localized infections

These are infections of epithelial surfaces: the skin, the conjunctiva, and the mucous membranes of the respiratory, gastrointestinal, and genital tracts. Some examples are given in Tables 4.1 and 4.2.

Localized infections of the skin by poxviruses result in papular lesions, usually proceeding to vesicle and then pustule formation (e.g. vaccinia, orf), or in proliferative lesions of the epidermis (molluscum contagiosum and papillomaviruses).

By contrast, infections of **mucous membranes** spread over comparatively large areas of the respiratory or gastrointestinal epithelium. The process is rapid, which means that such infections have a short incubation period, say 1–3 days. Although viral replication is restricted to these surfaces, the effects may be much more general, as anyone who has had influenza or even a bad cold knows only too well.

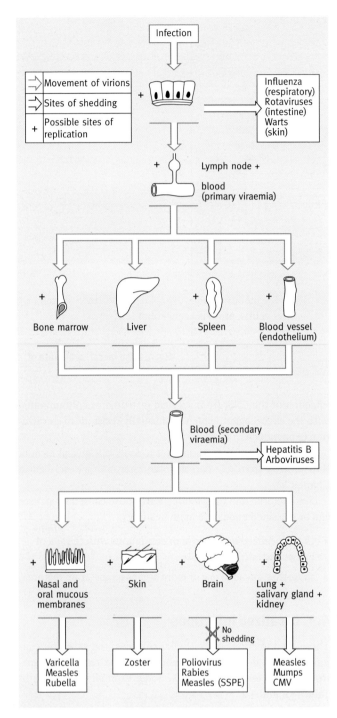

Fig. 4.5 Spread and replication of virus in a typical generalized virus infection. Modified from White D.O. and Fenner F.J. (1986), *Medical Virology*, p. 135. Academic Press, London.

4.4 Generalized infections

For various reasons, the pathogenesis of many generalized virus infections is not well understood: in some instances there is no suitable animal model; in others, such as the viral haemorrhagic fevers, the difficulty of working with dangerous pathogens under restricted conditions discourages extensive experimentation; and in others again, our lack of knowledge

results from inability to grow the virus in the laboratory. Nevertheless, a number of viruses, notably those causing the infectious fevers of childhood, follow a pattern of spread that was worked out by F. Fenner, in Australia, who studied a poxvirus infection of mice called ectromelia; the sequence of events, summarized in Fig. 4.5, is as follows.

(1) Virions enter through an epithelial surface, where they undergo limited replication. (2) They then migrate to the **regional lymph nodes** where some are taken up by macrophages and inactivated, but others enter the bloodstream. This is (3) the **primary viraemia**, which sometimes gives rise to prodromal malaise and fever. (4) From the blood, the virus gains access to the large reticuloendothelial organs—**liver**, **spleen**, **and bone marrow**—in which it again multiplies. In this further cycle of amplification, a large amount of virus is produced, which again, in a manner of speaking, spills over into the bloodstream, causing (5) a secondary viraemia. Viruses in the circulating blood may be free, as in the case of hepatitis B, but are more often associated with lymphocytes or macrophages in which they can replicate, examples being measles, CMV, and HIV. (6) From the bloodstream, virus finally reaches its **target organ**, the nature of which depends on the tissue tropism of the virus concerned, and mainly determines the clinical features of the illness. All this takes time, which explains why the incubation periods of infections of this type are of the order of 2 weeks.

In other infections, viruses reach their target organs by more direct routes, stage (3) being omitted. This may happen in, for example, certain arbovirus infections.

4.5 Some important target organs

The skin

A rash, or **exanthem**, features in a number of virus infections (Table 4.3). Dental students in particular should note that such

Table 4.3 Examples of virus diseases associated with a skin rash (exanthem)

Disease	Type of rash
Rubella, erythema infectiosum (parvovirus), entero- and ECHO virus infections, dengue	Macular
Measles, infectious mononucleosis, entero- and ECHO virus infections	Maculopapular
Herpes simplex, chickenpox/herpes zoster, poxvirus infections,	Vesicular or vesiculopustular
Coxsackie virus infections (especially type A9 and A16), entero- and ECHO virus infections	
Congenital rubella	Purpuric
Viral haemorrhagic fevers	Petechial/haemorrhagic

Table 4.4 Virus diseases associated with a rash (enanthem) on the buccal mucous membrane

Disease	Main features of the enanthem
Herpesvirus infections	
Herpes simplex (usually primary infection)	Gingivostomatitis, with vesicles and ulcers on an intensely inflamed mucosa, primarily affecting the **anterior** part of the buccal cavity
Chickenpox	Vesicles, rapidly ulcerating, especially on fauces and palate
Infectious mononucleosis	Petechiae occasionally seen on palate
Coxsackie A virus infections	
Herpangina	Small vesicles usually confined to **posterior** part of the buccal cavity (soft palate and fauces)
Hand, foot, and mouth disease	Vesicles and ulcers anywhere on buccal mucosa, but predominating in **anterior** part
Paramyxovirus infection	
Measles	Koplik's spots on congested mucosa near openings of parotid ducts; appear a day or two before the skin rash

Note. These and many other acute viral infections may be accompanied by pharyngitis.

an infection is sometimes accompanied by an **enanthem**, a rash affecting mucous membranes, which is of course best observed on the buccal mucosa (Table 4.4). There are several types, which are not necessary exclusive to particular viruses. Some viruses, notably the entero- and echoviruses, are notorious for causing almost any type of non-haemorrhagic rash.

Whereas the vesicular eruptions are due to replication of virus in the skin, with consequent damage to epithelial cells, other rashes may have other causes. Thus the characteristic maculopapular rash of measles is due to the destruction of infected cells by cytotoxic T lymphocytes; purpuric rashes are often associated with a fall in blood platelets; and some haemorrhagic rashes are the result of disseminated intravascular coagulation.

The lung

Most respiratory infections, even those of the lung, result from local spread of virus, as described in Section 4.3. Sometimes, however, the lung is involved as part of a generalized infection. This is particularly so in measles, in which some degree of pneumonitis is a constant feature. In patients whose immunity is damaged, both measles and varicella viruses may cause giant cell pneumonia, characterized by the appearance of syncytia (Section 3.2, and see Figs 32.2 and 32.3); this is a dreaded complication with a high mortality.

The liver

This organ is the target for the hepatitis viruses (Chapters 21–24). It may also be damaged as part of a more general infection of body tissues, the classical example being yellow fever (YF). Other virus infections come into this category and are listed in Table 21.2.

Kidney

The kidney is rarely infected by viruses. An important exception is CMV, one of the herpes group. Characteristic inclusions are found in the proximal renal tubules, from which the virus is shed into the urine. Certain hantaviruses (Chapter 28) cause a haemorrhagic fever with nephritis.

The central nervous system

Viruses gain access in one of two ways:

- from the bloodstream, during an episode of viraemia (e.g. poliomyelitis, arbovirus encephalitis); or
- via the nerves connecting the periphery with various parts of the CNS (e.g. herpes simplex, varicella-zoster, rabies).

See also Chapter 30.

4.6 Immunopathological damage

We have mentioned that some skin rashes are manifestations of the immune response rather than the result of tissue damage by virus

Table 4.5 Incubation periods of representative viral diseases

Disease	Usual period	Limits
Short incubation (times in days)		
Enterovirus conjunctivitis	1–2	
Common cold	1–3	
Influenza	1–3	
Arbovirus infections	3–6	2–15
Medium incubation (times in days)		
Poliomyelitis	7–14	2–35
Measles	13–14	8–14
Rubella	14–16	14–21
Varicella	13–17	11–21
Mumps	14–18	14–21
SARS	–	10–12
Long incubation (times in weeks)		
Hepatitis A	3–5	2–6
Hepatitis B	10–12	6–20
Infectious mononucleosis	4–6	2–7
Rabies	4–7	2–50
Very long incubation		
Subacute sclerosing panencephalitis (SSPE)		
Progressive multifocal leucoencephalopathy	Years	
Creutzfeldt–Jakob disease		

multiplication. This is often true of pathological changes in other organs infected by viruses (Chapter 5). Particular examples are damage to hepatocytes in the liver infected with hepatitis B virus and 'cytokine storm' (a sudden outpouring of various cytokines (e.g. tumour necrosis factor (TNF), IFN-α, interleukin (IL)-1) in response to a lung infection with influenza or SARS viruses.

4.7 Incubation periods

Knowledge of the incubation periods of the common virus infections is important not only as an aid to the diagnosis of individual patients, but also as an essential tool in tracing the spread of outbreaks (Chapter 7). They will be given in more detail in the chapters devoted to individual viruses, but for the moment, and as an aid to memory, we shall classify them

into four main groups: short, medium, long, and very long (Table 4.5).

Short means less than a week and primarily applies to viruses causing localized infections that spread rapidly on mucous surfaces. Some viruses injected directly (e.g. arboviruses transmitted by the bite of an arthropod) also, as a rule, have short incubation periods.

Medium incubation periods range from about 7 to 21 days; they are seen in generalized infections having the type of pathogenesis described in Section 5.2.

Long refers to periods measured in weeks or months (e.g. 2–6 weeks for hepatitis A and 6–20 weeks for hepatitis B). The pathogenesis of these infections has not yet been worked out, and we do not know what these viruses are doing between

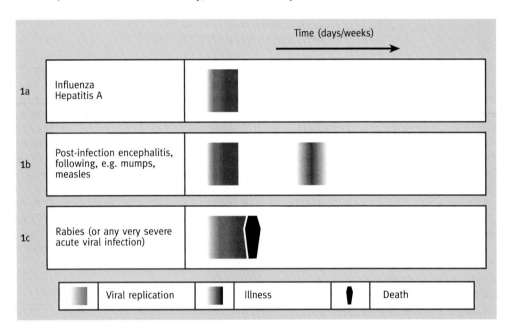

Fig 4.6 Patterns of viral pathogenesis. **Group 1**, acute non-persistent infections. Acute onset, usually with clinical signs, followed by **(a)** rapid recovery, **(b)** apparent recovery with early central nervous system complication, or **(c)** rapid death.

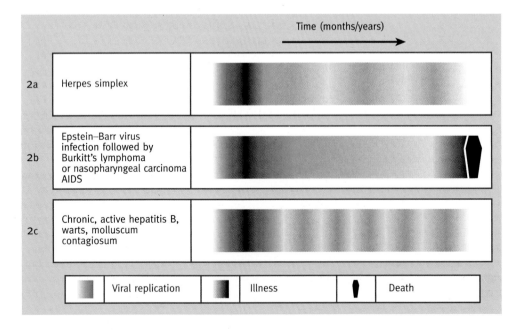

Fig 4.7 Patterns of viral pathogenesis. **Group 2**, primary infection, usually with physical signs, followed by persistent infection. **(a)** Symptom-free periods punctuated by reactivations; **(b)** long symptom-free period followed by illness and death; **(c)** chronic disease with periodic exacerbations.

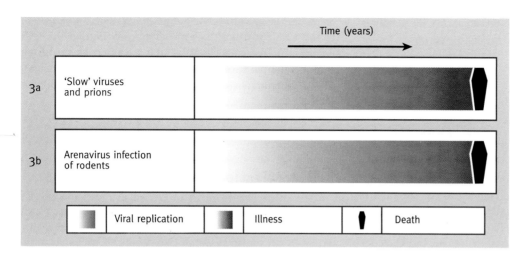

Fig 4.8 Patterns of viral pathogenesis. **Group 3,** insidious infections with fatal outcomes. **(a)** Long incubation period followed by illness lasting many months; **(b)** congenital infection followed late in life by acute illness.

entering the host and producing symptoms and signs of illness. Rabies may also have incubation periods extending for many months (Chapter 26), but in this instance we know that the time to onset depends on the rate at which the virus travels up neurons to the brain from the site of entry, and on the length of the nerves affected.

Very long incubation periods are measured in years, which is why the agents involved were originally termed 'slow' viruses. This group comprises the prions (Chapter 29) and a few 'conventional' viruses, such as papovaviruses (Chapter 15) and measles (Chapter 9), which very occasionally cause delayed disease of the CNS. These infections are invariably fatal. Why their incubation periods are so long remains a mystery.

5 Patterns of disease

Details of the pathogenesis of individual virus infections will be given in more detail in the relevant chapters; this section is intended just to give you a general idea of the variations that may occur. In Figs 4.6–4.8 they are classified into three main groups.

5.1 Acute non-persistent infections

Most acute virus infections resolve spontaneously (group 1a); sequelae are unusual unless the CNS is invaded, as for example in poliomyelitis and some arbovirus infections, but any very severe infection may, of course, be lethal. A comparatively rare complication of some of the infectious fevers of childhood is shown in group 1b; 10–14 days after onset, by which time virus can no longer be isolated, there may be an episode of encephalitis (Chapter 30). The pathogenesis of this condition is not clear; it may be due to an autoimmune response.

5.2 Persistent infections with acute onset

In this group, chronicity of infection is often due to **latency,** resulting from **persistence in the host cell of viral DNA;** clearly, this can only happen with DNA viruses or with retroviruses that form complementary DNA (cDNA) during replica-

Table 4.6 Latent virus infections

Virus	Site of latency
Herpesviruses	
Herpes simplex types 1 and 2; varicella-zoster	Neurons in dorsal root ganglia
Epstein–Barr virus	B lymphocytes
Cytomegalovirus	Lymphocytes; macrophages (?)
Human herpesvirus type 6	Probably lymphocytes
Hepadnavirus	
Hepatitis B	Hepatocytes
Papovavirus	
Papillomavirus	Epithelium
Retroviruses	
Endogenous oncornaviruses	Somatic and germ cells
Lentiviruses	
Human immunodeficiency viruses	T lymphocytes, macrophages, brain cells

tion. The viral DNA may be integrated into that of the host cell or be present in **episomal** form (i.e. as a circular molecule separate from the host DNA).

The cells affected vary according to the virus concerned (Table 4.6). Such latent infections may be established very soon after the primary infection, as with the herpesviruses, or be delayed by a matter of 2 or 3 years, as in some chronic carriers of hepatitis B. Subsequent events depend on the nature of the virus and sometimes on whether the patient's immune responses are adequate.

Note that:

- Latent infections may never cause signs of disease.

- They may reactivate on one or more occasions, causing an episode of illness.

- Infective virus may not be demonstrable while the patient is asymptomatic, but is produced in quantity during reactivations.
- Some latent infections lead to malignant disease.

With regard to the last-mentioned point, infections caused by the endogenous oncornaviruses (Chapter 6) are now of intense interest both to molecular biologists and to oncologists; they differ from the others mentioned in Table 4.6 because, being present both in somatic and germ cells, they can be transmitted vertically through many generations.

Chronic infection is the term applied to the situation in which **infective virus is continually being produced**, with or without integration of viral DNA into the host cell (group 2c). True chronic infections with certain viruses can be induced in cultured cells, which continue to generate infective virus without being destroyed. Such infections have their counterparts *in vivo* (group 3b). Unlike latent infections, they may be caused both by DNA and RNA viruses and the end result for the host is often determined by an abnormal or defective response of the immune system, as may be the case in subacute sclerosing panencephalitis, a fatal but fortunately very rare late complication of measles; chronic active hepatitis B is another example. Other chronic but more trivial infections are caused by the papillomaviruses responsible for warts and by the poxvirus that gives rise to molluscum contagiosum. In both these skin conditions, the viruses evade the immune response by remaining within their safe haven in the avascular epidermis. Papillomavirus genome may also integrate with host-cell DNA.

5.3 Insidious infections with fatal outcomes

The two types of infection in this group resemble each other only superficially. The 'slow' virus infections (group 3a) have already been mentioned in Section 4.7. The other type of infection (group 3b) is not known to occur in humans, but is of great interest both to virologists and to immunologists. Indeed, it was the study of lymphocytic choriomeningitis (LCM), an arenavirus infection of mice, which led the late Sir Macfarlane Burnet to the idea of **immunological tolerance** and a Nobel prize. In brief, every member of a mouse colony in which this virus is present becomes infected at birth and continues so for the rest of its life. In such mice, the immune system fails to recognize the virus-infected cells as 'foreign'. Some antibody is produced, but forms virus–antibody complexes; these are not dealt with in the normal way, and a proportion of infected mice eventually die because of their deposition in the kidney.

6 Shedding of virus from the host

Microbes only live to fight another day by getting out of one host and into another; the means of escape is therefore very important. Viruses may be shed from the **primary site of multiplication** or, in the case of generalized infections, from the target organ. Viruses can escape readily in one way

or another from all the main body systems, with the exception of the CNS, in which they are effectively bottled up. It is important to remember that many viruses may be shed from clinically normal people: they include herpes simplex (saliva), CMV (urine, breast milk), and the viruses that infect the gut (faeces).

We shall see in Chapter 7 what happens when viruses escape into the community.

7 How infectious is a virus?

Infectiousness is a well observed characteristic of viruses. We all can see how influenza can speed through a community, but why did SARS not spread so widely? Epidemiologists now quantify infectiousness and assign viruses a **reproduction number (Ro)**. This is the average number of secondary cases generated by one primary case in a susceptible community. The higher the number, the more persons can be infected from one case. The Ro value of SARS and smallpox would be about 2, whereas influenza may reach 6–8 and measles 10. But the incubation period is also important. Beware the virus, like influenza, with a high Ro value and short incubation period.

8 Reminders

- Viruses gain access to the host through **skin** and **mucous membranes**, and via the **respiratory, gastrointestinal,** and **genital tracts**.
- Their virulence or lack of it may be determined by very small mutations in the genome.
- Viral infection of cells may result in **lysis, fusion** and **syncytium formation**, the appearance of **inclusion bodies**, or, in some instances, **transformation** to cells with characteristics of malignancy.
- Infections caused by viruses are **localized** at or near the site of entry or **generalized** to involve one or more target organs. In generalized infections a common pattern of spread during the incubation period is **site of entry? local lymph nodes? primary viraemia? liver, spleen, bone marrow? secondary viraemia? target organ.**
- In humans, viral infections follow various basic patterns: **acute non-persistent, acute followed by persistent latent infection,** and **chronic with continued shedding of virus**.
- Very rarely, papovavirus, measles virus, and prions cause long-lasting, fatal disease of the CNS.
- During the course of infection, viruses are **shed** from the primary site of multiplication, or—with the exception of the CNS—from target organs, and are then free to infect other susceptible hosts.
- The Ro number is the average number of secondary cases generated by one primary case in a susceptible community; it may be useful in predicting the course of an epidemic.

Chapter 5

Resistance to virus infections

1 Introduction: innate and adaptive immunity

The scientific investigation of immunology started about a century ago with Metchnikoff's studies of phagocytosis of foreign particles, including micro-organisms. This early interest in what we now refer to as **cell-mediated immunity (CMI)** was soon overtaken by researches on **antibody-mediated (humoral) immunity**, which was for long regarded as the primary defence against microbial disease. We now know that, although the presence of antibody is important in preventing virus infections, cellular immunity plays a major role in the immune response once infection has been established.

An understanding of the immune responses to virus infections is important because the relationship between viruses and the immune system is much more intimate than it is for most bacteria: viruses often modify the cells within which they replicate, thereby rendering them 'foreign' and susceptible to attack by sensitized lymphocytes; furthermore, some viruses can multiply within the very lymphocytes and mononuclear phagocytes that are important components of the immunological defences. A good example is HIV, which attaches to and destroys the CD4+ 'helper' lymphocytes that are so important to the integrity of the immune system (Chapter 25).

So far, the emphasis of these opening chapters has been almost entirely on the ingenious means adopted by viruses to invade and damage their hosts (Chapter 5). On its part, however, the animal world has developed efficient and highly complex mechanisms for combating infection by parasites, which can be considered under the headings of **innate** ('general' or 'non-specific') immunity and **adaptive** (or 'specific') immunity (Table 5.1). The latter term refers to the array of immune responses directed against particular microbes, but it is not always possible to make a hard and fast distinction between this type of resistance and the more general innate defences, which will be dealt with first.

By 'innate' we mean those defence mechanisms with which we are born and form the first line of protection against microbial invasion. They can be regarded as 'built-in' defences, and fall into two categories: those that protect the individual (Sections 2.1–2.5) and others, genetically mediated, that determine the resistance or susceptibility of populations (Sections 2.6 and 2.7). Innate resistance mechanisms differ from adaptive mechanisms in having no immunological 'memory' (Section 4.2).

Table 5.1 Some properties of IFNs

IFN	Derived from	Principal functions
IFN-α	Most nucleated cells, especially fibroblasts. 12 species, produced by infected leucocytes and macrophages	Antiviral Enhances MHC class 1 expression
IFN-β	One species, produced by fibroblasts and epithelial cells	
IFN-γ	Th1 cells, NK cells	Enhances MHC class 2 expression

2 General factors in resistance

2.1 Mechanical and chemical barriers

The importance of the skin as a barrier to infection was mentioned in Chapter 4 (Section 4.2). The retrograde movement of epithelial cilia acts to prevent infection of the respiratory tract, and damage to these cells by influenza and paramyxoviruses may open the way to secondary bacterial infection. The gastrointestinal tract is to some extent protected against ingested viruses by the low pH in the stomach; although viruses that regularly infect by this route are resistant to acidity; this applies to most enteroviruses, but it is interesting that the rhinoviruses, a subgroup causing the common cold, do not have to survive passage through the stomach and are not acid resistant.

The secretions from mucous membranes, e.g. eyes, mouth, respiratory, genital, and gastrointestinal tracts, offer a means of transporting various elements of the immune systems (cytokines, antibodies, lysozyme, etc.) to where they are needed.

2.2 Fever

A high temperature is naturally regarded by patients as an unpleasant effect of a virus infection; but a body temperature much above 37°C is inimical to the replication of a number of viruses and is thus a defence mechanism. The febrile response seems to be triggered by soluble factors, notably IL-1, TNF, and IFNs, all of which are produced by macrophages (see Section 3.2).

2.3 Age

This factor is an example of the way in which the general overlaps with the particular, as age-related resistance is, in part at least, mediated by immune responses. An infant is sent into the world with a useful leaving present from its mother in the form of a package of IgG antibodies directed against infections from

which she has suffered. IgG antibodies to these predominantly viral infections, supplemented by IgA antibodies in colostrum and breast milk, helps to tide the baby over the first 6 months or so, after which its susceptibility to viral infections increases. The protection conferred by maternal milk is a good reason for breast feeding, especially in Third World countries where the energetic sale of manufactured substitutes is not in the best interest of babies born into a particularly hostile environment. Another great advantage of breast milk is that it is bacteriologically sterile.

The most obvious effect of ageing on the immune system is atrophy of the thymus gland, which starts in adolescence and continues for the rest of life. As might be expected, this process is accompanied by failures of function in both B- and T-cell immunity and in disturbances of cytokine traffic.

Virus infections in childhood are not usually serious, but become increasingly so with the advance of age; for example, poliomyelitis usually causes mild or even subclinical infection in children, but adults are often hit harder and the incidence of paralytic disease is higher. Some virus infections in elderly people can be very severe, herpes zoster (shingles) being a case in point.

2.4 Nutritional status

Poor nutrition may exacerbate the severity of some virus infections, an often-quoted example being measles in African children, which has a much higher mortality rate than in developed countries; but assessment of the importance of malnutrition is complicated by other factors such as intercurrent infections, particularly malaria, which is immunosuppressive.

2.5 Hormones

It is well known that treatment with steroids exacerbates the severity of herpes simplex and varicella-zoster infections but their precise role in natural resistance or susceptibility is unknown. The severity of hepatitis E may be exacerbated by pregnancy, presumably because of hormonal influences, but again, the mechanism is not yet understood.

2.6 Genetic factors

In experimental animals there is clear evidence that genetic factors influence resistance, or conversely, susceptibility to virus infections. Thus some highly inbred lines of mice are killed by very small inocula of HSV, whereas others withstand enormous doses with no sign of illness. In this case, resistance is dominant, and is mediated by only four genes: with other viruses, susceptibility may be the dominant genetic factor. The genes involved are sometimes, but not always, part of the major histocompatibility complex (MHC; Section 3.2).

The influence of genetic factors can to some extent be determined by these artificially controlled experiments involving inbred animals and well-defined virus strains. Needless to say, the assessment of such factors in humans is at present far more difficult, but is being helped by progress in our understanding of the genes that mediate immune responses.

2.7 Species resistance

The host range of many viruses is restricted, probably because the cells of resistant species do not possess appropriate receptors. The best understood example is poliovirus, the receptors for which are present only in humans and other primates. Others, notably the human immunodeficiency viruses and some hepatitis agents, are equally selective; by contrast, others again, such as rabies, are capable of infecting most or all warm-blooded animals

3 Local non-specific defences

The ways in which the above responses are mediated are for the most part poorly understood. We are on firmer ground when we examine what weapons are brought into play by local non-specific defences in the earliest phases of infection. These include **soluble factors** such as the IFNs, complement and C-reactive protein, and phagocytic cells, particularly **natural killer (NK) cells**, all of which are important components of the **innate immune system**. The various elements of these responses can be mobilized very quickly—within a matter of hours. They may be thought of as built-in defences, standing by, but ready for action until the more powerful and specific adaptive elements can be brought into play. It is clear that the many components of these elaborate systems need equally elaborate provision for recognition. **Pattern recognition systems** are groups of molecules, e.g. the so-called Toll-like receptors and CD14 (Fig. 5.1), that, among other activities, enhance the expression of MHC molecules and are thus important in the immune response.

These interactions between cells of the immune system are mediated by a substantial variety of small (about 20 kDa) glycoproteins referred to collectively as **cytokines**. *This is an umbrella term that encompasses a wide range of molecules. The cytokines act as chemical messengers, stimulating or inhibiting the activities of the various cellular components of the immune system. As such, they form an important component of innate immunity and can provide links between this and certain of the adaptive components. They contain several subgroups, of which the most important as far as viral infections are concerned are the* **IFNs**. *Other categories include the* **chemokines**, *which act as chemical attractants of leucocytes to sites of inflammation, and yet others that induce growth and differentiation or enhance cytotoxicity (note that a number of these activities relate to infections by bacteria rather than viruses). Cytokines secreted by and acting on leucocytes are referred to as* **ILs**. *The number of known ILs runs well into double figures. and they play an important part in regulating both T-cell and B-cell activities. For example, the binding of antigen to an immature CD4 cell is followed by differentiation of the latter into one or other of two main subsets of helper cell, Th1 or Th2. These subsets are*

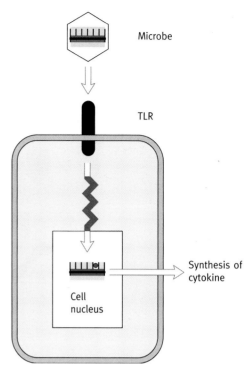

Fig. 5.1 **Molecular basis of innate immunity involving newly discovered toll-like receptors (TLRs).**

distinguished by the patterns of ILs that they secrete. Thus Th1 cells secrete IL-2 and IFN-γ, with stimulation of T cells leading to CMI, whereas IL-4, -5, -6, and -10 are secreted by Th2 cells (see also Section 5) leading predominantly to B-cell and antibody-mediated immunity.

3.1 Interferons

These cytokines are the most important to virologists, having found several clinical applications, so we shall deal with them at some length.

The discovery by Isaacs and Lindenmann in 1957 that virus-infected cells produce a soluble factor that protects other cells from infection seemed to herald a new era, as the substance was effective against a wide range of viruses and apparently non-toxic. At a time when rapid strides were being made in the chemotherapy of bacterial infections, IFN seemed like the answer to virologists' prayers. These early hopes were soon to turn to disappointment, but now, with better understanding and technology, IFNs have made something of a comeback.

There are several IFNs, which differ in the way they are produced, in chemical composition, and in mode of action. They are proteins with molecular weights of about 20 kDa, manufactured by leucocytes or fibroblasts in response not only to viral infection, but also to stimulation by natural or synthetic dsRNA and some bacteria (e.g. chlamydia). **These molecules are not virus-specific**, so that IFN induced by one virus is effective against others; on the other hand, they are **species-specific**, so that IFN produced by, say, a guinea-pig, is ineffective in mouse or human cells. IFN-γ differs in a major way from the α and

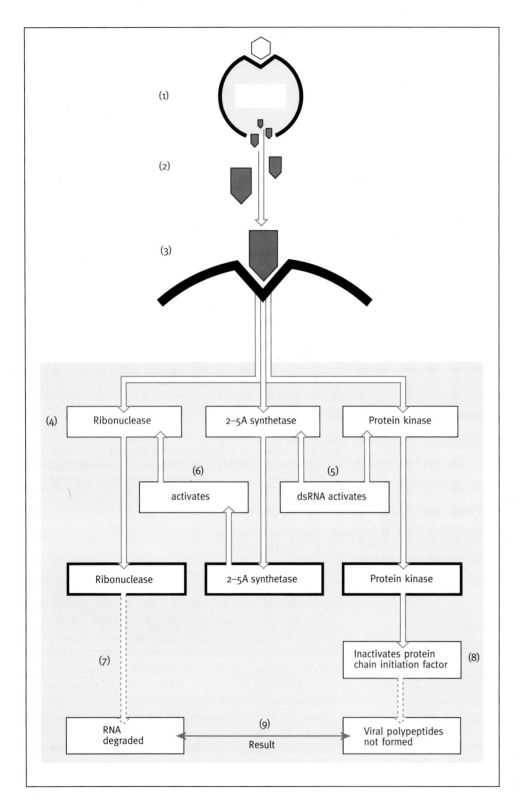

Fig. 5.2 **Mode of action of interferon.** For explanation, see text.

β varieties as it is produced by a subset of T memory cells in response to stimulation by an antigen previously encountered IFNs do not kill viruses, nor do they act like antibodies. The mechanisms are complex and indirect; one of them is summarized as simply as possible in Fig. 5.2.

(1) Viruses attach by a specific receptor to a cell that is stimulated to produce IFN molecules (IFN). The cellular transcription factor IRF3 is phosphorylated and activated by virus infection and by the presence of dsRNA. IRF3 moves to the nucleus where it switches on the expression of IFN and other genes. Some

viruses such as smallpox and hepatitis C viruses (HCVs) have evolved mechanisms to block IRF3 activation. These IFNs diffuse out from the cell (2) and induce an **antiviral state** in neighbouring cells. First, IFN molecules attach to receptors on the nearby cells (3) and induce the formation of three enzymes, a **ribonuclease** (RNase), a **protein kinase**, and **2–5A synthetase** (4). The two last-mentioned enzymes are activated by dsRNA (5). The activated 2–5A synthetase in turn activates the ribonuclease (6), which degrades RNA (7). The activated protein kinase is capable of phosphorylating, and thus inactivating, a factor that initiates synthesis of proteins (8). The end result (9) is inhibition of viral replication.

As well as blocking viral replication, IFNs have profound effects on cells, some of which also help indirectly to control infection. One of the most important is **enhancement of the display on cell surfaces of histocompatibility antigens**, which are essential to antigen-driven activation of T cells. Others involve modulation of both B- and T-cell activities, including enhancement of the cytotoxicity of the NK and cytotoxic T cells (T_c).

In addition to their antiviral effects, IFNs can inhibit cell division and this property, in conjunction with the immunomodulating activities just described, has been used to some effect as an adjunct to immuno- or chemotherapy of cancer.

How important are interferons in preventing or treating virus infections?

Although the effects of IFN are clear in experiments using cell cultures, it is quite difficult to disentangle them from all the other components of the immune response in intact animals. IFNs are generated very quickly—within hours of the start of infection—and help to hold the fort in the interval before clonal proliferation of T and B cells and antibody production get under way. This view is supported by the finding that treatment of animals with anti-IFN serum exacerbates virus infections; furthermore, some people, who have a natural defect in IFN production, are abnormally susceptible to upper respiratory tract infections.

With hindsight, the early attempts to use IFN for treatment were doomed to failure, because the amounts available were minuscule by today's standards. Now that genes coding for IFN can be cloned (e.g. in yeast cells), very large quantities can be produced and have been used with fair success in treating chronic hepatitis C; this will be dealt with in Chapter 24, but at this point it is interesting to note that part of the therapeutic effect may be due to IFN-mediated enhancement of MHC display on infected liver cells, resulting in their more efficient destruction by T_c cells. IFNs are also used for treating various malignancies, including Kaposi's sarcoma.

3.2 Complement

The complement system is an important component of the innate immune response to infection and is present in all vertebrates. It consists of about 20 glycoproteins of MW 80 000–200 000, of which nine are numbered C^1–C^9. The latter, appropriately stimulated, are capable of reacting sequentially, rather like a set of dominoes collapsing. Some of these components are enzymes capable of catalysing the next step, the whole cascade terminating in lysis or opsonization of the organism. The 'classical' pathway to destruction of a microbe is stimulated when an IgM or IgG antibody binds to an antigen. The 'alternative pathway' is triggered by component C3, which is present on the microbe, and its cleavage into two molecules, C3a and C3b, which initiates the next step in the cascade. The end result is attraction of immune cells to the area and lysis of the organism.

3.3 Acute-phase proteins

These comprise several plasma proteins which by and large are more important in immunity to bacterial than to viral infections. They are mostly produced in the liver and include C-reactive protein.

3.4 Collectins

These proteins bind to carbohydrate molecules on microbial surfaces and activate the alternative complement pathway.

4 The adaptive immune system

The two fundamentals of the specific immune responses are as follows.

1. The ability to distinguish between 'self' molecules that properly belong to the body and are ignored by the immune system; and 'non-self' molecules (e.g. those of microbes), against which the system is capable of reacting. The latter are known as **antigens.**

2. **Memory**, whereby an enhanced response is evoked to an antigen previously encountered. Specific immunity is also referred to as **adaptive** or **acquired** immunity, as opposed to the non-specific mechanisms with which we are born and were described in the first part of this chapter. **Acquired immunity may be passive**, as when preformed antibody is injected for prophylaxis of, say, rabies; or **active** as in the antibody response to an infection or vaccine.

Let us now take a look at the main components of the specific immune response. It will have to be brief because the adaptive immune system is fearsomely complicated; nevertheless, a knowledge of the basic features is essential. It should be remembered that many of its activities apply also to microbes other than viruses.

4.1 Antigens

Antigens are molecules, or groups of molecules, capable of eliciting an immune response. Within limits, the larger the molecule the stronger the immune response to it. Although antigens are usually large molecules such as proteins, only small sequences of, say, half a dozen amino acids actually induce the formation of antibodies and react with them. These sequences are known as **antigenic determinants**, or **epitopes**.

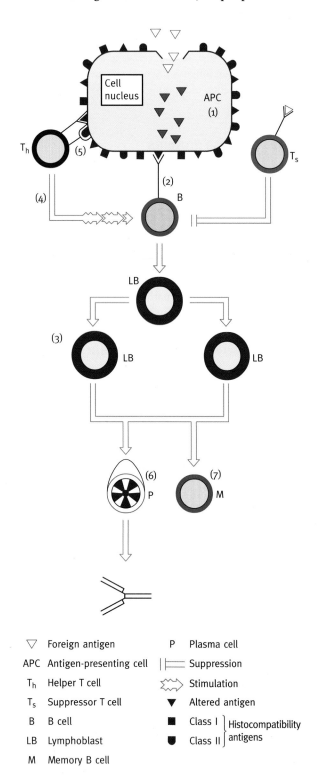

▽	Foreign antigen	P	Plasma cell
APC	Antigen-presenting cell	‖⊏	Suppression
T$_h$	Helper T cell	⟨⟩	Stimulation
T$_s$	Suppressor T cell	▼	Altered antigen
B	B cell	■	Class I ⎱ Histocompatibility
LB	Lymphoblast	▉	Class II ⎰ antigens
M	Memory B cell		

Fig 5.3 The B-cell response to viral infection. For explanation, see text.

4.2 Immunological memory

This is mediated by **lymphocytes**, each of which is capable of responding to a single antigen specific for that particular cell. It is astonishing that during the course of evolution we have developed a range of lymphocytes that can react to virtually any one of the myriads of molecules capable of evoking an immune response. There are two main classes, **B and T cells** that mature in the bone marrow and thymus respectively. Both types react with antigens by means of **cell-surface receptors**. Although respectively responsible for antibody- and CMI, the two main classes of lymphocyte should not be thought of as occupying separate compartments of the immune response. On the contrary, they co-operate closely with each other and with dendritic cells and macrophages that process antigens and 'present' them to the lymphocytes.

4.3 B cells and antibody-mediated immunity

The role of **B lymphocytes** is summarized in Fig. 5.3 (numbers in this section refer to steps in this figure). Note that in this figure and in Fig. 5.6, the nuclei of B and T lymphocytes are respectively stippled lightly and heavily.

B lymphocytes originate from stem cells in the **bone marrow**, enter the circulation and mature in the liver, spleen, and lymphoid tissue. Their surface receptors are **antibody molecules** that react on encountering their specific antigen, which usually has to be processed (1) by **antigen-presenting cells (APCs)**. These are **dendritic cells** present in the germinal centres of the lymph nodes and spleen; along with mononuclear phagocytes (macrophages and monocytes), they process foreign antigenic material in a way not fully understood, and present it on their surfaces in a form that is recognized by a B lymphocyte bearing the corresponding antibody receptors (2). This encounter stimulates the *B cell* to proliferate, thus forming a **clone** of cells with the same antigenic specificity (3). The process is assisted by ILs, notably IL-4, secreted by T-helper cells (4), which themselves are stimulated by reacting with the altered antigen, this time in association with class II antigens on the surface of the APC (5).

Many of the cells in the clone differentiate into **effector cells**, in this instance **plasma cells** (6) that secrete more antibodies capable of combining with that antigen and that antigen only. Some of the sensitized B lymphocytes persist for long periods as **memory cells** (7) that respond rapidly to further encounters with the antigen by clonal proliferation and production of more of the appropriate antibody. The amount of antibody generated is controlled by T cells, of which more later.

The five classes of immunoglobulin, IgA, IgM, IgG, IgD, and IgE, are each produced by particular clones of plasma cells; only the first three seem to be important in virus infections (Table 5.2). Each consists of one or more units made up of four polypeptide chains, two 'heavy' and two 'light', which together form a Y-shaped molecule (Fig. 5.4). The tips of the two prongs of the 'Y' are the **variable regions**. Within the population of lymphocytes, the extremely wide variation of amino-acid

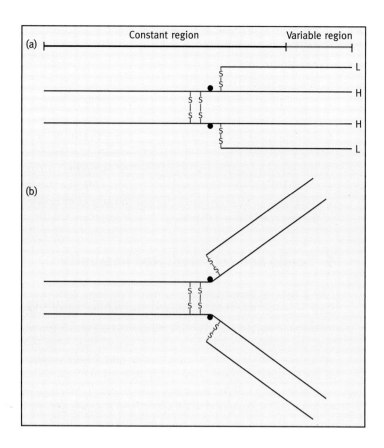

Fig. 5.4 Structure of an immunoglobulin molecule. **(a)** Basic structure: two identical 'heavy' polypeptide chains (H) are linked to two identical 'light' chains (L) by disulphide bonds. **(b)** The molecule opens at the hinge region. This is the position in which it combines with an antigen.

Table 5.2a Innate and adaptive immunity

Innate	Adaptive
Rapid response	Slow response
Little or no memory	Highly specific memory

Table 5.2b Representative cytokines

Cytokine	Examples of activity
IL-1α and -β	Inflammatory; pyrexia
IL-2	T-cell activation
IL-4	B- and T-cell activation
IL-5	B- and T-cell activation; eosinophil differentiation
IL-8	A chemokine: attracts polymorphonuclear leucocytes
IL-9	Mast cell growth factor
IL-12	Induces Th1 cells
IL-13	Suppresses Th1 cells
IFN-α	Antiviral
IFN-β	Antiviral
IFN-γ	Antiviral; activates macrophages; inhibits Th2 cells

sequences in these regions ensures that there will be a few cells capable of reacting with any antigen encountered for the first time. The variable regions thus confer upon each immunoglobulin molecule its individual **antigenic specificity**.

IgA antibodies

IgA antibodies are produced by lymphoid tissue underlying the mucous membranes at whose surfaces it acts; they are found in secretions of the oropharynx, gastrointestinal and respiratory tracts, and are thus important in defending against viruses that enter by these routes (Chapter 4). The IgA secreted at mucous surfaces consists of two immunoglobulin units (a dimer) attached to a 'secretory piece' that aids its passage through cells. IgA is also produced during lactation, particularly in the colostrum, and it is the specific antibodies provided in this form by the mother that help to protect against infections in early infancy (Section 2.3).

IgM antibodies

IgM antibodies are the first to be produced in systemic infections and are particularly avid in combining with antigen and complement. IgM is a large molecule and cannot cross the placenta; hence specific IgM antibody in a fetus or neonate indicates intrauterine infection. Production of IgM antibody is a fairly short-term process, lasting for a few weeks or months. **The finding of a specific IgM is thus evidence of a recent or current infection** and is used widely for diagnosis.

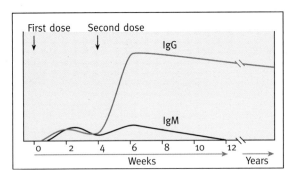

Fig. 5.5 Primary and secondary antibody responses to spaced doses of an inactivated vaccine.

Eventually, however, a negative feedback mechanism operates whereby the manufacture of IgM is switched off and replaced by production of specific IgG antibody.

IgG antibodies

By contrast with IgM, IgG antibodies continue to be produced for very long periods—often during the entire life span—and thus afford **long-term protection** against subsequent encounters with the same virus. As their presence is evidence of past infection, they are useful in epidemiological surveys (Chapter 7). IgG antibodies cross the placenta and, as mentioned above, provide protection during the first few months of life, thus supplementing the action of IgA antibodies.

The time course of antibody production can be observed most clearly during immunization with a non-living antigen such as an inactivated vaccine (Fig. 5.5). The **primary response** to the first injection results from the initial clonal expansion of B lymphocytes on first encounter with the antigen: it is comparatively slow and of low magnitude. By contrast, the **secondary responses** to subsequent injections given some weeks later reflect the presence of sensitized memory cells that are now available to undergo a greatly amplified clonal expansion; the resultant antibody response takes place very quickly (i.e. within a day or so), and much greater quantities are produced. This clear-cut picture is blurred when a replicating antigen such as live polio vaccine is given, or during the course of a naturally acquired virus infection: in this instance the primary stimulus continues for some time and other immune mechanisms relating to recovery are brought into play.

4.4 Mode of action of antibodies

There are several possible ways in which a specific immunoglobulin can act against a virus, the exact mechanism depending on the virus concerned.

- It can **neutralize** by agglutinating the virions and thus stop them attaching to susceptible cells or by blocking the receptor binding site, namely the virus docking protein. Some antibodies can block the functioning of an internal viral protein when, for example, it is expressed on the cell surface like the influenza M2 protein.

- Antibody may act as an **opsonin**, combining with virions and increasing the ability of macrophages to phagocytose and destroy them.

- **Macrophages** coated with specific antibody are **activated** or 'armed' to destroy infected cells expressing on their surfaces viral antigens with the same specificity.

- Antibody plus **complement** can combine with viral antigen expressed on the surface of an infected cell, which they lyse. This effect is known as antibody-dependent-cellular cytotoxicity (ADCC).

- Antibody can **interfere with the uncoating sequence** after the virus has entered the cell.

5 T cells and cell-mediated immunity

Like B cells, **T lymphocytes** originate from stem cells in the bone marrow, but then migrate to the thymus where they mature and acquire their specific antigen receptors. These cells are responsible for CMI; there are various subsets, some that operate by secreting ILs, of which more than 20 are involved in the immune response, some with production of antibodies and others with cellular responses. Like B cells, T lymphocytes undergo clonal expansion when appropriately stimulated, with the production of both effector and memory cells.

5.1 Regulatory cells

These either promote or inhibit the activities of other T cells and production of antibody by the B cells; they are known respectively as **T-helper** and **T-suppressor** (T_s) cells, or, according to surface markers identified by monoclonal antibodies, in a number of laboratories, as CD4 and CD8. In the blood, their normal ratio is about 2 : 1. Most viral antigens are T-dependent, which means that B cells can make antibody to them only in cooperation with T lymphocytes.

5.2 Cytotoxic cells

These cells (T_c) express CD8; they are particularly important in virus infections, as they recognize virus-specified antigens on the surface of infected cells, which they attack and lyse.

5.3 Delayed hypersensitivity

T_{dh} cells, as their name indicates, secrete cytokines that mediate delayed hypersensitivity.

5.4 Mononuclear phagocytic cells (MPs)

MPs comprise blood monocytes, fixed macrophages in the tissues (e.g. Kupffer cells in the liver, microglia in the brain), and populations of free macrophages in the lungs, peritoneal cavity, and other tissues. These cells are real busybodies in the immune system: as well as acting as APCs and phagocytosing antigen–antibody complexes they can lyse infected cells, produce IFN, and secrete other cytokines that modulate the behaviour of T cells. In turn, their own behaviour is affected by activating or inhibiting factors produced by T cells.

5.5 Major histocompatibility complex restriction

The MHC is a closely associated cluster of genes that encode various cell-surface and other antigens. In humans, it is known as the HLA (**h**uman **l**eucocyte **a**ntigen) system. There are three classes of antigen, of which only classes I and II concern us here. Class I antigens are expressed on the surfaces of all cells, whereas those of class II are present only on those of APCs (i.e. dendritic cells in the spleen and macrophages). The great variability in the alleles coding for MHC antigens is responsible for differences in the susceptibility of individuals to a number of diseases, both infective and non-infective.

The operations of T cells are intimately related to these antigens. Recognition of 'foreign' antigens takes place only if they are presented by the dendritic cell or macrophage in association with the correct MHC antigens: thus T_c and T_s cells act only when antigen is presented with class I antigens identical with their own, whereas the activities of T-helper lymphocytes are

restricted by the need for homologous class II antigens on the presenting cell surface.

Now look again at Fig. 5.3. The B cell is being assisted in its functions by cytokines secreted by the T-helper cell on the left, which itself is activated by interaction with altered viral antigen on the surface of the APC. Note particularly that this interaction can take place only in association with a class II MHC antigen normally present on the surface of the APC. On the right of the B lymphocyte, a T-suppressor cell stands by, ready to damp down overproduction of antibody by the B cell. This is the interface between antibody- and CMI.

Figure 5.6 illustrates some important interactions between T cells. An APC similar to that in Fig. 5.3 is shown; as a reminder, a B cell being helped by a T-helper lymphocyte (1) is depicted on the left, but this time the centre of the stage is occupied by various T cells.

A cytotoxic T cell (T_c) is stimulated by reaction with viral antigen on the surface of the APC (2) to undergo clonal proliferation (for clarity this is not shown). In association with class I histocompatibility antigens, T_c cells attach to viral antigen on the surface of infected ('target') cells and lyse them (3). These activities are assisted by T-helper cells acting through **IL-2** (4).

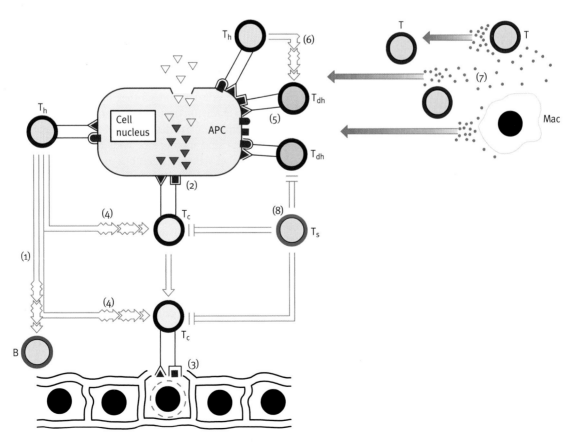

Fig. 5.6 The T-cell response to viral infection. For explanation, see text.

Another subset of T cells that mediates delayed hypersensitivity (T_{dh}) reacts with viral antigen on the surface of the APC in association either with class I or class II histocompatibility antigens (5); these, too, are assisted by T-helper cells (6). The stimulated T_{dh} cells secrete chemotactic cytokines that attract more T cells and some macrophages (7) to help at the site of infection.

As in the B-cell response, T_s cells stand by to moderate overenergetic behaviour by the T cells (8).

This diagram illustrates the central role of T lymphocytes in immunity to virus—and many other—infections; it has been likened to that of a conductor orchestrating the entire immune response.

Apart from mopping up antigen–antibody complexes, polymorphonuclear leucocytes are relatively unimportant in virus infections. This can be inferred readily from tissue sections or exudates in which, by contrast with bacterial infections, the overwhelming majority of cells are lymphocytes. An example is shown in Fig. 22.7 (a).

5.6 Natural killer cells

In addition to T_c cells and macrophages, about 10 per cent of circulating lymphocytes are larger than average, have electron-dense granules in their cytoplasm and are known as 'natural killer' cells or 'large granular lymphocytes'. They are produced in the bone marrow. They have no immunological specificity but can kill cells that they recognize as 'foreign', e.g. cells bearing microbial or tumour antigens on their surfaces. They can also recognize and kill cells coated with virus-specific IgG, a process known as antibody-dependent cell cytotoxicity. Their activity is greatly enhanced by IFN, but their role in recovery from infection is still uncertain.

6 Harmful immune responses

6.1 Enhanced T-cell responses

The destructive potential of the immune system is considerable and can sometimes be dangerous to the host. This was well illustrated during the outbreaks of hepatitis B that used to occur in renal dialysis units before the hazards posed by this infection were properly understood and guarded against. The immunity of the patients was impaired by their illness and by treatment; therefore those who contracted hepatitis B could not provide an effective defence against the infection, which tended to develop into the chronic carrier state in these patients (Chapter 22). By contrast, members of staff, healthy but presumably exposed to large amounts of virus, mounted vigorous cytotoxic T-cell responses, resulting in autoimmune destruction of their own infected hepatocytes, and illness that was, on average, more severe than that suffered by their patients. Similar mechanisms operate in the liver cirrhosis seen in some types of chronic active hepatitis.

6.2 Depressed T-cell responses

Immune responses to virus infections are complicated by the ability of some viruses to infect and damage the very cells that mediate these reactions. The best example is that of AIDS (Chapter 25), in which the HIV infects and destroys the T-helper subset which, as we have seen, is crucial in the activation of B cells and of other T lymphocytes. The resultant havoc in the immune system opens the way to so-called opportunistic infections by other viruses and bacteria and sometimes to tumour formation, resulting in death.

Measles is also a good example of the importance of an intact T-cell response. In children with a defect in CMI there is no rash, which, as explained in Chapter 4, is the result of cytotoxic T cells destroying virus-infected cells in the skin. The presence of a rash is thus a good sign that the patient is recovering; its absence is sinister, because the likely outcome is uncontrolled viral replication, resulting in giant-cell pneumonia and death.

Another example is infection with EBV, a herpesvirus that causes infectious mononucleosis (Chapter 20) and then becomes permanently latent in B cells. Because of efficient immune surveillance by T cells, the latent infection is usually without effect on the health of the host; but an upset of this balance by immune suppression (e.g. in renal transplant patients) can result in transformation of the infected B cells by the virus, with uncontrolled proliferation and death from lymphoma.

6.3 Viral infection of mononuclear phagocytes

Many viruses can replicate within these cells, which, as mentioned in Section 3.2, play a major role in regulating immunity. Because of the diversity of viruses involved, of the types and functions of MPs and of the cells with which they interact, the influence of viral infection of MPs on the immune response is extraordinarily complex. From the above description of the immune system you will appreciate that interference with MPs by viral infection can, among other activities, affect phagocytosis, antigen presentation, interactions with T cells, chemotaxis, and antibody-dependent cytotoxicity. A few examples of virus–MP interactions that have been elucidated in the laboratory follow.

- The age of the MP may be important: newborn mice are highly susceptible to herpes simplex because the virus multiplies readily in their macrophages; however, a pronounced increase in resistance develops about 3 weeks after birth and is related to a decreased ability of the virus to replicate in these cells.

- Genetic resistance to certain viruses may be partly mediated by MPs.

- Influenza and CMV infections may depress the function of lung macrophages and increase susceptibility to bacterial infection.

- Arginase secreted by macrophages may interfere with the replication of HSV, which has a requirement for arginine; this, however, is an unusual type of effect.

The precise role of these and other factors in the immune response cannot as yet be quantified, but they do provide some pointers to the part played in pathogenesis by viral infection of these important cells.

6.4 Immune complex disease

In certain chronic infections of animals, immune complexes between virus and antibody lodge in small vessels, particularly in the kidneys, causing glomerulonephritis. This sequence of events does not seem to be an important feature of infections of humans; nevertheless, immune complexes may be the trigger for the disseminated intravascular coagulation seen in some of the viral haemorrhagic fevers (Chapter 28). They may also be implicated in dengue haemorrhagic shock syndrome (DHSS), which occurs in people, mainly children, with antibody to dengue virus who subsequently become infected with another serotype (Chapter 27).

7 Resistance and recovery

At the start of this chapter it was emphasized that the mechanisms whereby we resist infection differ from those involved in recovery.

By and large, **resistance to invasion by viruses** is mediated by **antibodies**. These may be:

- **acquired passively** by infants from the mother, or by older people given passive immunization (e.g. immunoglobulin to protect against rabies (Chapter 26) or hepatitis A (Chapter 23);
- **acquired actively** as the result of an earlier encounter with the same virus. In this case, the comparatively small amount of existing antibody (**IgG or IgA**) is supplemented rapidly by clonal proliferation of antibody-secreting B lymphocytes.

Recovery from infection, once acquired, is a more complicated affair and the responses brought into play depend to some extent on the virus concerned. In Chapter 4 cytopathic viruses were classified as 'bursters', lysing cells with liberation of large numbers of virions into the circulation, or as 'creepers', moving directly from cell to cell. During the viraemia resulting from 'burster' infections, such as poliomyelitis or YF, the virions are susceptible to antibody, notably the IgM induced early in a primary infection. Antibody thus plays a larger part in recovery from 'burster' than from 'creeper' infections, the latter being caused by enveloped viruses such as herpes and influenza. 'Creepers' readily induce specific antigens on the surfaces of infected cells, thus evoking powerful cell-mediated responses. However, even with lytic virus infections, CMI is an important factor in recovery.

Experimental evidence for the relative roles of antibody and CMI in resistance and recovery is powerfully supported by observations of infections in patients with deficiencies in these responses. This subject will be dealt with in Chapter 32.

8 Reminders

- Protection against microbial infection is conferred both by **innate** (built-in non-specific) and **adaptive** (acquired) mechanisms. Innate factors include **mechanical** and chemical barriers in individuals, and **genetically determined** resistance or susceptibility in populations. Many of the activities within the immune system are mediated by leucocytes, of which there are two main classes, (1) B cells, which mature within the bone marrow; and (2) T cells, which mature within the thymus.

- The mechanisms of **innate immunity** come into play very quickly in response to microbial infections, and act as a stopgap until the adaptive mechanisms come into play. **IFN, cytokines**, and **other molecules such as complement and C-reactive protein form part of innate immunity** and help to suppress virus replication during the **early stages of infection** before antibodies and CMI are fully mobilized.

- **Adaptive immunity** is characterized by (1) its ability to **distinguish between 'self' and 'non-self'** molecules, and (2) **memory**, whereby an enhanced response is evoked to an antigen previously encountered.

- The two main components of adaptive immunity to virus infections are (1) **antibodies** produced by B lymphocytes in cooperation with APCs and T lymphocytes, and (2) **CMI** conferred by a variety of cells, mostly T lymphocytes, including particularly helper, suppressor, and cytotoxic cells.

- Acting as a bridge between the innate and adaptive systems is a highly diverse system of molecules known as **cytokines**, which form a network of intercellular messengers that help to regulate the response to infection. This general class includes the IFNs, which have antiviral activity but only in the species of animal in which they were produced.

- The operations of T cells are intimately related to the **MHC antigens**; thus T_c and T_s cells act only when antigen is presented with class I antigens identical with their own, whereas the activities of T-helper lymphocytes are restricted by the need for homologous class II antigens on the presenting cell surface.

- The responses to infections by some viruses are complicated by their ability to replicate in **lymphocytes** and **macrophages**.

- As a generalization, **protection** against virus infections is largely mediated by antibody, whereas in recovery CMI is relatively more important, especially in the case of the enveloped 'creeper' viruses.

- Immune responses can sometimes be **harmful**; for example, several manifestations of virus infections are caused by the cytotoxic effects of T cells or by immune complexes of antigen with antibody.

Viruses and cancer in humans

1 Historical note

If any one topic can be regarded as the leading edge in molecular biology, it is the relationship between viruses and malignancy, or viral oncogenesis (Greek, *ongkos* = tumour). Its ramifications are wide, and extend to the fundamental mechanisms by which growth and other activities of cells are controlled at the molecular level. Since the first edition of this book, the literature on the subject has grown exponentially and there are now literally thousands of papers dealing with a huge variety of molecular controls on the proliferation, differentiation, and inhibition of cells and on the ways in which these activities are influenced by viruses. The student attempting to make head or tail of this mass of information will be struck both by the variety of these control mechanisms, and the difficulty of deciding what is relevant to the role of viruses in causing cancers, particularly those of humans. Clearly, observations on people are much more limited than those on animals and birds, and extrapolations from one species to another may well be misleading. We shall try to present this subject intelligibly, but it must be emphasized that doing so involves considerable simplification.

Having given due warning about drawing conclusions from animal experiments, it is true to say that much of our knowledge of oncogenesis has been gained in this way. A brief review of the history of the subject serves as a useful introduction to some of its important features. Table 6.1 lists some of the major advances, which can be divided into two phases.

1.1 Early researches

This period covers the half century from about 1910 to 1960; it began with the finding by Rous that a fowl sarcoma could be transmitted to normal chickens by injecting them with cell-free filtrates of the tumour. A quarter of a century later, Bittner described a mouse mammary tumour virus that was transmitted to newborn animals in their mothers' milk. This was followed by the identification by Gross and Friend of the two mouse leukaemia viruses that are named after them; it later proved significant (Section 3.1) that Gross leukaemia had an incubation period of about 2 years, whereas the Friend agent induced the disease in a matter of weeks.

Many other basically similar agents were identified in a variety of animals and birds, usually causing various types of leukaemia or sarcoma. These agents were referred to as

Table 6.1 Some milestones in the association of viruses with cancer

Early researchers

1911	Peyton Rous	Demonstrated that fowl sarcoma is caused by a transmissible agent (Nobel Prize—but not until 1966!)
1927	H.J. Muller	Ionizing radiation mutagenic in *Drosophila*
1936	J.J. Bittner	Discovered mouse mammary tumour virus
1944	O.T. Avery, C.N. MacLeod, and M. McCarty	Showed (in bacteria) that genetic information is contained in DNA
1951	L. Gross	Discovered a 'slow' murine leukaemia virus
1957	C. Friend	Discovered a 'fast' murine leukaemia virus

The modern era

1962	J.D. Watson, F.H.C. Crick, and M.H.F. Wilkins	Worked out the structure of DNA and discovered the genetic code (Nobel Prize)
1963	M. Vogt and R. Dulbecco	Transformed normal cells to tumour cells *in vitro* by exposing them to a virus
1969	G.J. Todaro, R.J. Huebner, and H. Temin	Oncogene hypothesis
1970	D. Baltimore, H. Temin, and S. Mituzani	Discovered reverse transcriptase (Nobel Prize)
1976	D. Stehelin, H.E. Varmus, J.M. Bishop, and P.K. Vogt	Discovered the oncogene Nobel Prizes for Varmus and Bishop
1980	B.J. Poiesz, F.W. Ruschetti, M.S. Reitz, V.S. Kalyanaraman, and R.C. Gallo	First isolation of a human T-cell leukaemia virus (HTLV-I)

'oncornaviruses' (i.e. oncogenic RNA viruses) and classified as type B, C, or D, according to their morphology and growth characteristics. As with other viruses, infection could be transmitted by passage of infective virions from one host to another. This mode was termed **horizontal** transmission, even when, as with mouse mammary tumour virus, it involved transfer from a parent to its offspring, either *in utero* or shortly after birth. Viruses transmitted in this way to previously uninfected cells are termed **exogenous**. But then a new mode was discovered—the transmission of infection from parents to off-spring via the germ cells. Part of the viral genome becomes incorporated into all cells—both somatic and germ line—of the host, so that it continues to be passed by **vertical** transfer from generation to generation. Viruses transmitted like this are **endogenous**. This type of infection can remain silent, or result in a high incidence of tumours in a particular strain of laboratory animal. Furthermore, such viruses may, under different conditions, be transmitted either horizontally or vertically. These infective agents are not cytolytic, which helps to ensure their survival.

In addition, it was appreciated early on that papovaviruses (Chapter 15), which contain DNA, could also give rise to tumours, both malignant and benign.

Meanwhile, other discoveries were being made, not directly involving viruses. It was known that ionizing radiation and various chemicals (e.g. small amounts of mustard gas) are oncogenic, and these treatments were also found to induce mutations in fruit flies (*Drosophila*). This led to the idea that cancers might be caused—at least to some extent—by mutations in cellular genetic material, shown in 1944 by Avery and his colleagues to be DNA.

1.2 The modern era

This period was heralded in 1962 by the scientific equivalent of a fanfare of trumpets—the discovery by Watson, Crick, and their collaborators of the structure of DNA and the way in which genetic information is encoded within it. Research on the molecular mechanisms of oncogenesis—and on so much else—could now begin in earnest.

At about this time, Vogt and Dulbecco in the USA found that normal cells cultured *in vitro* would, after infection with polyomavirus, take on many of the characteristics of malignant cells (Table 6.2 and Fig. 6.1). This laboratory manipulation, known as **transformation**, was to play a key role in the study of virus-induced cancer.

During the two decades following these researches, more viruses were added to the list of those able to induce malignant changes in cell cultures or in animals. They included adeno-

Table 6.2 Properties of transformed cells

Only one oncogenic virus particle needed to induce a focus of abnormal (transformed) cells
Foci are therefore **clonal**, i.e. they originate from a single infected cell
Can often be **propagated indefinitely** *in vitro*
Increased rate of **metabolism** and **multiplication**
Change in karyotype from diploid to **polyploid**
Lack of contact inhibition, with consequent **disorderly growth**
Possess new **tumour (T) surface antigens**
May give rise to **malignant tumours** when injected into animals

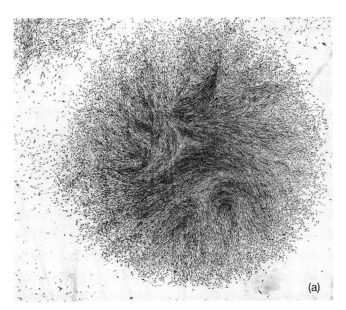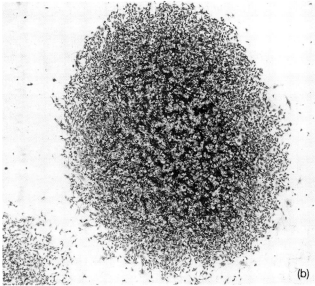

Fig. 6.1 Transformation of a cell line by a DNA virus. **(a)** Normal hamster cells. The colony is flat and the cells are aligned in parallel arrays. **(b)** After infection with polyomavirus the cells are piled up and disorientated. (Reproduced, with permission, from Wyke, J. (1986) in *Introduction to Cellular and Molecular Biology of Cancer* (1st edn) (ed. L.M. Franks and N. Teich), p. 179. Oxford University Press.)

viruses, papillomaviruses, herpesviruses, and hepatitis B. By contrast, none of the RNA viruses had this property, with the single and obvious exception of the oncornaviruses. The reason became clear with the discovery in 1970 by Baltimore and others of the method by which the oncornaviruses replicate their nucleic acid. This was described in Chapter 3, but in brief, viral RNA is transcribed into a DNA copy by an enzyme, RT, so-called because it reverses the usual direction of information transfer (i.e. from DNA to RNA).

As a result of this discovery, the oncornaviruses were redesignated as the family *Retroviridae*, subfamily *Oncovirinae* (we shall meet other retroviruses when we discuss AIDS in Chapter 25).

By this time, it was possible to start fitting parts of the jigsaw puzzle together, and, also in 1970, Todaro and others formulated the **oncogene theory**, which was proved to be fundamentally correct by later experimental work, and provided the basis for much of our current thinking about oncogenesis.

2 General features of viral oncogenesis

2.1 Genetic control of cell behaviour

In order for our various tissues to develop and function normally, their cells must be regulated by complex systems governing replication, differentiation, repair, and many other activities. Growth must be regulated in such a way that organs conform to a certain shape and size, and do not hypertrophy uncontrollably when cells damaged by disease or trauma are replaced; thus mechanisms are needed for suppressing growth

as well as stimulating it. These activities are largely mediated by chemical signals, which, in turn, are under genetic control; in other words, their production is determined by whether particular genes are active or inactive. It follows that the introduction, deletion, or mutation of genes coding for the polypeptide signals may have profound effects on cell activity, including the possible development of malignant changes. **Carcinogens** such as radiation, various chemicals (including nicotine), and certain mycotoxins may induce oncogenic mutations. These may be very small; experimentally, a c-*onc* gene was made oncogenic by a single base change—a point mutation—in its DNA. However, it is often uncertain whether these agents act alone, or whether they work in combination with other mutagenic agents, such as viruses. Furthermore, oncogenic mechanisms are not mutually exclusive; several may operate together in the induction of a particular malignancy.

There is more than one stage in oncogenesis. The establishment of a cancer requires first an initiation event. This is an irreversible change in a cell, which does not, by itself, necessarily result in tumour formation: insertion of an oncogene or other viral DNA is an example. The next step is the action of a promoter (i.e. some influence that pushes the cells toward the malignant state). Some or all of the possible cofactors listed in Table 6.3 may act in this way.

2.2 Integration of viral DNA

We saw in Section 1 how certain viruses were implicated in causing at least some malignancies. How do they do it? The basic mechanism is the integration of all or part of a viral genome into the DNA of a host cell. It follows that only dsDNA viruses, or retroviruses that synthesize DNA during replication,

Table 6.3 Viruses implicated in human cancers

Virus	Tumour	Possible cofactors
DNA viruses		
Human papillomaviruses (HPV)	Carcinomas of skin and genitalia, larynx	Sunlight, smoking
Epstein–Barr virus (EBV)	Burkitt's lymphoma	Malaria
	Nasopharyngeal carcinoma	Nitrosamines in diet; taking of snuffs containing phorbol esters; genetic factors
	B-cell lymphoma	Immunosuppression
Kaposi's sarcoma herpesvirus (HHV-8)	Kaposi's sarcoma	Human immunodeficiency virus (HIV) infection
Hepatitis B (HBV)	Primary liver cancer	Liver cirrhosis/alcoholism; food contaminated with aflatoxin
RNA viruses		
Human T-cell lymphotropic virus (HTLV-I)	Adult T-cell leukaemia/lymphoma	
Human immunodeficiency virus (HIV)	B-cell lymphoma, invasive cervical carcinoma	Immunosuppression
Hepatitis C (HCV)	Primary liver cancer	Liver cirrhosis

are oncogenic. The mode of action of retroviruses is the best understood, and is described in the next section. However, it must be emphasized that this model is not the only, or indeed the most frequent, method by which viruses cause cancers of humans; once integrated, the means by which oncogenesis is effected varies with the virus concerned. For example, unlike retroviruses, integration of the DNA of some other viruses may be quite transient—the so-called 'hit and run' action.

This may result in a latent infection that reactivates with the production of infective virus (e.g. herpes simplex) or, if the conditions are suitable, initiates oncogenic changes.

3 Viral oncogenes

Knowledge of how retroviruses replicate (see Chapter 3) is essential for following this section. Some, but not all of them, possess a special gene—an **oncogene**, *onc* for short—that is capable of conferring the properties of malignancy on a host cell. Many oncogenes are known, and there are certainly more waiting to be discovered. They work in a variety of ways and there is no point in detailing all of them here. The fundamentals of the process can be illustrated by reference to the first transmissible tumour to be described—the Rous sarcoma (Table 6.1).

3.1 Mode of action

Oncogenes are named after the tumours they cause. The one discussed here is *src*, for sarcoma. Figure 6.2 shows the possible outcomes of infection of a chicken fibroblast with Rous virus; note that provirus DNA must be circularized before integration with host DNA, but for simplicity is shown here in linear form.

The sequence of events (numbered steps as in Fig. 6.2) is as follows.

1. A retrovirus attaches to specific receptors on the host cell.
2. The virion uncoats in the cytoplasm.
3. Viral ssRNA is transcribed to dsDNA by **RT**.
4. Viral DNA (now termed a **provirus**) is integrated into the host-cell genome.

The sequence of events from (1) to (4) is similar to that for any retrovirus. At this point, however, one of three courses may be taken:

- The integrated provirus often remains quiescent, giving rise to a silent but persistent infection.
- It may (5) be translated by a host-cell polymerase to mRNA. Then either (6A) the *gag*, *pol*, and *env* genes are translated to form new viral components which are assembled with RNA in the cytoplasm to form (7) progeny virus, released by budding from the cell surface; or
- The oncogene may become activated and transcribed to an mRNA coding for the oncogene product (6B), in this example a phosphorylating enzyme (protein kinase). This and other gene products, of which there are a considerable number, modify the activity of various cell proteins concerned with suppression or stimulation of cell growth. Such modifications may have as their end result a transformed cell, which, by clonal expansion, forms a malignant tumour. During this process, the transformed cell acquires new tumour (T) antigens in its cell membrane, which may also help to change its growth characteristics.

There are pronounced differences in the time taken for the transforming viruses to exert their oncogenic effects. The Gross

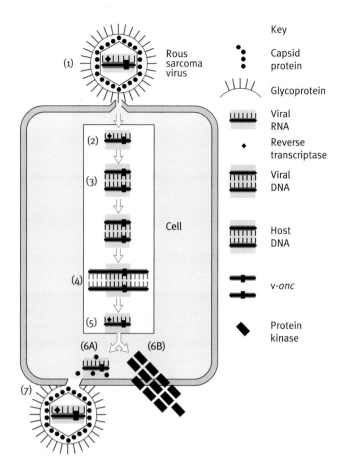

Key

Capsid protein

Glycoprotein

Viral RNA

Reverse transcriptase

Viral DNA

Host DNA

v-*onc*

Protein kinase

Fig. 6.2 Integration of the Rous sarcoma provirus and oncogene into host-cell DNA. For description, see text.

are unable to produce new virions without the aid of a 'helper' virus capable of supplying the missing gene(s).

4 Cellular oncogenes

During their research on the *src* oncogene, Stehelin and his colleagues (Table 6.1) made a most remarkable discovery. They found that normal cells of birds, fishes, and mammals contain a counterpart of *src*, having a rather different molecular structure, but coding for the same protein kinase. The same applies to other oncogenes, so that we have to specify whether we are referring to viral oncogenes (v-*onc*), or their cellular counterparts (**proto-oncogenes**, or c-*onc*). It appears that during the course of evolution, certain viruses have **transduced** (captured) host genes that in their cellular form participate in the normal activities of the cell, but in their viral form behave as described in Section 3.1. Cellular oncogenes are present in the germ cells of animals, birds, fishes, and even insects.

4.1 Can c-*onc* genes be oncogenic?

As they occur with such frequency, this question is of crucial importance to our understanding of how cancers in general, not only those related to viral infection, are initiated. The answer is yes; a number of different stimuli may have this effect.

- Figure 6.4 shows a viral oncogene, with its *gag*, *pol*, and *env* genes inserted into host-cell DNA. The genes are flanked by long sequences of repeated nucleotides (long terminal repeats, LTRs), which have regulatory functions. Insertion of the viral LTR may activate an adjacent cellular oncogene (c-*onc*), thus giving rise indirectly to malignant change in the host cell. This mechanism is known as **insertional mutagenesis**.

- Another way in which cellular genes may be involved is by loss or mutation of a growth suppressor gene, normally concerned with controlling cell proliferation. One of the best characterized gene products in this category is p53, a nuclear protein that binds to specific DNA sequences and functions as a transcriptional regulator, arresting cell

virus (Section 1.1) is an example of a weakly transforming ('slow') retrovirus. These have a full complement of *gag*, *pol*, and *env* genes and thus replicate normally; integration of provirus only infrequently results in transformation. However, some exogenous viruses have in the past acquired an oncogene that displaced one or more replicative genes (*pol* in the example shown in Fig. 6.3). Such 'fast' viruses are rapidly oncogenic, but

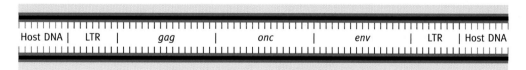

Host DNA | LTR | *gag* | *onc* | *env* | LTR | Host DNA

Fig. 6.3 Loss of a replicative gene (pol) by recombination and consequent displacement with an oncogene (onc). For explanation, see text.

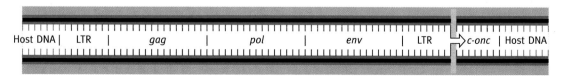

Host DNA | LTR | *gag* | *pol* | *env* | LTR | c-*onc* | Host DNA

Fig. 6.4 Activation of a cellular oncogene by insertional mutagenesis. For explanation, see text.

growth so as to allow repair in the case of damage to DNA. The induction of p53 may also lead to apoptosis, or 'programmed cell death', a normal mechanism for restricting cell growth; thus loss of the *p53* gene may lead to unrestricted proliferation and development of a tumour. Another well-known cellular suppressor protein is Rb.

- Carcinogens such as **radiation** and various chemicals—including nicotine—may induce oncogenic mutations, which may be very small: experimentally, a c-*onc* gene was made oncogenic by a single base change—a point mutation—in its DNA.

- Another way in which cellular genes may be involved is by loss or mutation of a **growth suppressor gene**, normally concerned with controlling cell proliferation.

5 Indirect mechanisms

5.1 Cell regeneration

Hepatitis B differs from most oncogenic viruses in that fragments of its DNA—normally a circular molecule—are integrated into the host hepatocyte genome at variable sites; the usual process of insertional mutagenesis (Fig. 6.4) cannot therefore operate and it is difficult as yet to define the oncogenic role of the viral nucleic acid. It may be that with both hepatitis B and C viruses, abnormal cellular proliferation associated with cirrhosis is a factor in tumour formation. It is also possible that proliferation of mucosal cells due to infection with papovaviruses viruses may, in combination with other factors, give rise to carcinoma of the cervix.

5.2 Immunosuppression

In thinking of oncogenesis at the cellular level, we must not forget the influences exerted by the responses of the host as a whole. Thus immune mechanisms play a major part in determining the course of malignant disease. It is noteworthy that immunodeficient patients have an increased liability to cancer (Chapter 32), perhaps because the immune surveillance system loses its capacity to recognize cells with new tumour antigens as 'foreign'. Some forms of immunosuppression are themselves due to viral infection, both by retroviruses and others. In this way, viruses can promote oncogenesis by indirect means. The human immunodeficiency viruses provide an example (Chapter 25). They do not themselves possess oncogenes, but, by inducing profound immunodeficiency, permit the growth of tumours that would otherwise be suppressed (see Section 6.2).

5.3 Other factors

Genetic influences determine susceptibility to some forms of cancer; for example, nasopharyngeal carcinoma following EBV infection is particularly liable to occur in people of southern Chinese origin (Chapter 20). Dietary and hormonal factors may also be implicated in some malignancies (Table 6.3), but their modes of action are not fully understood.

6 Viruses implicated in cancers of humans

You will encounter various examples of virus-induced oncogenesis in Parts 2 and 3 of this book; Table 6.3 lists the viruses for which there is good evidence of oncogenicity in humans. Three families of DNA viruses do *not* cause malignant disease: the adenoviruses (except when injected into new-born rodents), the poxviruses, and the parvoviruses.

6.1 DNA viruses

Papillomaviruses (Chapter 15)

In recent years, papillomaviruses have to a large extent superseded herpes simplex as the prime suspect for causing cervical cancer. Some 'high-risk' genotypes, notably 16 and 18, are particularly liable to cause carcinomas. An important factor seems to be the ability of their E6 and E7 proteins to bind to the cell-suppressor proteins Rb and p53 (see Section 4.1).

Epstein–Barr virus (Chapter 20)

This virus is almost ubiquitous as a latent infection of humans, although the age of acquisition varies in different populations, as does the frequency and type of associated malignancies.

Burkitt's lymphoma

In the zone of Africa where is BL is endemic, EBV can be detected in 95 per cent of the tumours. Its oncogenic effect has been ascribed, at least in part, to the translocation of certain immunoglobulin genes to positions at or near the location of c-*myc*, an oncogene whose consequent deregulation may result in malignant change. The mechanism of oncogenesis in the remaining 5 per cent of EBV-negative tumours in Africa, and in similarly virus-negative tumours elsewhere, is unknown.

Nasopharyngeal carcinoma

As in endemic BL, EBV is constantly present in the tumour cells, but its implication in formation of the tumour has not been worked out. It is, however, interesting that the age distribution differs from that of BL (4–12 years), in that adults are also affected. Furthermore, the cofactors differ in the two diseases (Table 6.3).

B-cell lymphoma

These tumours are liable to occur in immunosuppressed patients, including those suffering from AIDS. Their causation seems to be much more straightforward than that of other EBV-associated tumours: they result from the uncontrolled proliferation of latently infected B lymphocytes when freed from surveillance by EBV-specific cytotoxic T lymphocytes.

Human herpesvirus type 8 (HHV-8) (Chapter 20)

This is the latest herpesvirus to be identified—not actually isolated—because the evidence for its existence is based on the finding of DNA sequences resembling those of a type B herpesvirus in Kaposi's sarcoma (see Chapter 25). This form of cancer is particularly, but not exclusively, found in AIDS patients. The possibility that HHV-8 is causally related to the tumour is now under investigation.

Hepatitis B virus (Chapter 22)

Hepatocellular carcinoma (HCC) following chronic infection with hepatitis B virus is one of the most prevalent forms of cancer. Worldwide, there are about 300 million people chronically infected, with more than 250 000 new cases being reported annually. It is also the only malignant disease of humans preventable by immunization against the causal agent. Unfortunately, however, the pathogenesis of this major cause of cancer is still poorly understood. It is often associated with cirrhosis, and is thought by some simply to result from cellular proliferation during regeneration of damaged tissue. However, this explanation seems too simplistic. We do know that viral DNA is present in most of the tumours, and is integrated at random sites within the chromosomal DNA. As we have seen, such insertions are liable to cause perturbations of functions of the host genome. Among the possible oncogenic mechanisms for HCC that have been suggested are insertional mutagenesis, with destabilization of the host genome, including deregulation of c-*myc*; and inactivation of tumour-suppressor genes. Consumption of food contaminated with aflatoxins, such as occurs in areas of Africa, seems to play an accessory role. These are produced by *Aspergillus* spp. and contaminate groundnuts and cereals. They can cause liver cancer in animals, apparently without the presence of hepatitis B virus.

6.2 RNA viruses

Human T-cell lymphotropic virus (Chapter 25)

Human T-cell leukaemia virus type 1 (HTLV-I), a retrovirus, is the cause of adult T-cell leukaemia, a malignant proliferation of CD4+ lymphocytes. The basic model for oncogenesis by HTLV is that portrayed in Fig. 6.2. In the case of this virus, the v-*onc* component of the provirus contains the genes *tax* and *rex* encoding two phosphoproteins, tax (40 kDa) and rex (21 kDa), which are respectively transcriptional and post-transcriptional regulators. Tax *trans*-activates a wide variety of genes and appears to be intimately involved in cell transformation, which can be accomplished *in vitro*.

The involvement of HTLV-II in disease of humans seems to be minimal, and little is known of its role in oncogenesis.

Human immunodeficiency viruses (Chapter 25)

These retroviruses contain no oncogenes, and although their RNA integrates readily with the host genome, they do not appear to cause malignant disease directly. Nevertheless, the profound immunodepression afflicting AIDS patients opens the door to the formation of various tumours normally held in check by immune surveillance (see Chapter 25).

Hepatitis C virus (Chapter 24)

Since its discovery in 1989, HCV, a flavivirus, has emerged as an important cause of HCC. This is surprising, in view of the obvious impossibility of its RNA genome reacting with host-cell DNA. The answer probably lies in the tendency of HCV infections to become chronic, and to lead to cirrhosis. Most of the associated liver cancers do not develop until about 30 years after the infection is acquired. For want of a better explanation, the tendency to malignancy has been ascribed to uncontrolled cell proliferation following inflammation, destruction, and repair of damaged hepatocytes. It is worth noting that concurrent infections with hepatitis B (HBV) and deltavirus (hepatitis D virus, HDV) are quite frequent.

7 Reminders

- Many cellular activities, including replication, differentiation, and death are governed by chemical signals, which in turn are controlled by genes.

- Some viruses that possess a **DNA genome**, or that **synthesize DNA during replication (the retroviruses)**, are able to induce malignant changes in cells, both *in vivo* and *in vitro* (transformation).

- Transformed cells have an **increased rate of multiplication,** grow in a **disorderly fashion**, and can be **propagated indefinitely** in the laboratory; they possess **tumour (T) antigens** on their cell surfaces.

- Malignant changes can be initiated by a variety of **mutagenic stimuli**, including radiation, chemical carcinogens, and insertion of viral DNA into the host-cell genome.

- In the case of **retroviruses**, the DNA is a copy of the RNA genome—the **provirus**. Oncogenic retroviruses possess an additional gene—the **oncogene**—which may either remain quiescent or be translated to proteins that affect the normal growth characteristics of the host cell; it does not participate in synthesis of viral components.

- Viral oncogenes (v-*onc*) possess almost identical **cellular counterparts** (c-*onc*) from which they were derived in the distant past. These c-*onc* genes can also be activated by mutagenic stimuli to induce malignancy.

- Some DNA viruses are oncogenic; in their case the integrated DNA is not a specialized oncogene, but encodes viral components in the normal way.

- The main oncogenic DNA viruses are papillomaviruses, EBV, and hepatitis B. Most of the oncogenic RNA viruses are retroviruses; long-term infection with hepatitis C, a flavivirus, may result in liver cancer, but the mechanism is probably indirect.

- Viral oncogenesis may be assisted by **host factors**, including immunosuppression, genetic make-up, dietary habits, and exposure to mutagenic influences such as ionizing radiation or chemical carcinogens.

Viruses and the community

1 Introduction

In Chapters 2 and 3, we considered viruses at the molecular level, after which we went on to discuss them in relation to individual cells, to organs of the body, and thence to their effects on individuals. It is now time to stand back and look at a much broader canvas—the way in which viruses affect whole communities. This is the province of **epidemiology**, a word of Greek derivation meaning 'upon (i.e. affecting) the people'; the corresponding term for disease in animal communities is **epizootology**.

The story of the way in which microbes and other parasites affect communities is one of a constantly shifting balance of power between parasite and host, both of which, during their evolution, evolve quite elaborate means of attack and defence, and hence of survival. The results of such battles—which determine the effects of microbes on individuals and hence on the community—are the outcomes of a highly complex interplay of factors. These were neatly summarized by the American epidemiologist John Paul under the headings of *seed*, *soil*, and *climate*, the first referring to the parasite, the second to the host in which it grows, and the third not just to the weather, but to all the other environmental factors involved.

2 Definitions

2.1 Prevalence

The number of cases of a given disease—clinical or subclinical—recorded **at a particular time** and expressed as a proportion of the population under study.

2.2 Incidence

The number of cases recorded **during a particular period** (e.g. 1 year). This measurement is often given in terms of **an attack rate** (i.e. the number of cases per thousand or per hundred thousand of the general population (or of a subgroup within it) during the period in question).

2.3 Endemic

This term refers to a disease that is constantly present at a significant level within a community. Herpes simplex is an example. Endemicity may be high or low. The corresponding term for infections of animals is **enzootic**.

2.4 Epidemic

An unusual increase in the number of cases within a community. In this context, 'unusual' is defined arbitrarily: 100 cases of measles in London might not be regarded as an epidemic, but 100 cases of poliomyelitis certainly would be. The corresponding term for infections of animals is **epizootic**. Localized epidemics are usually referred to as **outbreaks**.

2.5 Pandemic

An epidemic involving several continents at the same time. The corresponding term for infections of animals is **panzootic**.

3 What use is epidemiology?

There is much more to this science than dry tables of statistics; it is the key to four major clinical activities, the first three of which may be aided by the application of mathematical models.

- **Predictions of trends in diseases**; for example, knowledge of the behaviour of an infection in the past helps to predict the course of an epidemic.
- Guide to the **introduction, improvement, or modification of control measures**; for example, immunization programmes, control of insect vectors, or improvements in hygiene.
- Evaluation of the success of such measures, locally, nationally, or worldwide.
- **Aids to diagnosis**. A knowledge of what infectious diseases are currently prevalent is very useful to the physician as a diagnostic pointer; it may also suggest to the laboratory the need for certain specific tests.

4 Epidemiological methods

It is not possible to discuss epidemiological techniques in detail here. For our purposes, it is enough to know that for infective diseases, the two principal methods of surveillance are **clinical** and **microbiological**, both of which must be tied in with an adequate system of **data collection** and **processing**.

4.1 Clinical observations

Well before bacteria and viruses were discovered, clinical observations alone, carefully recorded, and made major contributions to epidemiology. The story is well known of how, many years before the cholera vibrio had been identified,

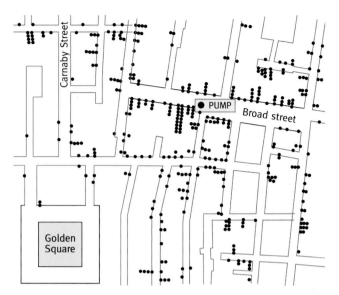

Fig. 7.1 The clustering of cholera deaths around the Broad Street pump in Soho, London, during 1854. (Data from *Medicine International*, 1984; by courtesy of Dr N.S. Galbraith.)

Dr John Snow determined which water companies supplied different parts of London, and concluded that this infection was waterborne. In 1854, he identified the Broad Street pump in Soho as the source of a major outbreak of cholera and dealt with the situation very successfully by persuading the parish authority to remove the pump handle (Fig. 7.1). There are many examples of equally acute observations of viral infections, one of the most striking being P.L. Panum's study of measles in the Faroe Islands in 1846. During that year there was a major epidemic in this isolated community, which, not having been exposed to the infection since 1781, consisted almost entirely of non-immune people. Within the next 6 months, more than 6000 people in a total population of 7782 contracted measles, an extraordinary attack rate of over 770 per 1000. Panum noted that none of the elderly people who had had measles in the previous epidemic acquired it on this occasion. By meticulously recording the dates of contacts and of the onset of disease, this young Danish doctor established that measles is infective for others only at about the time of appearance of the rash. He found the incubation period to be 13–14 days and confirmed by personal investigation that cases with significantly longer or shorter incubation periods either were suffering from something other than measles, or had had a contact outside this period.

Nearer our own time, N.M. Gregg noticed that during 1941 there was a high incidence of cataract in newborn babies in Sydney, and that this abnormality was often associated with deformities of the heart. He then made the acute observation that the mothers of most of these infants had had rubella (German measles) while pregnant during an epidemic in the previous year. The making of this association, purely by clinical methods, was fundamental to the recognition that several virus infections acquired during pregnancy may damage the fetus. We shall return to this subject in Chapter 31.

4.2 Laboratory studies

Good clinical observations are useful, provided that an adequate **case definition** is established at the outset; this means laying down the criteria by which a case is accepted or rejected as suffering from a particular disease. Purely clinical studies do, however, have the following disadvantages:

- Despite the use of case definitions, some syndromes, such as respiratory infections or diarrhoea, are often difficult to diagnose accurately on clinical grounds alone.
- They cannot reveal the extent of very mild or subclinical infections.
- They cannot usually provide accurate information about the prevalence of a particular viral infection in the past (which is often a good guide to the state of immunity to that virus possessed by the community as a whole).

For these purposes, laboratory investigations are brought into play, and are especially useful in viral infections, most of which induce a firm and long-lasting antibody response. As in general diagnostic work, the tests fall into two main categories:

- detection of virus in acutely ill patients;
- detection of specific antibody.

For epidemiological work, the first category is of limited value; it is useful for some purposes (e.g. identifying the prevalent strain of influenza during an epidemic), but such tests are normally carried out only on a limited sample of the population. Serological tests, many of which are now automated or semi-automated, are much more practical for large-scale surveys.

5 Serological epidemiology

This expression was also coined by John Paul, who wrote that serum antibodies 'represent footprints, either faint or distinct,

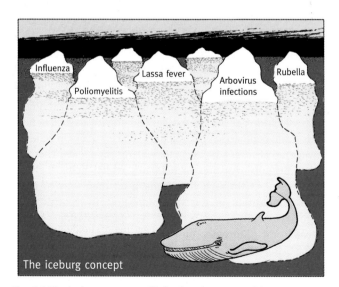

Fig. 7.2 **The iceberg concept of infections in communities.**

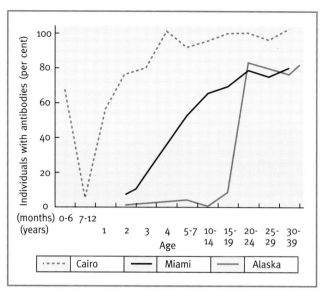

Fig. 7.3 Prevalence of poliomyelitis antibody in different populations. Percentages of individuals with antibodies to poliovirus type 2, surveyed during 1949–51. (Reproduced with permission from Paul, J.R. and White, C. (ed.) (1973). In *Serological Epidemiology*, p. 10. Academic Press, New York.)

of an infection experienced in the remote or recent past'. During the 1930s it was found, even with the crude methods then available, that antibodies to certain infections were present in much higher proportions of the study populations than was warranted by the amount of clinically apparent disease. This situation can be likened to that of an iceberg (Fig. 7.2) in which the part above water represents clinical illness, and that below, the prevalence of antibody in the population. The simultaneous discovery that the prevalence of antibody varies with age provided a powerful tool for studying the history of viral infections in communities.

Now look carefully at Fig. 7.3, which contains much more information than at first appears. These are the results of early studies on antibody to a poliovirus, carried out during 1949–51 in three locations differing greatly in socio-economic conditions. The first, in Cairo, included young infants and clearly shows that those aged less than 6 months still had maternal antibody, which was lost after this period; thereafter, however, it rapidly reappeared, reflecting an active immune response to early infection with the virus. This finding was surprising, because epidemics of *clinical* poliomyelitis were unknown—or at least unreported—in Egypt; it represented hitherto unsuspected infection—the part of the iceberg under water. The early acquisition of antibody is characteristic of societies with poor hygiene in which transmission of infections by the faecal–oral route occurs readily.

In Miami, a world apart both geographically and economically, hygienic conditions were such that exposure to the virus came later in life, and poliomyelitis tended to occur in clinically apparent outbreaks at intervals of 7–10 years. (We explain in Chapter 16 how at certain times and places poliomyelitis is more severe in older than in younger people.)

In the much more isolated Alaskan population, there had been an epidemic of poliomyelitis 20 years previously, but none since. Note that the percentage of people with antibody is insignificant in those aged less than 20 years, but rises steeply to nearly 80 per cent in those aged 20 years or more. If Dr Panum had had the benefit of serological methods, he would have found a very similar pattern 20 years after the measles epidemic in the Faroes in 1846.

5.1 Methods

In carrying out serological surveys it is important to **define the objectives**, to use a **suitable sample** of the study population, and to gather **adequate information** about those tested. If these conditions are met, it is often possible to use the sera for multiple studies, not only on different infections, but also, for example, on blood chemistry. Sera stored at −20 °C or below can be kept for many years and used for retrospective investigations. Drops of blood can be collected on discs or strips of filter paper, dried, and later eluted in buffer for antibody tests; this technique is especially useful for young infants.

The methods of measuring antibodies vary with the virus concerned; for example, those to polioviruses, measles, and influenza might be assayed respectively by neutralization, complement fixation, and haemagglutination-inhibition tests (see Chapter 36).

5.2 Monitoring an immunization programme

In addition to studying patterns of disease, serological tests are invaluable for monitoring the success of mass immunization programmes. Here, it is important to know what proportion of people in the target population is immune to the disease in question, whether as a result of the immunization itself or of natural infection. The following is an example of what can be done at a purely local level.

In the UK, sera from women attending antenatal clinics are routinely screened for rubella antibody; if negative, the patient is advised that she should be immunized soon after delivery, to avoid the risk of rubella in subsequent pregnancies, with consequent damage to the fetus (see Chapter 31). During 1983, it was noticed in two London virology laboratories that the prevalence of rubella antibody in women from the Indian subcontinent was significantly lower than that in the indigenous population. This finding indicated the need for a stepped-up information and immunization campaign directed at this particular group.

5.3 Processing of data

The collection of epidemiological information is pointless unless there is an efficient system for collating it and applying the results for the improvement of the public health. Such systems exist at the local, national, and international levels. It is not possible here to explain in detail the machinery for processing epidemiological information, but an important principle is that much of the traffic is two-way; data collected by clinicians and in laboratories are processed centrally, and the results are ultimately returned to these 'front-line' workers for action at the local level.

On the international level, much information is collected by the World Health Organization, an outstanding example being the monitoring, through national centres, of the incidence of influenza and identification of the prevalent strains of virus, an activity of prime importance to vaccine manufacturers.

In the USA, the surveillance and investigation of infective diseases is managed centrally by the Centers for Disease Control (CDC) in Atlanta, Georgia. In the UK, these functions are the responsibility of the Health Protection Agency (HPA) and, for Scotland, the Scottish Centre for Infection and Environmental Health (SCIEH).

In addition, clinical data are collected by panels of physicians who report on specified diseases through the Royal College of General Practitioners. There are also weekly reports on certain diseases to the Office of Population Censuses and Surveys; and certain infections must by law be reported to the appropriate authorities (Appendix B). Other countries have analogous systems, their scale and quality being governed largely by economic circumstances.

These sources of intelligence cater primarily for healthcare professionals. It should also be the job of governments to provide up-to-date and accurate information and guidance about current epidemiological problems in their respective countries (e.g. outbreaks of food poisoning, influenza immunization, AIDS, CJD[nv], and so forth). Such information is—or should be—disseminated by notices to doctors in general practice, and to the press.

6 Factors in the spread of viral infections

At this point, we must take stock of the 'seed, soil, and climate' factors mentioned at the opening of this chapter. First, the seed.

6.1 Characteristics of the virus

Table 7.1 lists the main features of viruses that determine how they are transmitted, and hence their potential for spread within communities.

First, how well does the virus survive in the environment on its way from one host to another? Enteroviruses such as hepatitis A and polioviruses can remain viable for weeks in water or sewage, an obvious advantage for waterborne agents. They are also unusually resistant to acid pH, which helps them to survive transit through the stomach on their way to their site of replication in the small intestine. By contrast, the rhinoviruses—also members of the *Picornaviridae*—being spread by the respiratory route, do not possess this property.

The existence of a **reservoir of infection** in a primary (alternative) host, usually a mammal but sometimes a bird, clearly has many implications for the mode of spread. Such infections are called zoonoses, among which are many infections by toga

Table 7.1 Properties of viruses that determine transmissibility

Property	Particular features	Examples
Survivability outside the host	Resistance to ambient temperatures, drying, ultraviolet light (in sunlight), pH	Enteroviruses, e.g. polio and Coxsackie viruses
Existence of an alternative host	If so, direct transmission? Via arthropod vector?	Rabies virus Arboviruses, e.g. yellow fever
Portal of entry	(see Tables 4.1 and 4.2)	
Evasiveness	Rapid multiplication on a mucous membrane before immune response can be mounted	Viruses infecting the respiratory tract, e.g. rhinoviruses, and conjunctiva, e.g. some adenoviruses
	Variability in antigenic structure, thus evading immune response to a previous infection	Influenza A and B viruses, human immunodeficiency virus (HIV)
Pathogenesis	Incubation period: short, medium, or long	See Chapter 4
Route by which virus is shed	Respiratory secretions	Viruses causing childhood fevers, e.g. measles, mumps, rubella; those causing respiratory infections
	Conjunctival secretions	Conjunctivitis viruses, e.g. some adeno-viruses, enterovirus 70
	Skin, epithelial mucosae	Warts, herpes simplex and zoster
	Faeces	Entero- and rotaviruses
	Blood transfusion, contaminated needles or instruments	Cytomegalovirus, hepatitis B and C, HIV

and flaviviruses (Chapter 27) and by those causing certain haemorrhagic fevers (Chapter 28). If—as is often the case—a vector such as a mosquito or tick is also involved, many more factors complicate the picture; these include its feeding and breeding patterns, range of mobility, length of time for which the virus persists within it, and whether the virus is transmitted to its offspring. The transmission of such infections to humans clearly depends on the degree of exposure of the latter to the vector, which in turn may be conditioned by the place of work or recreation.

The routes by which viruses enter and are shed from the body are obviously very important in transmission; and what happens to them within the host may be equally so. Much depends on how well the virus is able to evade the host's defences, in terms of either its site of replication or its ability to undergo mutations that give rise to new, antibody-resistant, strains. The ways in which viruses spread within their hosts were discussed in Chapter 4; they determine the incubation period of a given infection, and thus the rapidity with which it can be transmitted from person to person. To take two extremes, conjunctivitis caused by enterovirus type 70 has an incubation period of about 2 days, and causes explosive epidemics that sweep through whole communities like wildfire; the AIDS viruses, with incubation periods measured in years, spread correspondingly more slowly and insidiously.

6.2 Characteristics of the host and the environment

We have combined the 'soil' and 'climate' factors in Table 7.2 because one cannot consider host species apart from their environments. We have not given examples of how the various factors operate because there are so many that isolated instances would give a misleading impression. However, there is one very important point. The environment does, to a great extent, determine what sort of virus infections are most prevalent in given geographical areas; this means that there is a considerable difference between the patterns of infection in developed and developing countries (Table 7.3).

7 Herd immunity

This expression signifies the proportion of the population that is immune to a given infection, whether as a result of natural

Table 7.2 Characteristics of the host and environment that influence the pattern of viral infections

The host
Age
Sex
Ethnic group and genetic factors
Occupation and economic status
Nutrition
State of immunity

The environment
Geographical location
Urban or rural setting
Existence of zoonotic infections/vectors
Socio-economic status/state of hygiene/overcrowding

Table 7.3 High-prevalence viral infections: comparison between developed and developing countries

Developed countries

Upper respiratory tract infections

Paramyxoviruses

Influenza

Herpesviruses

Papillomaviruses

Human immunodeficiency virus (in certain population groups)

Developing countries
All the above, plus

Poliomyelitis

Gastroenteritis viruses

Hepatitis A

Hepatitis B

Yellow fever; haemorrhagic fevers and encephalitis due to arbo-, filo-, and arenaviruses

SARS

Rabies

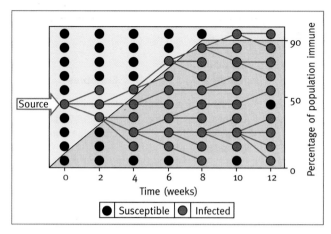

Fig. 7.4 Spread of measles in a highly susceptible population in the Faroe Islands, 1846.

in Fig. 7.4. The box represents the isolated community, all of whom, except for a small minority of elderly people, had never been in contact with this infection and were thus fully susceptible. The arrow at the left represents the cabinet-maker who imported the infection on returning from a trip to the mainland. The incubation period was 2 weeks, and on the assumption that those who became infected were immune after another 2 weeks, the increase in herd immunity can be plotted, and is shown as the shaded area. (Needless to say, epidemics do not behave as regularly as this in real life. Successive waves of infection soon get out of synchrony.) Note that some infections are 'dead-end' (i.e. are not transmitted to anyone else). The epidemic petered out when there were too few susceptible people left to keep the chain reaction going. In practice, not all the population must be immune for this to occur; it can happen when the proportion reaches 70–80 per cent.

7.2 Endemic infections

Look again at Fig. 7.3, in which the age-specific distributions of antibodies to poliovirus type 2 in different geographical areas during 1949–51 are compared. In Cairo, the majority of the population had been infected during infancy, an age when most polio infections are asymptomatic. As immunity following exposure to this virus is virtually lifelong, it follows that the proportion of susceptibles in the total population was very small (Fig. 7.5(a)). There may have been the odd sporadic case of clinically apparent disease, but the pie chart shows that there are certainly not enough susceptible people to sustain an epidemic. By contrast, the proportion of immune people in the various age groups in Miami did not much exceed 50 per cent until early adolescence, leaving a substantial proportion of children unprotected during a period of life when poliomyelitis is liable to cause severe paralytic illness. The situation in this age group is shown in Fig. 7.5(b), from which it can be seen that there has been a build-up of susceptibles to a point at which an epidemic could be initiated. Before the introduction of polio vaccine, such epidemics did, as mentioned in Section 5, occur at 7–10-year intervals in this community.

infection or artificial immunization. Most acute viral infections induce firm and long-lasting immunity; and infective but apparently healthy carriers are not usually a significant factor in the behaviour of endemic or epidemic viral infections.

There are two main methods by which viral infections are propagated in communities:

1. **from person-to-person**: viruses spread in this way are usually transmitted by the respiratory route, e.g. influenza, colds, measles, rubella, mumps;

2. **from an external source**: many viral infections are spread by the faecal–oral route (e.g. poliomyelitis, hepatitis A, gastroenteritis viruses) or by the bites of infected arthropods (e.g. tick-borne encephalitis, YF, dengue fever).

In both modes of spread, the degree of herd immunity is of paramount importance in determining patterns of endemicity and epidemicity. From what has been said, it will readily be appreciated that such patterns are governed by extremely complex factors, so much so that they are often difficult to predict even with the most elaborate mathematical models. Nevertheless, three simplified examples will give a good idea of the general principles.

7.1 An epidemic in an isolated community

First, let us go back to the 1846 measles epidemic in the Faroe Islands. The situation faced by Dr Panum is shown schematically

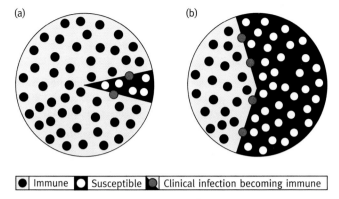

| ● Immune | ○ Susceptible | ◉ Clinical infection becoming immune |

Fig. 7.5 Herd immunity in poliomyelitis. **(a)** 'Cairo' model. Herd immunity is high and clinically apparent infection is rare: no danger of epidemic. **(b)** 'Miami' model. Herd immunity is only moderate and there are sporadic cases of clinically apparent infection: an epidemic is probable.

8 Hospital-acquired infections (HAIs)

Infections are classed as hospital-acquired if they become manifest more than 48 hours after admission or less than 48 hours after discharge. They are also known as **nosocomial infections.** HAIs present us with the paradox that some people who enter hospital to have their illness cured acquire another, possibly worse infection from other patients, their environment, or even medical or surgical equipment used for their treatment. Various factors contribute to this state of affairs, including, for example, the increasingly rapid turnover of staff and patients, the complexity of modern instruments and the difficulties in sterilizing them, and the emergence of antibiotic-resistant pathogens. All this is compounded by the fact that the immunity of some hospital patients is impaired by their illness.

8.1 Sources of infection

HAIs may be **exogenous,** transmitted from :

1. contamination of the environment, e.g. food, water, air, dirt and dust, ward equipment, bedclothes and other fomites; or

2. **cross-infection** from another patient, member of staff, or visitor.

The possibility of an **endogenous infection**, i.e. one arising from within the patient, must also be remembered, for example reactivation of a herpesvirus infection following a transplant. There have also been several reports in recent years of transmission from organ donors who were incubating the infection. The earliest of these involved recipients of corneal transplants, but in 2004 four patients in the USA were infected in this way by donations of lung, liver, and kidney from the same donor, who later died of rabies.

8.2 Microbial causes of HAI

The pride of place, if that is the right expression, must be given to bacterial rather than viral infections, headed by those of the urinary and lower respiratory tracts and bacteraemia. With shifting patterns of antibiotic resistance the relative prevalences of particular bacteria have varied over the years, the most notable being the methicillin-resistant *Staphylococcus aureus* (MRSA). This dangerous pathogen flourishes particularly where hygienic conditions are not of the best and has been implicated in many deaths in the UK. A major factor in spreading these infections is the failure of staff to wash their hands thoroughly between moving from one patient to another.

8.3 Viral infections

Viral infections account for a substantial proportion of illnesses contracted in hospitals. The chances of acquiring one are the result of several factors including:

- good staff discipline, especially in relation to hand washing
- cleanliness of the wards
- length of stay
- whether surgery involved
- prevalence of the virus
- transmissibility of the virus
- state of immunity of the patient
- age of the patient (risk greater for very young or very old people)
- care and cleanliness of apparatus such as air-conditioning systems.

Needless to say, these general precautions apply not just to the transmission of viruses, but to all microbial infections.

Table 7.4 Control of infection in individuals and communities

Individual measures	Community measures
Personal hygiene, especially hand washing	Surveillance of food/milk/ water supplies and blood products
Personal behaviour, e.g. 'safe sex', avoidance of injected drug abuse	Maintenance of hygiene and avoidance of overcrowding in residential institutions
Isolation of patients with dangerous infections	Where appropriate, control of insect vectors and immunization of animals
Appropriate individual immunizations for travellers	Routine immunization programmes
	Dissemination of information
	(a) to professional colleagues
	(b) to the public

Table 7.5 Examples of control measures for infections transmitted from insects and animals.

Disease	Transmitted by	Control measures
Yellow fever (Ch. 27)	Mosquitoes	Antimosquito measures: insecticides; spraying or elimination of breeding grounds; use of mosquito nets and insect repellants Immunization (for yellow fever)
Dengue (Ch. 27)	Mosquitoes	Antimosquito measures
Viral encephalitides (Ch. 27)	Mosquitoes, ticks	Antimosquito and tick measures
Crimean and Omsk haemorrhagic fevers (Ch. 27)	Ticks	Antitick measures
Lassa and other arenavirus infections (Ch. 28)	Contact with infected rodent urine or faeces	Rodent-proofing of living quarters
Hantavirus haemorrhagic fevers, pulmonary and renal infections (Ch. 28)		Rodent-proofing of living quarters
Filoviruses: Marburg and Ebola (Ch. 28)	Contact with infected monkeys or bats (may also be transmitted by contact with human blood and body fluids)	Avoidance of contact in hospitals, isolation, and barrier nursing
Rabies (Ch. 26)	All warm-blooded animals, especially dogs, foxes, bats, raccoons	Immunization (humans, dogs, foxes) Quarantine where appropriate
Poxviruses, e.g. cowpox, orf, monkey pox (Ch. 14)	Cows, monkeys	Avoid contact with skin lesions
Pandemic influenza	Contact with chicken	Close live markets
SARS	Contact with civet cats	Close live markets
New variant CJD	Eating beef	Cull contaminated herds

Table 7.6 Examples of hospital-acquired infections (HAIs) caused by viruses

Body system	Virus
Respiratory tract	Influenza
	Parainfluenza
	Respiratory syncytial virus
Gastrointestinal tract	Noroviruses (Norwalk)
	Rotaviruses
Skin	Varicella-zoster
Contamination with blood	Hepatitis viruses
	HIV
	Filoviruses
Generalized infections	Measles
	Rubella

Table 7.6 lists the most important viruses causing HAI. Note, however, that the same virus may have several routes of entry.

A special situation arises when a patient has a reactivation of herpes zoster, particularly if immunocompromised, in which case he or she may shed virus and be a danger to other patients, and a potential hazard to the medical and nursing staff. To avoid this problem, the immune status of the attendants should be ascertained before rather than after they take up their duties and any without antibody should be offered varicella-zoster virus (VZV) vaccine. The patient should be transferred to an isolation facility forthwith.

There have been several instances of patients acquiring rabies from transplant donors (Chapter 26).

9 The periodicity of epidemics

In the absence of interference with the natural order (e.g. by introducing vaccines, improvements in hygiene, or campaigns against arthropod vectors), the pattern of acute infections may alternate between endemic and epidemic. Epidemics create highly immune populations, which, however, steadily become diluted with susceptibles as new babies are born into the community. When the proportion of non-immune people reaches a 'critical mass', contact with an infectious person may start a 'chain reaction' epidemic; water- or vector-borne diseases may also occur in epidemic form as a result of waning immunity in the

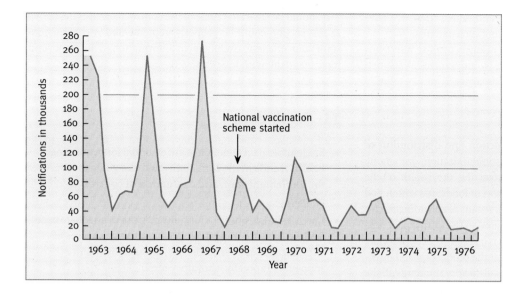

Fig. 7.6 The periodicity of measles epidemics. Typically, this pattern occurs when the infection is transmitted from person to person and confers long-lasting immunity. The effect of introducing mass immunization is apparent. (Reproduced by permission of the Public Health Laboratory Services Communicable Disease Surveillance Centre.)

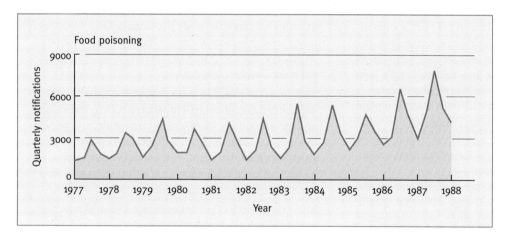

Fig. 7.7 The periodicity of food-poisoning epidemics. This pattern results from periodic outbreaks of 'common-source' infections. (Data from Figure A, OPCS Monitor, MB2 89/1 of April 1989. Reproduced by permission of the Office of Population Censuses and Surveys.)

general population. In areas unaffected by immunization, epidemics of acute infections such as measles or rubella may recur at regular intervals. Figure 7.6 shows such a pattern, and also illustrates the effect of introducing immunization. Another type of periodicity, superficially similar but basically different, is shown in Fig. 7.7. Here, regular annual epidemics result from infections transmitted from an external source—in this case food—and not from person to person. The peaks are due not so much to a build-up of susceptibles, but to the increased opportunities for bacteria to multiply and be transmitted during the warmer months.

10 Control measures

So far, we have described the factors involved in the spread of infective agents in the community and the methods for collecting epidemiological data. Clearly, such information is of little value unless it can be used both to combat outbreaks as they occur and to provide guidelines for preventing them in the future. Such control measures fall into two main groups: those directed respectively at individuals and at the community

(Table 7.4). Almost by definition, most of them cannot be implemented adequately in Third World countries, although within recent years there has been a welcome increase in the number of mass immunization programmes in the less affluent areas.

10.1 Individual measures

It goes without saying that personal hygiene is important for everyone, but particularly for those whose occupations carry the risk of spreading infections to others. They include food handlers, healthcare workers, and laboratory staff. **The single most important measure is probably hand washing**, especially after defecation, and, for clinical personnel, between contacts with patients with infective illnesses.

Infections transmitted by blood and body fluids, such as hepatitis and HIV and, of course, bacterial STD, can be prevented by avoiding both unprotected penetrative intercourse and sharing of syringes and needles used to inject drugs.

The control of dangerous infections such as the haemorrhagic fevers (Chapter 28) to the community at large is possible only when cases are few in number (e.g. importations from an infected to a non-infected country) and where there are adequate containment facilities for nursing such patients.

Finally, travellers can protect themselves against infections not prevalent in their own countries by immunization against, for example, YF and some encephalitis viruses.

10.2 Community measures

Constant **surveillance of the production and distribution of food and water**, together with mass immunization, are among the most important elements in protecting the health of the community at large. The rapid transport of foodstuffs within and across national boundaries is a potent means of spreading microbial infection. Objections are often raised to the intrusion of government into our daily lives, but there is no doubt that appropriate legislation is essential for ensuring that the production and distribution of food, milk, and water meet satisfactory standards all the way from production to the point of sale.

Although contamination of blood and blood products such as plasma, immunoglobulins, and clotting factors is comparatively rare and affects much smaller numbers of people, the consequences for individuals may be very serious. Virtually all such episodes involve viruses rather than bacteria, and a high degree of technical expertise may be needed to identify them. It is far better that blood products originate from healthy, unpaid donors rather from those giving blood for money, who are more prone to infections such as HIV and viral hepatitis and may be drug addicts. Furthermore, where paid donors are used, screening facilities may well be inadequate.

Hygienic measures in institutions such as those housing the mentally subnormal may be difficult or impossible to maintain, with resultant outbreaks of gastrointestinal and respiratory infections.

In some areas, often tropical or subtropical, **certain infections are transmitted to humans from animals,** with or without the participation of an insect vector. Control measures often involve counter-attacks on the animals or insects involved. Some of these infections are caused by arboviruses (Chapter 27) and a number fall into the 'exotic and dangerous' category (Chapter 28). Table 7.5 gives some examples.

A most important weapon in the control of infective illnesses is the **mass immunization** of susceptible people, the great majority of whom are young children (Chapter 37). By this means alone, smallpox was eradicated from the planet by 1977, and we are in sight of doing the same for polio and measles, which have already been eliminated from several countries. This hopeful prospect is reinforced by the fact that the whole vast area of the Americas now seems to be free of wild poliovirus.

It should be clear that none of the control measures described in this section could be properly implemented without a constant and efficient exchange of information. This important topic was dealt with in Section 5.3.

11 Reminders

- Epidemiological techniques are essential for **predicting health trends** in the community and as a guide to the **implementation and evaluation of control measures**.

- Careful clinical observations, making use of adequate **case definitions**, are important in establishing patterns of endemic and epidemic disease, but usually require supplementation by laboratory tests.

- **Serological surveys** of communities must be well designed in terms of their objectives and collection of adequate information about the study population. They show that for many viral infections there are high ratios of antibody positivity—the 'footprints' of past infections—to clinically apparent disease.

- The control of infection in communities depends on the implementation of **control measures** both by individuals and the community. They include maintenance of personal hygiene, immunization, surveillance of food and water supplies, control of insect and animal vectors, and dissemination of epidemiological information at local, national, and international levels.

- Many factors affect the **transmission** of viral infections, among which are **survivability** outside the host, the existence of **reservoirs of infection** in alternate host species, the need for an **arthropod vector**, the routes by which the virus **enters** and is **shed** from the host, and **incubation period**. Hospital-acquired infections pose their own epidemiological problems. It is most important that hospitals have **written control of infection policies** in place and that the medical and nursing staff implement them meticulously.

- The prevalence of the various viral infections differs with **socio-economic status**, and between developing and developed countries.

- The degree of **herd immunity** is important in determining the balance between endemicity and epidemic disease. In turn, shifts in this balance may result in recurrences of epidemics of a particular disease at regular intervals.

Part 2

Special infections

Upper respiratory tract and eye infections due to adenoviruses, coronaviruses (including SARS CoV), and rhinoviruses

1 Introduction

This chapter introduces three groups of viruses that, although differing greatly in structure and genetic organization, all cause disease of the respiratory tract or eye.

2 Adenoviruses

These viruses were first isolated from human adenoids, hence their name; they cause disease of both the respiratory tract and the eye and give rise to an estimated 5–10 per cent of respiratory viral infections.

2.1 Properties of the viruses

Classification

Members of the family *Adenoviridae* are icosahedral, non-enveloped DNA viruses some 80 nm in diameter. The name derives from the fact that they were first isolated from human adenoids. There are two genera, *Mastadenovirus* and *Aviadenovirus*, each of which possesses its own genus-specific antigen and affects mammals and birds respectively. Forty-seven serotypes of human adenoviruses are now known, distinguished on the basis of cross-neutralization tests, but this number will undoubtedly creep slowly upwards as time passes. In general, their host range is confined to one species. Various syndromes are associated with particular serotypes (Table 8.1).

The only reason to remember some of the avian adenoviruses is that they may inadvertently be present in eggs used for virus vaccine production, and at least one, CELO (chick embryo lethal orphan virus), causes cancer in animals.

Table 8.1 Some clinically important human adenoviruses

Disease	Predominant serotypes
Infantile gastroenteritis	40, 41
Upper respiratory tract infections	3, 7, 11, and others
Lower respiratory tract infections	3, 4, 7, 21
Pharyngoconjunctival fever	3, 4, 7
Epidemic keratoconjunctivitis	8, 19, 37
Acute haemorrhagic conjunctivitis	11
Acute haemorrhagic cystitis	7, 11, 21, 35
Genital ulcers; urethritis	2, 19, 37
Gastroenteritis and pneumonia in immunocompromised patients	Many serotypes

Morphology

When the first EM pictures of adenoviruses were published by Horne and his team at the National Institute for Medical Research in London, they caused a minor sensation, revealing as they did an architecture of remarkable beauty and precision (Figs 8.1 and 2.3). The capsid is formed from 252 capsomeres, which are arranged in a icosahedron with 20 sides and 12 vertices. A unique morphological feature is a slender fibre projecting from each of the 12 vertices of the icosahedron, giving the virus something of the appearance of an orbiting satellite.

Genome

The genome is linear dsDNA, 36–38 kbp with inverted terminal repeats and a protein primer at each 5′ terminus.

Replication

The virus binds to the host-cell receptor via the fibre and enters by endocytosis. After uncoating, the outer capsid is removed; the core containing the genome and associated histones is transported to the nucleus where replication takes place.

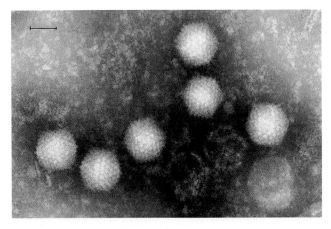

Fig. 8.1 Electron micrograph of an adenovirus. (Courtesy of Dr David Hockley.) Scale bar = 50 nm.

Transcription of both strands of the viral DNA by cellular RNA polymerase II leads to sequential formation of early and late mRNAs, coding respectively for 'early' and 'late' proteins. RNA is transcribed in a precisely controlled order from nine promoters. Splicing is an essential mechanism, first discovered in adenovirus-infected cells to expand the genome coding. About 12 NS proteins are formed before the genome is replicated. The viral structural proteins are synthesized late, following DNA replication. Viral DNA replication is initiated from both ends of the DNA by a strand displacement mechanism.

New virus particles are assembled in the nucleus, often in such vast numbers that they form crystalline aggregates. Not unexpectedly, with this amount of viral synthesis the synthetic machinery of the cell is progressively shut down. First, cellular DNA synthesis stops, followed in the latter part of the viral cycle by cellular RNA and protein synthesis. The cell then dies.

2.2 Clinical and pathological aspects

Endemic respiratory infections in children

Most children are infected with adenoviruses early in life, but probably fewer than half these infections result in disease, the frequency of symptomatic illness depending on the type of virus; adenovirus 2, for example, causes comparatively little illness. In young children the symptoms include a stuffy nose and cough, whereas in older children pharyngitis is common. In some colder areas of the world, for example China and Canada, adenoviruses type 3 and 7 can cause pneumonia in infants younger than 2 years.

A good proportion of these infections result not from aerosols, but from faecal–oral spread on cups and utensils. This mode of spread is not uncommon with other respiratory viruses.

Epidemic disease in military recruits

Adenoviruses are notorious for causing outbreaks of upper and lower respiratory tract infections in military recruits, probably because of crowding and stress. The illness usually lasts for about 10 days and pneumonitis is not uncommon.

Immunosuppressed patients

Severe infections, including pneumonias, may occur in AIDS patients and in persons receiving organ transplants.

Pharyngoconjunctival fever

This syndrome is characterized by pharyngitis and conjunctivitis, mainly in children and young adults. Many outbreaks have been associated with swimming pools, and the possibility of an adenovirus infection should be considered in any patient with conjunctivitis developing about a week after using a communal pool.

Epidemic keratoconjunctivitis ('shipyard eye')

Why 'shipyard eye'? This form of keratoconjunctivitis, which may leave permanent corneal scars and impaired sight, first occurred in epidemic form during the Second World War in American shipyards, which were, of course, very busy. Foreign bodies (e.g. flakes of rust) often had to be extracted from the workers' eyes and the infection was spread both within and without the clinics that they attended. In one shipyard, a particular employee acquired a high reputation for removing foreign bodies more skilfully than the local doctors; unfortunately, he never sterilized his home-made instruments and thus spread adenovirus type 8 to many hundreds of his workmates. Any criticism of this amateur operator should be tempered by the knowledge that, on a number of occasions, adenovirus infections of the eye have been transmitted by medical staff using infected solutions or inadequately sterilized instruments, notably tonometers.

Gastrointestinal infections

Symptomatic adenovirus infections of the gut occur mainly in infants and are caused by types 40 and 41. These agents do not grow in cell cultures (see Chapter 11).

Other syndromes

Adenoviruses have been implicated in acute intussusception in infants, necrotizing enterocolitis, haemorrhagic cystitis, and meningoencephalitis. They may also cause life-threatening pneumonia and other infections in immunocompromised patients, including those with AIDS.

Pathogenesis

Infections in humans are rarely lethal and the pathogenesis of adenovirus infections is difficult to study. However, infected cotton rats develop a similar pulmonary syndrome, characterized by replication in the bronchiolar epithelium and infiltration with lymphocytes. In this model, disease appears to be due more to the immune response than to direct effects on the pulmonary tissues; one should, however, be cautious in extrapolating these results to the disease in humans.

Epidemiology

All 47 serotypes are endemic in the community and some may cause explosive outbreaks of disease, usually respiratory, but also involving the eye. Another feature of the epidemiology of adenoviruses is the degree of seasonal variation. As an example, most outbreaks of pharyngoconjunctival fever in school-age children occur in the summer, perhaps because they use swimming pools more often. Eye infections may also be acquired following infection of the respiratory or alimentary tracts and, as we have seen, by inadequately sterilized instruments or other fomites. Epidemics of respiratory disease in military recruits occur almost exclusively in the winter. In general, of the 47 adenovirus serotypes, infections with types 2, 3, 5, and 7 are most common throughout the world. Type 1 and 2 infections occur in early childhood, whereas types 3 and 5 predominate late in life. The virus is known to infect persons by aerosol and by direct contact, but is probably also spread by the faecal–oral route, especially where hygiene is poor.

The vigorous humoral and cell-mediated **immune responses** account for the generally mild diseases caused by adenoviruses,

except of course in immunocompromised patients, in whom they may be lethal.

Laboratory diagnosis

Few laboratories carry out serological investigations with adenoviruses; thus laboratory help depends on virus isolation or on rapid identification of virus-infected cells in clinical samples by immunofluorescence.

Viral isolation from faeces, pharyngeal swabs, conjunctival swabs, or urine is slow, taking at least a week and perhaps as long as a month with some serotypes.

Human diploid, HeLa, or Hep-2 cells can be used for viral isolation and observed for typical CPE. The pH of the medium usually falls rapidly as the virus-infected cells become swollen, rounded, and refractile, clustering together like bunches of grapes.

Once a virus has been isolated it may be subgrouped by agglutination patterns with rat or rhesus monkey erythrocytes or by haemagglutination inhibition (HI) tests with specific antisera.

Prophylaxis

Because of the disruptive effects of large outbreaks of respiratory disease in army camps, the US military as long ago as the 1960s encouraged the development of a vaccine. Live preparations of adenovirus types 4 and 7 were enclosed in a gelatine capsule and swallowed, bypassing the stomach and being released in the intestine. Here the virus replicates and induces immunity, but causes no overt disease. However, the problems for widespread use of such a vaccine in the community are formidable, not least of which being the variety of serotypes causing respiratory disease. Another worrying thought is that certain adenoviruses have oncogenic effects in animals, although there is no evidence of these in humans.

Molecular biologists have now taken a special interest in these viruses as potential viral vectors and are beginning to use them to carry other genes into the body, thus inducing immunity not only to adenoviruses but also to influenza and HIV.

3 Coronaviruses

Coronaviruses (Latin, *corona*: a crown) infect humans, birds, and other animals. The first two human strains infect the respiratory tract and are normally confined to the ciliary epithelium of the trachea, nasal mucosa, and alveolar cells of the lungs. Some of the first isolates were obtained in the UK from volunteers at the Medical Research Council (MRC) Common Cold Research Unit, Salisbury. More recently a third respiratory coronavirus was discovered and then a fourth (SARS CoV, see Section 4).

3.1 Properties of the viruses

Classification

The family *Coronaviridae* belongs to an Order of viruses named *Nidovirales* and contains two genera, *Coronavirus* and *Torovirus*.

Three serotypes of human coronavirus are known and around 15 more infect birds and animals.

Recently an entirely new virus was identified as the cause of SARS. It first emerged in Southeast Asia (see Section 4) and caused outbreaks of acute respiratory infection in 32 countries. It was isolated from civet cats and is placed in a grouping of its own. The other family in this Order, the *Arteroviridae*, do not cause disease in humans.

Morphology

Coronaviruses are pleomorphic, ranging from 60 to 220 nm in diameter, and have club-shaped glycoprotein surface spikes about 20 nm in length. These very large (200 kDa), heavily glycosylated spikes give the virions the appearance of a crown, hence their name (Latin *corona*, a crown) (Fig. 8.2).

In thin sections the envelope appears as inner and outer shells separated by a translucent space. Coronaviruses contain three major envelope proteins. The first, the matrix protein, is a transmembrane glycoprotein. The second is the protein S that constitutes the surface peplomer and is responsible for eliciting neutralizing antibodies, receptor binding, membrane fusion, and HA activity. The third protein, HE, has HA and esterase activities and so may have a role in virus exit, much like the NA of influenza virus. The internal RNP component has the appearance of a helix condensed into coiled structures of varying diameter.

Genome

The genome is the largest of all the RNA viruses of humans (Fig. 8.3). It is positive-sense ssRNA, 30 kb in size, is 5′ capped, 3′ polyadenylated, and is infectious.

Replication

Virions initially attach over the whole cell surface. Uptake into cells is rapid and temperature-dependent, probably involving endocytosis followed by a spike-mediated fusion in the cytoplasmic vacuole.

The viral RNA is translated directly into two polypeptides that are cleaved to form an RNA polymerase. The RNA polymerase transcribes a full-length negative RNA strand. This is transcribed

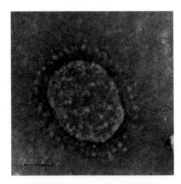

Fig. 8.2 Electron micrograph of a coronavirus. The surface spikes protrude through the lipid bilayer to give the appearance of a corona, or crown. (Courtesy of Dr Ian Chrystie.) Scale bar = 50 nm.

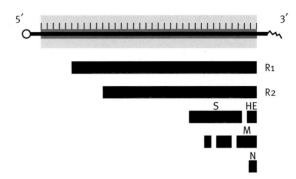

Fig. 8.3 Coronavirus genome and encoded proteins. Labelled proteins are S (surface glycoprotein), M (membrane protein), N (nucleoprotein), and R1, R2 the two replicase proteins. ○, cap (5′ end); ∿, poly (A) tail (3′ end).

both to a full-length virion plus (genome) strand and also to a unique 3′ coterminal nested set of subgenomic mRNAs. A number of NS proteins and virus-coded proteases are also synthesized.

This essential feature of coronavirus genomic replication allows the mediation of genetic information through multiple subgenomic mRNAs, each of which directs the translation of only one protein.

RNA replication and particle assembly take place in the cytoplasm of the infected cell, where progeny virions are formed by a budding process from membranes of the rough endoplasmic reticulum and not from the plasma membrane. The virions acquire their lipid envelopes from the cells, excluding host-cell proteins in the process, and are subsequently transported through and accumulate in the Golgi complex and smooth-walled vesicles. Virions are released by fusion of smooth-walled virion-containing vesicles with the plasma membrane.

3.2 Clinical and pathological aspects of coronaviruses other than SARS

It is thought that 2–10 per cent of common colds are caused by coronaviruses, typified by OC43 and 239E. Infection can precipitate wheezing in asthmatics and exacerbate chronic bronchitis in adults. In a typical case there is an incubation period of 3 days, followed by an unpleasant nasal discharge and malaise, lasting about a week. Patients excrete virus during this period. There is a little or no fever, and coughs and sore throat are not common.

Less is known about the toroviruses. They are often visualized in diarrhoea samples and may cause gastroenteritis.

Pathogenesis

Replication is confined to the cells of the epithelium in the upper respiratory tract. Inflammation, oedema, and exudation occur in the tract for several days following destruction of cells by the virus.

Epidemiology

Coronavirus colds occur in the colder months of winter and early spring with sizeable outbreaks every 2–4 years. Antibody surveys show that most people have been infected at some time in their lives and it is thought that reinfections are quite common, either because of the **poor immune response**, or as a result of antigenic mutations, or both.

Laboratory diagnosis

Most routine clinical virology laboratories are not equipped to isolate coronaviruses, which replicate poorly in cell cultures and require organ cultures of human embryo trachea or nasal epithelium. In any event, the trivial nature of the infection does not call for routine diagnostic tests. For epidemiological purposes, paired acute and convalescent sera can be tested by haemagglutination inhibition for a rising titre of specific antibody.

4 Severe acute respiratory syndrome (SARS CoV)

The first cases of a new syndrome emerged in November 2002 in the Guangdong Province of China. By April 2003 the virus had spread worldwide, affecting 3500 individuals and resulting in 182 deaths (Fig. 8.4). Unexpectedly, the virus was identified as a coronavirus (CoV), which emerged suddenly from a mammalian reservoir in China to infect humans, probably the civet cat, which is used for exotic foods, or a rat upon which the civet preys (Fig. 8.5).

Genome

Remarkably, the genome structure was established in a matter of weeks and was typical of other members of the family with 11 ORFs coding for 23 proteins. Most of the NS proteins are

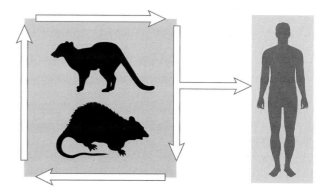

Fig. 8.5 Emergence of SARS from a civet cat or rat.

encoded in the first half (5′) end of the genome (such as the proteases nsp1, nsp2, and the RNA polymerase nsp9), whereas the structural protein spike (S), membrane (M) envelope, and nucleocapsid proteins are positioned towards the 3′ end.

Unlike most other coronaviruses, the SARS virus possessed no HE protein. This genetic analysis immediately indicated that the virus was not a recombinant, with portions of human and perhaps of avian or animal coronaviruses, but a completely novel virus.

Nucleotide sequence comparison of isolates in Hong Kong, Taiwan, Vietnam, and Canada showed them to have a local genetic fingerprint but they were all related to the original virus, indicating, fortunately, some genetic stability.

Clinical and pathological agents

The clinical symptoms included high temperature (over 38°C), dry cough, myalgia, and breathlessness. The incubation period

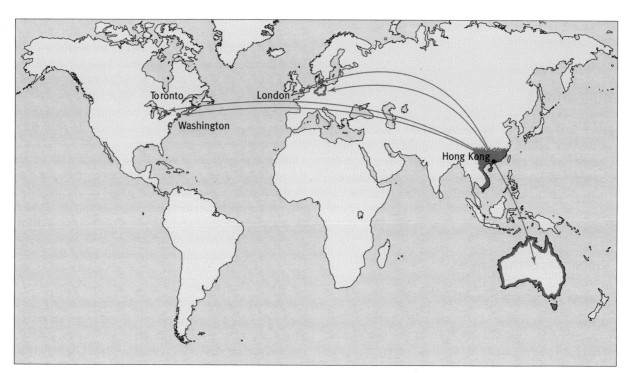

Fig. 8.4 Global spread of SARS.

could be as long as 10 days and virus excretion, at least in the throat, began with early symptoms and peaks 7–8 days later, followed by a slow decline. Person-to-person transmission was relatively inefficient and necessitated close contact, infection from cough droplets or via hand contamination or drinking cups. High levels of personal hygiene, hand washing, cleanliness of furniture and cooking utensils together with rapid quarantine were able to break the chain of transmission. The Ro value for the virus (Chapter 7) was quite low, about 2, and this, together with the long incubation period meant that the public health measures introduced to break the chains of transmission were successful.

New vaccines are being produced against SARS CoV and antiviral inhibitors developed but the most effective prevention is good virological surveillance to detect human cases quickly, and to quarantine them to prevent person-to-person spread. The most vulnerable sector in the community is the healthcare groupings, nurses and doctors. The virus is likely to persist either in humans or mammals in South-east Asia and to flare up: occasionally, during these episodes, it is liable to be carried to the rest of the world by persons incubating the disease.

Replication

Genome expression commences with the translation of two large polyproteins, ppla and pplab, encoded by the viral replicase gene. These two polyproteins are processed by two viral proteases to the smaller functional components of the viral replicase complex. This new enzyme then facilitates viral genome replication and transcription of a nested set of subgenomic mRNAs, which code for the structural proteins S, E, M, and N, and also a number of so-called accessory proteins. The viral replicase is probably the most complex of enzymes in the RNA virus families.

5 Rhinoviruses

A landmark in the study of the virology of the common cold came in the 1960s when, after years of patient investigation, David Tyrrell and his colleagues at the MRC Common Cold Research Unit in Salisbury isolated viruses in a simple cell-culture system. A chance observation that an alkaline pH in the culture medium favoured the growth of the viruses was the key to their success.

5.1 Properties of the viruses

Classification and general properties

Rhinoviruses (Greek, *rhinos*: nose) constitute a genus of the family *Picornaviridae* (see Chapter 16) and are small, non-enveloped RNA viruses some 18–30 nm in diameter; they possess icosahedral symmetry and are morphologically similar to other picornaviruses (Fig. 16.2). By conventional neutralization tests they fall into more than 150 serotypes. However, the more recently applied techniques of RNA–RNA hybridization (Chapter 36) define different patterns of genetic relationships between the viruses and suggest that rather fewer than 100 different rhinoviruses exist. These genetic differences may have practical implications since antiviral agents inhibit only viruses in particular groups.

In many properties, rhinoviruses resemble other members of the *Picornaviridae*. They differ, however, in their inability to withstand acid conditions, and in their low optimum temperature for growth (33°C). The latter characteristic is undoubtedly an evolutionary adaption to the comparatively cool environment of the nasal mucosa.

Genome

The genome is linear, positive-sense ssRNA, some 7–8 kb in size with a protein primer at the 5' end and a poly(A) tail at the 3' end. The genome is infectious.

Replication

The virus attaches to the intercellular adhesion molecule, ICAM-1, and penetrates the plasma membrane of the cell. The virion RNA acts directly as mRNA and is translated into a single, large polyprotein. This is cleaved into intermediates (P1–P2), which are themselves cleaved to form structural and NS proteins.

RNA is replicated via a double-stranded replicative intermediate. The viruses shut down translation of cellular mRNAs and new virions are released by destruction of the host cell.

5.2 Clinical and epidemiological aspects

Replication is restricted to cells of the upper respiratory tract. The infection is spread by aerosol, by hand contact, and from the surface of cups and plates. The incubation period is 2–3 days. Inflammation and copious exudation from the upper respiratory tract last for a few days. The symptoms are nasal congestion, sneezing, sore throat, and often headache and cough. There is rarely a fever. There are few serious sequelae except in chronic bronchitics, in whom attacks may be precipitated by infection with a common cold virus.

Rhinovirus colds occur throughout the year in all countries of the world. It is thought that several virus serotypes co-circulate for a year or so, to be displaced by a new group; one individual may experience two or three infections per annum. Children are more susceptible than adults, and one of the hazards of living in a large family is the risk of contracting colds from the younger members. The frequent occurrence of more than one cold per season in the same person is due to the large number of serotypes, which confer little or no cross-protection.

Although corona- and rhinovirus infections are trivial in themselves, the economic losses due to absences from work are enormous, a fact well recognized by the general public. Most medical students and doctors will have been asked the irritating question 'Have you found a cure for the common cold yet?', which brings us to the following question.

Antiviral chemotherapy or vaccines to prevent the common cold?

The potential antiviral effects of IFN were first established in volunteers infected with common cold viruses at the Salisbury experimental unit. This single experiment in 1973 used up almost all the world's supply of the new drug. Nowadays, with the arrival of recombinant DNA technology, a range of IFN molecules is available for clinical use. However, even cloned and highly purified IFN is not without side-effects, a particularly unfortunate one being the production of a stuffy nose after intranasal use. Therefore, the early promise of IFN as an effective antiviral compound has not yet been realized. A number of synthetic antiviral molecules, such as enviroxime and dichloroflavan (see Chapter 38), have good antiviral activity against certain rhinovirus serotypes in the laboratory, but only marginal effects have been noted in volunteer experiments.

Little progress has been made with vaccines because of the antigenic diversity of the rhinoviruses. Data from X-ray crystallography and nucleotide sequencing may help to delineate common amino-acid sequences among the capsid proteins of rhinoviruses, which could be used as peptide vaccines. However, the effective control of the common cold lies very much in the future.

6 Reminders

- **Adenoviruses** have a **linear dsDNA genome** some 36–38 kbp in size. The viruses have an icosahedral structure embellished by a projecting fibre at each apex.

- Shipyard eye is an **epidemic keratoconjunctivitis** caused mainly by serotype 8; many of the remaining 41 serotypes cause respiratory symptoms. Some adenoviruses cause outbreaks of **respiratory infection** in the winter, and others, **gastrointestinal illness**.

- **Coronaviruses** are **positive-strand RNA** viruses with a 30 kb genome. Three serotypes are known. They cause **upper respiratory tract** infections. These viruses are difficult to grow in the laboratory but spread readily and infect humans, causing up to 10 per cent of common colds. A new coronavirus (SARS) has emerged from an animal reservoir in Southeast Asia and can cause severe pneumonia. Fortunately it is not highly transmissible.

- **Rhinoviruses** or **common cold viruses** are picornaviruses with a positive-strand RNA genome 7–8 kb in size; there are 100 serotypes, explaining why repeated infections are not uncommon. The viruses cause **upper respiratory tract infection** at all times of the year throughout the world; they do not infect the lower respiratory tract.

- No universally effective vaccine or antiviral exists to counter the effects of these three groups of viruses, although experiments are in progress with live attenuated adenovirus vaccines and with specific drugs against common cold viruses.

Chapter 9

Childhood infections caused by paramyxoviruses

1 Introduction

The *Paramyxoviridae* cause a variety of diseases, predominantly involving the respiratory tract, in humans, birds, and other animals (Table 9.1). In humans, they include measles, respiratory infections caused by RSV and parainfluenza viruses, and the more innocuous salivary gland infection of mumps. Although few in number, they are responsible for half the cases of croup, bronchiolitis, and pneumonia in infants. These viruses, particularly RSV, cause fusion of infected cells with formation of multinucleated giant cells (syncytia).

The paramyxoviruses are worldwide in their distribution and cause measles and mumps in children and respiratory disease in all age groups, but predominantly in children. They are also responsible for a number of economically important infections in domestic and farm animals.

The viruses are transmitted by airborne droplets or hand contact, and spread is rapid among children in institutions.

2 Properties of the *Paramyxoviridae*

2.1 Classification

Members of the family *Paramyxoviridae* are enveloped, negative-stranded **ssRNA** viruses, 150–200 nm in diameter, with a nucleocapsid of helical symmetry. Two subfamilies are recognized: the *Paramyxovirinae*, containing the genera *Paramyxovirus*, *Rubulavirus*, and *Morbillivirus*; and the *Pneumovirinae*, with two genera, *Pneumovirus* and *Metapneumovirus* (Table 9.1). The morbilliviruses differ from those in the other genera in not possessing a NA.

2.2 Morphology and structural proteins

Because of the fragility of the lipoprotein envelope, the viruses often appear distorted or disrupted in the EM, with the nucleoprotein spewing out from inside the virion (Fig. 9.1). The structural polypeptides of the capsid include the HN (HA–NA) and F (fusion) glycoproteins, which form the surface spikes, and the internally situated M (matrix) protein. Three other proteins,

Table 9.1 The paramyxoviridae and their diseases

Subfamily and genus	Representative viruses	Diseases of humans	Economically important diseases of domestic animals
Subfamily *Paramyxovirinae*			
Paramyxovirus	Human parainfluenza viruses types 1, 3	URTI, notably croup (types 1, 2); pneumonia, bronchiolitis (type 3)	URTI in various species
Metapneumovirus	Type 1	Mainly targets children	URTI
Rubulavirus	Human parainfluenza viruses types 2, 4	URTI, including croup (type 2)	URTI in various species, including Newcastle disease in poultry
	Mumps	Mumps	
Morbillivirus	Measles virus	Measles	Canine distemper
			Rinderpest in cattle
Subfamily *Pneumovirinae*			
Pneumovirus	Human respiratory syncytial virus	URTI, notably bronchiolitis	Respiratory infections of cattle and poultry

URTI, upper respiratory tract infection.

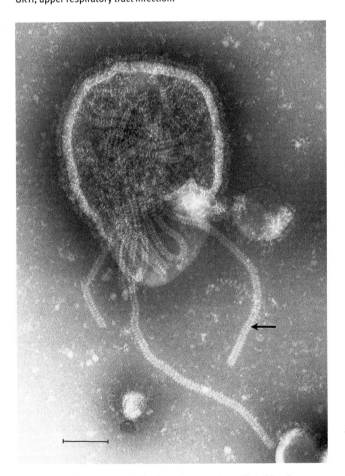

Fig. 9.1 Electron micrograph of a paramyxovirus. The virion has ruptured, spilling out coils of ribonucleoprotein (arrowed). (Courtesy of Dr David Hockley.) Scale bar = 100 nm.

together with the RNA, form the nucleoprotein core of the virion and the RNA transcriptase possessed by all negative-stranded viruses. There are two NS proteins.

The **F** or **fusion protein**, formed by proteolytic cleavage of a larger precursor polypeptide, is important, as it mediates the fusion of infected cells that then form the **syncytia** so characteristic of infections with this group of viruses.

2.3 Genome

The genome of the *Paramyxoviridae* is an **ssRNA** molecule of negative polarity of some 15 000 nucleotides, containing the 10 genes coding for the 11 known virus-specific proteins (Fig. 9.2).

There are many similarities in the genome structure of members of the family, although the large P gene has evolved differently. For example, the gene codes for four proteins by a curious dual mechanism of internal initiation of translation and insertion of a non-templated guanosine residue into mRNA to shift the reading frame. This guanosine is inserted into the mRNA during transcription by a so-called 'stuttering' of the polymerase.

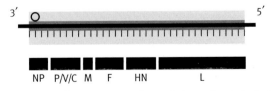

Fig.9.2 Paramyxovirus genome and encoded proteins. Labelled proteins are NP (nucleoprotein), M (matrix), F (fusion), HN (HA–NA), P (phospho protein) and V/C (non-structural proteins), and L (large polymerase).

Thus the large P protein is translated from an mRNA copy of the complete gene. The smaller C protein is read, following initiation from an internal initiation codon, in a different reading frame. The V (NS1) protein has an extra guanosine inserted into the mRNA during transcription, making this frame distinct from that utilized to translate the C protein.

2.4 Replication

The strategy of replication is that of a typical negative-stranded RNA virus (Chapter 3). These viruses replicate entirely within the cytoplasm of the cell. Viruses dock to the cell using a glycoprotein or glycolipid cell receptor and its own H or HN spike protein. The virion enters a cell by mediating fusion of its lipid envelope with the external plasma membrane of the cell and this vital event of catalysed 'fusion from without' is mediated by the F protein. The genome is released immediately into the cytoplasm. The intact negative-sense viral genome is transcribed by the viral RNA transcriptase to give 6–10 subgenomic, generally monocistronic (i.e. only one protein is encoded by a single mRNA species), mRNAs. The transcriptase binds at the 3' end and moves along the genome beginning with the first gene NP. After the gene has been transcribed the transcriptase enters the terminator region, stops transcribing, and there are now two alternatives. First, the transcriptase enzyme may fall off the gene and therefore must bind again at the 3' end and start transcription again. Secondly the transcriptase moves along the gene until it reaches the next transcription signal where it starts to transcribe the second gene, namely P/V/C. Therefore genes at the 3' end are transcribed to higher levels than those at the 5' end. Shortly afterwards gene transcription switches into gene replication, when full-length positive RNA strands are synthesized, which act as templates for RNA replication. Three viral proteins, namely H, NSI, and M, inhibit viral transcription and help the switch from transcription to replication. The newly synthesized negative RNA strands interact with N protein and the virion transcriptase, and these nucleocapsid structures then combine with viral M protein. The viral spikes already inserted into the plasma membrane of the cell interact with the M protein. The viruses are released from the infected cell by budding from the plasma membrane. Because of the tendency of infected cells to fuse, they may, under certain conditions, release hardly any new viruses into the extracellular environment; instead, the viruses may spread from cell to cell, behaving as typical 'creepers' (Chapter 4).

3 Clinical and pathological aspects of paramyxovirus infections

3.1 Measles

'Measles' derives from a Middle English word, *maseles,* and so has been with us for several centuries. Its Latin name, *morbilli,* is a diminutive of morbus, a disease, and thus signifies a minor illness. In temperate countries measles is a comparatively mild infection and serious complications are rare; however, in some tropical areas it is still a killer of children on a large scale.

Clinical features

The period from infection to appearance of the rash is fairly constant at about 2 weeks, but may be less by a few days. Before the rash there is a **prodromal stage lasting 2 or 3 days**, with running eyes and nose, cough, and moderate fever. At this time, careful examination of the buccal mucous membrane adjacent to the molar teeth may reveal **Koplik spots**, which resemble grains of salt just beneath the mucosa. They may be many or few in number, but when present, are pathognomic of measles.

The **rash** first appears on the face and spreads to the trunk and limbs within the next 2 days. It is a dull-red, blotchy, **maculopapular** eruption, usually characteristic enough to have its own designation, 'morbilliform' (see Fig. 4.1(a)). If severe, it may have a purpuric appearance.

Although the rash is one of the most obvious physical signs, it is but one manifestation of a generalized infection. The temperature rises sharply to about 40°C, and in every case there is evidence of **bronchitis** and **pneumonitis**, with cough and 'crackles' in the chest. Occasionally, diarrhoea in the early stages indicates inflammatory lesions in the gut.

Within 2–3 days of onset, the rash starts to fade, the temperature subsides, and the child feels better; recovery is usually uneventful.

Complications

Along with the fever and rash there are widespread lesions of various body systems (Table 9.2). Although they are listed as complications, it is arguable whether most of them should be referred to as such, as they are all part of the generalized infection and are thus present in most cases; whether they surface in the form of signs and symptoms depends on their severity. The exceptions are those in which the immune response of the host is abnormal. They include **postinfection encephalitis** (about 1 per 1000 cases), and giant-cell pneumonia, a life-threatening infection seen occasionally in immunodeficient children (Fig. 32.2). **Subacute sclerosing panencephalitis** is particularly insidious, becoming clinically apparent only years after the initial measles infection, perhaps in 1 per million cases (Chapter 30).

Table 9.2 Complications of measles

Site	Complication
Respiratory system	Croup (in prodromal stage); bronchitis; giant-cell pneumonia (in immunocompromised patients)
Eye	Conjunctivitis; corneal ulceration (rare)
Ear	Otitis media; possible secondary bacterial infection
Gut	Enteritis with diarrhoea
Central nervous system	Febrile convulsions (acute phase); postexposure encephalitis (rare) (Chapter 30); subacute sclerosing panencephalitis (very rare) (Chapter 30)

Pathogenesis and pathology

Infection is acquired via droplets that enter the respiratory tract or eye. Measles is one of the most highly infectious viruses known. The genome of the virus is shown in Fig. 9.3. The pathogenesis is that of an acute generalized infection (Chapter 4), the secondary viraemic phase corresponding to the height of the fever. After a minor burst of replication in the cells lining in the respiratory tract, the virus multiplies in local lymph nodes and infects mononuclear cells, which release virus into the blood whence the virus reaches most epithelial surfaces of the body. Cells of the respiratory tract and conjunctiva are particularly susceptible to destruction and, coincident with this phase, 10 days postinfection there is an abrupt onset of symptoms of a chest infection.

The rash is not due to a direct CPE of virus on cells but to a reaction by cytotoxic T cells against viral antigen appearing in the skin cells. In addition, antigen–antibody complexes form on the capillary endothelium with consequent cell damage, vasodilatation, and leakage of plasma. The rash is thus a clear sign that a satisfactory immune response is in progress, and that recovery is on the way; conversely, its failure to appear (e.g. in immuno-deficient patients) is a bad prognostic sign. In these patients giant-cell pneumonia may occur, often many weeks after the acute infection.

During the prodromal and acute phases, **virus is shed in body fluids**, including **respiratory secretions**; it replicates in leucocytes, causing **leucopenia**. During the acute phase, virus-infected giant cells containing up to 100 nuclei have been found in the pharynx and tonsils, skin, respiratory epithelium, lymph nodes, and Peyer's patches. The virus is widespread in the skin but disappears quickly with the onset of the rash and the appearance of circulating antibody.

Immune response

IgM, IgA, and IgG antibodies appear at the same time as the rash, the first two disappearing within a month or so, the latter persisting for life. During the acute phase, replication of virus within monocytes and other white cells depresses cell-mediated responses to other antigens, although cytotoxic T lymphocytes specifically directed against measles M protein in infected cells are important in the recovery process and also provide protection against subsequent infection.

Epidemiology

Measles virus is highly infectious and has a worldwide distribution. It becomes endemic only in countries with popula-

tions large enough to provide a continuing supply of susceptible children; in small, isolated communities it dies out until a fresh importation causes a major epidemic (see Chapter 7). In the past, and before widespread use of measles–mumps–rubella (MMR) vaccine in countries with high standards of living, endemic infection was punctuated every 2–3 years by epidemic infections that attack predominantly 3–5 year olds, in whom the illness is relatively mild. Because of vigorous vaccination campaigns epidemics are now unknown in most European countries and the USA. In Third World countries, on the other hand, measles still has a high incidence in infants less than 2 years old and is much more severe, with unusual clinical features such as blindness, and a high case fatality rate of 3–6 per cent (see 'Measles in developing countries', below).

Laboratory diagnosis

In day-to-day practice, laboratory confirmation of the clinical diagnosis is not needed because the rash is so typical. In atypical cases, usually seen in hospitals, serological diagnosis can be made by detecting specific IgM or a fourfold or greater rise in antibody titre, usually by enzyme-linked immunosorbent assay (ELISA).

Prophylaxis

Passive protection with **normal immunoglobulin**, in a dose sufficient to modify but not completely prevent measles, is valuable for protecting debilitated or immunodeficient children who have been exposed to infection.

Modern **attenuated vaccines** are very effective and, ideally, are given in combination with mumps and rubella vaccines (MMR) at 13–15 months of age (see Chapter 37), by which time there is no risk of neutralization by maternal antibodies. The preparation of vaccine is simplified by the fact that there is only one virus serotype and no evidence of marked antigen variation. In the USA, and to some extent in Europe, an attempt is being made to eradicate measles by achieving vaccination rates approaching 100 per cent. As part of the campaign, in the USA children are not admitted to state schools without a certificate of vaccination. These efforts are now bearing fruit: measles deaths have declined from about 400 per annum in 1960 to fewer than 10 per annum at present. Similarly, cases of measles encephalitis, reported annually, have fallen from about 300 to single figures. The economic saving in medical care and hospital beds is enormous. But isolated outbreaks still occur in ethnic minority groups and, in some cases, university students. To maintain high levels of immunity, children are now given a booster vaccine at age 3–5 years (11–12 years in the USA). This has been a setback in the UK where flawed data were published attempting to show that the vaccine virus was associated with autism. In fact there is no sound evidence of such an association but meanwhile parental confidence has been seriously undermined.

Measles in developing countries

Over 1 million malnourished children die each year of measles in the developing world. Two host factors seem to be of primary

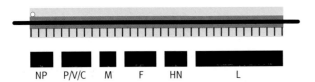

Fig. 9.3 Measles virus genome. Labelled proteins are NP (nucleoprotein), M (matrix), F (fusion), HN (HA–NA), P (phospho protein) and V/C (non-structural proteins), and L (large polymerase).

importance in explaining why measles is much more severe in developing countries than in the USA and Europe:

1. on average, children acquire the infection at a younger age;

2. these children are poorly nourished; during the Nigerian civil war, when there was severe famine, at least 15 per cent of children infected with measles died.

In these children, measles differs considerably from the relatively benign illness described above, and more nearly resembles the disease as it existed in Europe 100 years ago. The **rash is more severe** and exfoliates extensively, exposing large areas of skin to bacterial invasion. **Stomatitis** interferes with eating and drinking. **Vitamin A deficiency** and measles infection combine to cause **corneal ulceration** and blindness. The virus is cleared less rapidly than in well-nourished people; this results in

1. more damage to leucocytes with depression of CMI and increased susceptibility to bacterial infections; and

2. prolongation of the period of virus shedding by a week or more.

Bronchopneumonia and **persistent diarrhoea** with protein-losing enteropathy often result in death, mortality rates being of the order of 10 per cent.

Measles vaccine in developing countries

Inoculation of infants at 9 months of age is a top priority of the WHO. The heat lability of measles vaccine complicates its distribution in tropical climates and maintaining the 'cold chain' is essential. The freeze-dried vaccine has to be held at 2–8°C until minutes before injection and, unless this temperature range is maintained, the vaccine rapidly loses its potency. The other problem in providing effective immunization for children in developing countries is reaching them during the brief interval between the loss of maternal antibodies and the acquisition of natural disease (the so-called 'window of opportunity'). It was thought that this could be solved by the use of more concentrated ('high-dose') vaccine, which is not swamped by maternal antibody and is effective in babies less than 9 months old. However, field trials showed that suppression of T-cell immunity to other diseases could occur and so the new strategy is to use the standard Schwartz strain of virus at 9 months.

3.2 Respiratory syncytial virus infections

This virus—RSV for short—is highly contagious and causes sharp outbreaks of respiratory disease throughout the world, particularly in infants. It is spread by aerosol and hand contact. It may cause death in the young and also the elderly and immunocompromised. In the northern hemisphere the outbreak usually occurs in December.

Clinical aspects

The illness often starts like a common cold but within 24 hours the baby may be acutely ill with cyanosis and respiratory dis-tress. Typically, there is **bronchiolitis**, with or without involvement of the lung parenchyma causing **pneumonitis**. There is some evidence that RSV infection in infancy may cause long-term respiratory problems. Severe illness carries a significant risk of death at both extremes of age and, in the elderly, the infection may be confused with influenza, which is also prevalent at the same time of year.

Pathogenesis and pathology

The incubation period is about 5 days. There is a necrotizing bronchiolitis in which partial blocking of the bronchioles leads to the collapse of areas of lung. Peribronchial infiltration may spread to give widespread interstitial pneumonitis. Inapparent infections also occur.

Immune response

As infants as young as 6 weeks are often infected, maternal antibody does not seem to provide protection for very long after birth. RSV induces both antibody- and cell-mediated responses; impairment of the latter in immunocompromised patients may lead to **persistent infection**. The **IFN response** is noticeably worse than in other paramyxovirus infections. It has been suggested that harmful immune responses (e.g. formation of antigen–antibody complexes) plays a part in pathogenesis, but this has not been proved. In later life, **reinfections** are comparatively frequent, suggesting that first infections do not always induce long-term immunity. Antigenic variation between strains of RSV may also contribute to reinfections.

Epidemiology

The causative viruses fall into two serological groups, A and B, which can be distinguished by specific antisera.

RSV infections are transmitted by infected **respiratory secretions**, in this case, not mainly by small droplets but by **contamination of hands** or **fomites** such as bedding. In temperate climates, they occur annually in epidemic form during the winter months, but in the tropics, the incidence may be highest during the summer months or rainy season. Babies aged from 6 weeks to 6 months are predominantly affected; indeed, RSV is the most important respiratory pathogen in young infants.

During epidemic periods, spread within hospitals, crèches, and day nurseries (**nosocomial infections**) often takes place, facilitated by close personal contacts and the liability of those infected to shed virus for up to 3 weeks after the acute phase. Adults may also acquire RSV, particularly the elderly, in whom it may exacerbate existing bronchitis and cause an increase in deaths, easily misdiagnosed as influenza.

Reinfections are common, although they may often be subclinical. These subclinical infections maintain a huge reservoir of infective virus. In a unique study at the Antarctic base at the South Pole, parainfluenza viruses were isolated continuously, although the personnel were completely cut off from the outside world for several months during the winter.

Laboratory diagnosis

The virus can be isolated in continuous lines of human cells (e.g. HeLa), in which CPEs with formation of syncytia appear after 2–10 days. The method of choice is demonstration by **indirect immunofluorescence** of viral antigen in cells from a nasopharyngeal washing, which gives an immediate result or detection of viral antigen in nasal fluid using enzyme immunoassay kits. Detection of viral RNA by RT PCR is also used. The technique of sampling has to be precise and the sample must reach the laboratory quickly.

Prevention

Attempts to develop attenuated vaccines have so far met with little success; the use of recombinant DNA technology for making RSV vaccine is now being studied.

In the absence of a vaccine, limitation of spread within paediatric units, nurseries, and the like depends on good hygienic practice, such as hand washing, covering of the mouth when coughing or sneezing, and careful disposal of paper handkerchiefs.

Treatment

Small-scale trials of the nucleoside analogue ribavirin (Chapter 38), given by continuous aerosol inhalation to babies with serious RSV infections, met with some success, but not enough to make it a routine treatment. At present, ribavirin should perhaps be reserved for infants with pre-existing cardiopulmonary disease, who succumb readily to chest infections.

High titre human immunoglobulin or humanized monoclonal antibodies are efficacious in high-risk infants but the treatment is expensive and is used only in emergencies.

3.3 Mumps

The name probably originates from an old word meaning 'to mope', an apt description for the miserable child afflicted by this common illness. Mumps was one of the first infections to be recognized and was described by Hippocrates as early as the fifth century BC. Robert Hamilton in *An Account of a Distemper by the Common People of England Vulgarly Called the Mumps*, noted in 1790 that 'The catastrophe was dreadful; for the swelled testicles subsided suddenly the next day, the patient was seized with a most frantic delirium, the nervous system was shattered with strong convulsions, and he died raving mad the third day after'. Fear of orchitis and consequent sterility, in reality greatly exaggerated, explains the continued interest in immunization against what is otherwise a comparatively benign disease.

Clinical aspects

The onset is marked by malaise and fever followed within 24 hours by a painful enlargement of one or both parotid glands; the other salivary glands are less often affected. In most cases, the swelling subsides within a few days and recovery is uneventful. Inapparent infections are common.

Complications

Orchitis develops in about 20 per cent of males who contract mumps after the age of puberty; it may develop in the absence of preceding parotitis. Typically, there is pain and swelling of one or both testicles 4–5 days after the onset of parotitis. The pain is often severe enough to demand strong analgesics. There is often an accompanying general reaction with high temperature and headache. Symptoms tend to subside after 3–6 days. Although some degree of testicular atrophy follows in about 30 per cent of cases, sterility following mumps orchitis is rare.

Inflammation of the **ovary** (oophoritis) and **pancreas** has been reported, but these complications do not seem to have serious long-term effects.

Central nervous system

The incidence of 'aseptic' **meningitis** is higher after mumps than after any other acute viral infection of childhood. Rates of 0.3–8.0 per cent have been reported in the USA. This complication almost always resolves without sequelae. Postinfection **encephalitis** is, however, more serious and carries an appreciable mortality. These syndromes are described in Chapter 30.

Some degree of **deafness** is a residual complication in a small percentage of cases.

Pathogenesis

The infection is spread in saliva and secretions from the respiratory tract, and is acquired by the **respiratory route**, either by aerosol or hand contact. The incubation period is 14-21 days. Viraemia during the acute phase is followed by generalized spread to various organs, including the parotid gland. Virus is shed for several days before and after the first symptoms, not only from the respiratory tract but also in the urine.

Immune response

The appearance of specific IgM, IgA, and IgG antibodies follows the sequence usual for these acute viral infections. CMI is probably important in the recovery process.

Epidemiology

Mumps has a worldwide distribution and mainly affects those aged less than 15 years. In temperate climates, sporadic cases occur all year round although the incidence is highest in winter, but there is no seasonal variation in tropical countries. Mumps is highly infectious; outbreaks in institutions are common and there have been a number of epidemics in military recruits in barracks.

Laboratory diagnosis

Virus can be isolated in various cell lines and in monkey kidney cells and identified by haemadsorption or haemagglutination inhibition (Chapter 36). Serological tests are, however, more widely used; they include **ELISA** tests for **specific IgM** and **complement fixation tests**.

Prevention

Live mumps vaccines prepared either from the Jeryl Lynn or Urabe attenuated strains are available. They are both highly effective, but there is an appreciable incidence of postvaccination meningitis with the latter, which has now been abandoned in the UK. In the UK and USA mumps vaccine is combined with measles and rubella vaccines (MMR). Where uptake rates are high, there have been very substantial reductions in the number of cases of mumps and its complications; immunity can last for 20 years.

3.4 Parainfluenza viruses types 1–4

Parainfluenza viruses cause up to one-third of all respiratory tract infections and nearly one-half of respiratory infections in pre-school children and infants (Table 9.1). Types 1 and 2 are most often associated with laryngotracheo bronchitis (croup), boys being affected more often than girls; type 3 usually causes infection of the lower respiratory tract (e.g. bronchiolitis and pneumonia).

What little is known of the pathogenesis and immune response suggests similarities with those of RSV infections. The epidemiology is also broadly similar to that of other respiratory infections due to paramyxoviruses. The methods of laboratory diagnosis are similar to those for RSV infections, in particular, the use of RT PCR or indirect immunofluorescence for detecting antigen in nasopharyngeal washings.

Prevention

Inactivated vaccines for use in humans have so far proved unsuccessful. Nevertheless, the efficacy of an attenuated vaccine for the related and economically important virus infection of poultry, Newcastle disease, suggests that similar vaccines may eventually be prepared for use in humans.

3.5 Human metapneumovirus

This newly discovered virus has now been shown to cause acute respiratory illness in children in many countries of the world and also in the elderly and immunocompromised. It causes peak numbers of infections in the winter months. Two major lineages of the virus have been described along with antigenic differences in the G spike protein. There are at present no vaccines or antiviral drugs against these viruses.

4 Reminders

- The family *Paramyxoviridae* contains two subfamilies: *the Paramyxovirinae,* containing the genera *Paramyxovirus, Rubulavirus,* and *Morbillivirus*; and the *Pneumovirinae,* with one genus, *Pneumovirus.* The viruses are about 200 nm in diameter, of **helical** symmetry.

- The ssRNA genome of negative polarity is 15 kb in length with 6–10 genes. The genome is transcribed into 6–10 subgenomic monocistronic mRNAs encoding glycoprotein spikes (G, H, or HN), fusion protein (F), and transcription related proteins (N, P, and L).

- All the viruses code for a **fusion protein** (F), which causes adjacent infected cells to fuse and form multinucleate giant cells (**syncytia**).

- Morbilliviruses cause **measles** in humans and other generalized infections, including canine distemper, in animals. Measles is an acute febrile illness of childhood associated with a characteristic **maculopapular rash**, which results from cell-mediated cytotoxicity and an interaction of virus in capillary endothelium with newly formed antibody. Complications include **encephalitis, subacute sclerosing panencephalitis** (very rare), and, in patients with defective immunity, **giant-cell pneumonia. Severe forms** of measles with high mortality rates are seen in some developing countries and are associated with **malnutrition**.

- **Passive protection** with normal human immunoglobulin is used to protect immunodeficient children exposed to infection. **Active immunization** with attenuated measles vaccine, alone or in combination with mumps and rubella vaccines (MMR), is highly effective.

- **RSV** affects the **lower** respiratory tract in infants and probably the elderly; it may cause **necrotizing bronchiolitis** and **pneumonitis**. RSV is spread more by contamination of hands and fomites than by droplets and, in the absence of an effective vaccine, prevention in institutions depends on good hygiene. For rapid **diagnosis**, the best method is RT PCR or demonstration by **indirect immunofluorescence** of viral antigen in cells from nasopharyngeal washings.

- **Mumps** is a generalized infection of childhood, in which the salivary glands, especially the **parotids**, are attacked. It is a comparatively benign illness. In 20 per cent of infected adolescent and adult males **orchitis** develops, but rarely results in sterility. Other complications include 'aseptic' **meningitis, postexposure encephalitis,** and **deafness.**

- Laboratory diagnosis depends on isolation of the virus, or, preferably, serological tests. A positive enzyme immunoassay (ELISA) for IgM antibody indicates current or recent infection.

- Parainfluenza viruses types 1–4 are a major cause of respiratory tract infections, especially in infants and children. Types 1 and 2 are particularly liable to cause **croup**, and type 3, **bronchiolitis**. All four serotypes also cause upper respiratory infections. The pathogenesis, epidemiology, and methods of diagnosis are similar to those of RSV. A new human virus, a metapneumovirus, has been discovered that causes acute respiratory disease in children and also in the elderly and immunocompromised.

Chapter 10

Orthomyxoviruses and influenza

1 Introduction

Influenza has long been with us; indeed, the name itself refers to the ancient belief that it was caused by a malign and supernatural influence. In Florence during the time of the Renaissance, astrologers linked a curious juxtaposition of stars with an outbreak of infection in the city and attributed it to the 'influence' of the stars, hence influenza. Known in the sixteenth century as 'the newe Acquayntance', influenza still causes major outbreaks of acute respiratory infection. It has indeed been described as 'the last great uncontrolled plague of mankind' and in this chapter we shall show how the property of causing epidemics and even pandemics is related directly to the ability of the causal viruses to undergo antigenic variation ('drift') or massive genetic reassortment ('shift'), and thus evade their hosts' immune defences. The virus is a so-called emergent virus because originally, at the time of the Ice Age 10 000 years ago, it crossed the species barrier from birds to humans. It is still predominantly an avian virus spread silently around the world by migrating geese and chickens.

Meanwhile the human version has evolved. Massive problems can still occur when the avian and human viruses coinfect a human or pig and result in a brand new pandemic virus.

In 1918, after the Great War, influenza emerged and spread rapidly around the world, killing over 50 million people: *the so-called Forgotten Plague*.

But health authorities did not forget and by 1948 WHO had established a global network of laboratories to track new influenza variants. We are experiencing the benefit of this investment now because those same laboratories were able to identify chicken (H5N1) virus quickly and also, totally unexpectedly, an entirely new virus—SARS—in 2003; this discovery allowed preventive and quarantine measures to be introduced quickly.

2 Properties of the orthomyxoviruses

2.1 Classification

Although laymen (and some doctors who should know better) refer to many incapacitating respiratory infections as 'flu', true influenza is caused by the small family of the *Orthomyxoviridae*. *Myxo* derives from the Greek for mucus and refers to the ability of these viruses to attach to mucoproteins on the cell surface;

ortho means true or regular, as in orthodox, and distinguishes these viruses from the paramyxoviruses (Chapter 9).

There are four genera, distinguished serologically on the basis of their matrix (M) and nucleoprotein (N) antigens. They are:

- influenza virus A;
- influenza virus B;
- influenza virus C;
- 'thogoto-like viruses', which do not infect humans and are not considered here.

Influenza C differs significantly from A and B and is of much less importance in infections of humans; the descriptions that follow relate only to the A and B viruses.

Influenza A viruses have been designated on the basis of the antigenic relationships of the external spike HA and NA proteins. H1–H16 and N1–N9. Of these, only viruses with H1, H2, H3, and N1 or N2 are known to infect humans or to cause serious outbreaks. The avian viruses, H5, can infect humans but do not appear to spread from person to person. You may also see, for example, in descriptions of the latest influenza vaccine, the designations of the individual strains from which it was prepared: these follow the pattern A/Wisconsin/2003 (H3N2), where A is for influenza A, followed by the place where it was isolated, the laboratory number, the year of isolation, and the H and N subtypes. Type B strains are designated on the same system, but without H and N numbers as major changes in these antigens have so far not been observed.

2.2 Morphology

The virions are 100–200 nm in diameter and are more or less spherical. The lipid envelope is covered with about 500 projecting spikes, which can be seen clearly under the EM (Fig. 10.1). About 80 per cent of them are **HA** antigen and the remainder are another antigen, **NA**, and have a mushroom-like shape. The HA

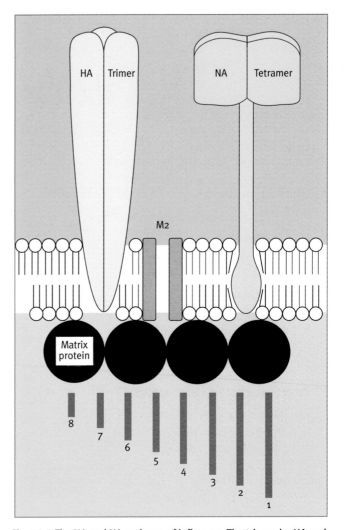

Fig. 10.2 The HA and NA antigens of influenza. The triangular HA and mushroom-shaped NA spikes protrude from the viral lipid in a ratio of 5:1. A layer of matrix protein underlies the lipid membrane and encloses the eight segments of viral RNA, which are closely associated with PA, PB1, PB2, and NP proteins. M2 forms an ion channel, which penetrates through the lipid bilayer.

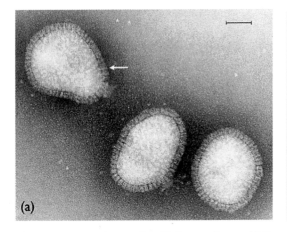

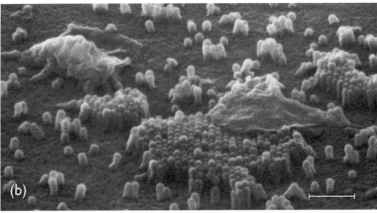

Fig 10.1 Electron micrographs of influenza viruses. **(a)** Negatively stained virions. The surface HA and NA antigens are arrowed. Scale bar = 50 nm. **(b)** Scanning electron micrograph of virus particles budding from the cell surface. Many thousands are present on an infected cell. (Courtesy of Dr David Hockley.) Scale bar = 500 nm.

is a rod-shaped glycoprotein with a triangular cross-section (Fig. 10.2). It was first identified by its ability to agglutinate erythrocytes, hence its name, but it is now apparent that it also has important roles in the attachment and entry of virus to the cells of the host and in determining virulence.

The NA can remove neuraminic (sialic) acid from receptor proteins. Its main function seems to be connected with release of new virus from cells.

Penetrating the lipid membrane of the virus are molecules of M2 that form ion channels, allowing protons to enter the interior of the virus during replication in the cells. Inside the matrix shell are the **nucleoprotein** and an **RNA transcriptase**, which are essential for transcription of viral RNA to mRNA during replication (Section 2.4).

2.3 Genome

The eight discrete fragments of the negative-sense ssRNA genome, approximately 13 kb in size (see Fig. 3.6) are complexed with proteins (NP, PA, PB1, and PB2) to form a RNP arranged in a helix.

2.4 Replication

After attachment to the specific receptors on the cell membrane (Fig. 10.3), virions are taken into the cell by endocytosis and then transported to vacuoles (endosomes), where the acid pH induces a change in the configuration of the HA. This structural rearrangement of the HA brings a special set of catalytic amino acids, the 'fusion sequence', in contact with the lipid of the vacuole wall of the cells.

Simultaneously, protons pass along the M2 ion channel to the interior of the virion and cause the M1 protein to be released from the ribonucleoprotein complex. Thus 'released' the RNP : RNA complex can enter the cell nucleus for transcription and replication. Uniquely, influenza can use its endonuclease to cleave 10–13 nucleotides and the 5'-methyl guanosine cap from the normal nuclear RNA of the cell. This 'snatched' cap and associated nucleotides is then used as a primer for transcription of each of the eight negative-sense RNA gene segments. Six newly transcribed mRNAs are translated immediately into viral structural proteins, while two primary RNA transcripts are each spliced into two mRNAs coding for NS proteins.

The new influenza virions are assembled at the host-cell surface membrane and released by a process of budding in which both HA and NA are involved. Viral NA has the important function of cleaving sialic acid from viral and cellular glycoproteins, thus preventing virus aggregation and allowing individual virions to be released from the cell. Some cells die but others may allow many viral replication cycles to occur without specific damage to themselves.

2.5 Genetic variation in influenza viruses

Influenza A viruses readily undergo gene 'swapping' or **reassortment** (Fig. 10.4), so that, in a cell infected simultaneously with two different viruses, the progeny virions may contain mixtures of each parent's genes. Add this property to the ability of influenza A virus to infect animals such as pigs and

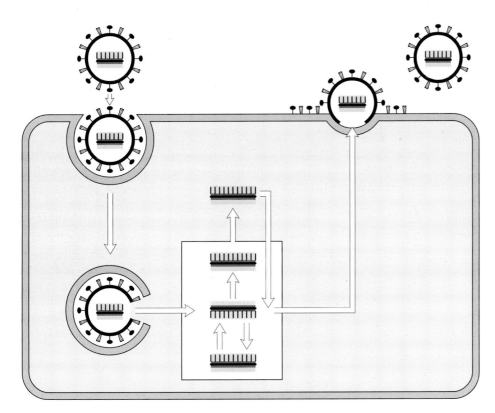

Fig. 10.3 Cellular replication of influenza virus (simplified version).

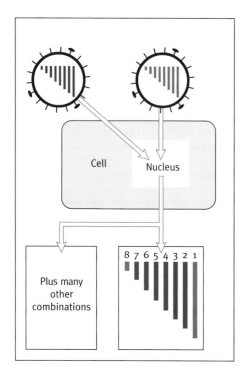

Fig. 10.4 Genetic reassortment with influenza A virus. Infection of a single cell by two different influenza A viruses could result in exchange of any of the eight genes of each parent to create a 'new virus' with genes from both parents.

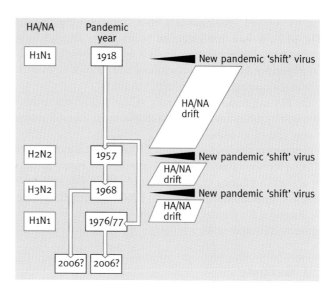

Fig. 10.5 Antigenic shift and drift. For explanation, see text.

birds that often live in close association with humans, and we have a situation in which double infections with viruses of human and non-human origin may result at unpredictable intervals in the formation of new strains with genetic compositions differing from those in general circulation. This reassortment of genes, known as **antigenic shift**, can, of course, also take place between two influenza A viruses of human origin. It cannot occur between influenza A and B viruses.

RNA viruses tend to have high mutation rates—more than 10 000 times higher than that of human or viral DNA—and this is true of all the influenza viruses. The viral RNA replicase is a low-fidelity enzyme, so transcription errors accumulate. Moreover there are no proof-reading or corrective enzymes. These mutations give rise to changes in the viral polypeptides, such as HA which, out of a total of 250 amino acids, undergoes two or three amino-acid substitutions each year.

Both influenza A and B are subject to antigenic drift but only A viruses undergo antigenic shift and hence have the potential of causing pandemics.

2.6 Pandemic influenza

Figure 10.5 shows the relationship between antigenic drift, shift, and epidemics and pandemics of influenza A.

The great pandemic of Spanish influenza in 1918 was especially terrible in its effects in Europe; worldwide, it killed about 50 million people, far more than lost their lives in the whole period of the First World War (Fig. 10.6(a)). An influenza

pandemic that occurred nearly 30 years later in 1957, when a strain differing completely in both HA and NA appeared in China, was less virulent. In 1968 there was another pandemic (Fig. 10.6(b)), again originating in the Far East; the virus, first isolated in Hong Kong, had now undergone a partial shift that affected only the HA and not the NA.

In 1976 there was considerable alarm in the USA when the dreaded swine-type H1N1 influenza A virus appeared in a military barracks. This was a drifted variant related to the 1918 virus; it could have arisen again by genetic reassortment, but it is more likely that the strain circulated for many years in an animal reservoir, such as pigs, before resurfacing in humans. An H1N1 virus re-emerged in China in 1977 and is still spreading round the world. At present chicken influenza A (H5N1) is spreading widely in 10 countries in Southeast Asia.

2.7 The origin of pandemic or shifted strains of influenza A

Why do pandemic strains of influenza A seem to originate in southern China—or do they? The answer may lie in the close association of humans with domestic animals and birds. Migrating geese and ducks are the end source of all 16 antigenic subtypes of influenza and most often the infection is silent. The birds excrete virus from their respiratory tract and also in their droppings. Domestic birds become infected and the virus soon mutates to a virulent form, killing chickens by the tens of thousands. Largely unremarked except by farmers and veterinarians, influenza A viruses are constantly circulating in pigs, horses, and birds, including poultry; and it is a reasonable assumption that, in areas of very intensive small-scale farming, the chances of interchange of viruses between humans and other species—and hence of genetic reassortment—are considerable. Another factor that may be important is the very high human population density in that area, in which lives half the world's population and most significant of all, live chickens are

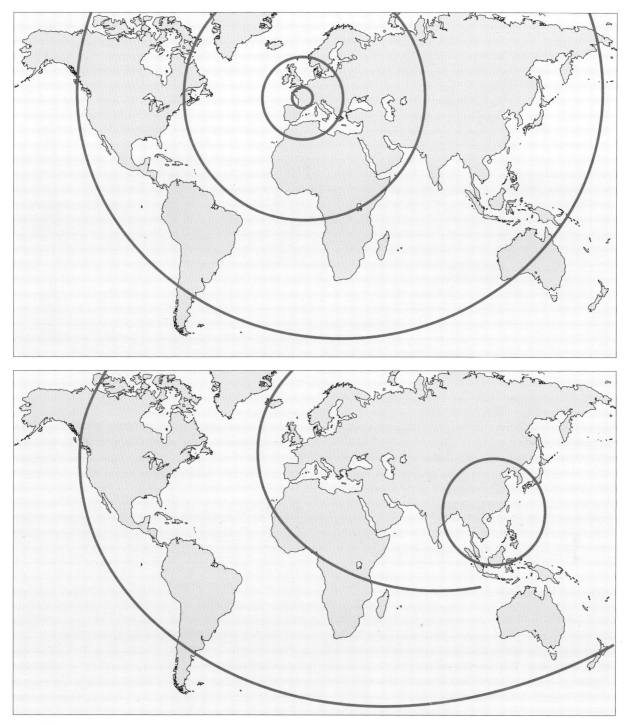

Fig. 10.6 **(a)** The emergence and spread of the great Spanish influenza virus pandemic in 1918 from Europe to the rest of the world. **(b)** The emergence and spread of the 'Asian' or Hong Kong pandemic in 1957 and 1968 from Asia to the rest of the world.

sold in the markets where purchasers can inadvertently become infected.

Live bird markets in Hong Kong, or indeed in the USA or anywhere else in the world, give a particular opportunity for mutated avian influenza A virus to cross the species barrier to infect persons (Fig. 10.7). In the last few years there have been outbreaks of avian H5 and H9 viruses in Hong Kong and H7 in

the Netherlands. Pandemic viruses can arise anywhere that the particular juxtaposition of infected birds, pigs, and humans coexists.

A less accepted but still possible explanation of the origin of these pandemic strains is that influenza A viruses continually recycle in humans and 'new' pandemic viruses are really old viruses re-emerging from a previously infected individual. Time

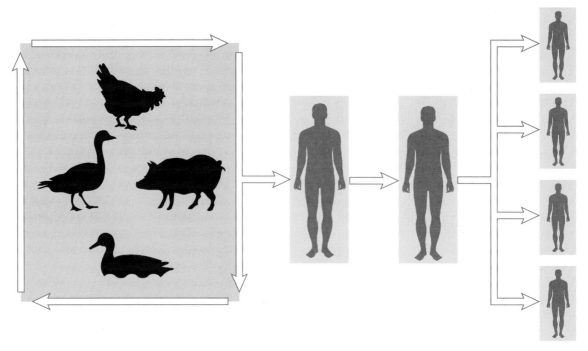

Fig. 10.7 Origin of pandemics—the cycle.

will tell which hypothesis is correct but everything is in favour of the bird ecosystem theory.

Virologists expect a new pandemic within the next few years and many countries have formal plans to cope with such an emergency. WHO has urgently requested all 250 countries of the world to plan now before it is too late.

3 Clinical and pathological aspects

3.1 Clinical features

After an incubation period of 2–3 days there is usually a very **abrupt onset,** with shivering, malaise, headache, and aching in the limbs and back. Characteristically, the patient is prostrated and has to take to bed. The temperature rises rapidly to about 39°C. Influenza is **not** characterized by runny noses or sore throats at the beginning, as are common cold infections.

Fortunately, influenza is usually short-lived in younger persons. In older people and the 'at-risk' group, however, recovery may take much longer, with persistent weakness and lassitude sometimes for 3–6 months. In general, the severity of influenza is proportional to age. *There are no differences between influenza A and B as regards the clinical picture. There is one important caveat here:* babies are as much at risk of complications as the elderly. This is a virus that strikes at both ends of the age spectrum.

Apart from the only important and sometimes life-threatening secondary bacterial infection caused by *Streptococcus pneumoniae* there are few complications, but one rare condition, **Reye's syndrome**, is sometimes associated with influenza in children, often of the B type. The taking of aspirin has also been implicated in the causation of this syndrome, which involves encephalopathy with fatty degeneration of the liver and other viscera; it is often fatal (see also Chapter 30).

3.2 Pathogenesis

Infection is acquired by the respiratory route and is usually an infection of the upper respiratory tract. Virus multiplies in the epithelial cells in the nose and sinus passages and destroys the cilia, which are an important element in the defence of the respiratory system. This is accompanied by production of IFN and other cytokines such as IL-6 and TNF—the so-called cytokine storm—which accounts for the severe malaise.

Viral infection of the lower respiratory tract, in the form of influenzal pneumonia, sometimes occurs, presenting as an overwhelming toxaemia with a high mortality. The virus replicates in epithelial cells of the alveoli, causing exudation into the air sacs and pneumonia. Pneumonia is, however, often due to **secondary infection with bacteria**. Of these, *Strep. pneumoniae* and *Staph. aureus* are both the most frequent and the most dangerous, leading to respiratory distress, cyanosis, and collapse within 2–3 days of the onset of infection. More recently there is strong evidence that infection with influenza enhances the chance of stroke and heart disease.

3.3 Immune response

We have seen that protection against infection is mediated by antibodies, the **anti-HA** being the most important in this respect. **Anti-NA antibody** prevents the release of newly formed virus from the host cells. Antibody of the IgA class is probably important in preventing infection, acting as it does at the mucous surfaces of the respiratory tract where the virus first attaches.

In addition to these humoral factors, CMI, in the form of cytotoxic T cells and alveolar macrophages, plays an important part in recovery. Cytotoxic T cells may have a wider response against all influenza A viruses, particularly if they are directed towards epitopes of the type-specific NP or M proteins. This is the subject of intense research to make a more universal influenza vaccine protecting against a wider range of variants.

3.4 Laboratory diagnosis

In general practice, the diagnosis of influenza is made on the evidence of the characteristic clinical picture, backed up by the knowledge that an outbreak is in progress. In the UK, figures of influenza-like illness are published weekly by the Health Protection Agency (HPA).

If isolation of influenza virus in culture for further examination is not essential, it can be identified rapidly by **immunofluorescence** staining of cells in nasopharyngeal aspirates, a useful method in hospital practice. However, this method is being replaced by rapid **ELISA-type tests**, which can be carried out at the bedside in 30 minutes, and by RT–PCR in the laboratory. Both NIs and M2 blockers may be used in the family unit to prevent spread from an index case, perhaps the youngest child. As long as the drugs are taken within 36 hours of the first symptoms the disease is less severe and less prolonged and virus excretion is diminished. WHO has recommended that every government should develop a pandemic plan in preparation for the first global pandemic of the twenty-first century. It would be wise to stockpile antivirals and archetype vaccines in advance of any outbreak.

4 Prevention and cure

4.1 Drugs against influenza

Influenza A viruses—but not B or C—are inhibited by **amantadine**, a primary amine, and **rimantadine**, a methylated derivative (Chapter 38). Two anti-NA drugs, which inhibit viruses from budding from the cell surface, are being used in many countries. The anti-NA drugs (oseltamivir and zanamivir) have the big advantage, compared with amantadine, of inhibiting influenza B as well as influenza A viruses.

These two drugs have to be given to the patient within 36 hours of the onset of influenza symptoms, when they reduce virus excretion, alleviate symptoms, reduce hospitalization and the misuse of antibiotics. In the family environment, once an index case of influenza is identified, rapid distribution of antivirals can reduce transmission by at least 80 per cent. Experience over the next years will show how the drugs can be used with greatest benefit. At present and given the impact of influenza, both personally and in the community, they are under-

used and the most important reasons appear to be economic rather than the needs of public health *per se*.

4.2 Vaccines

At present, immunization rather than chemoprophylaxis is the method of choice for preventing both influenza A and B. Even so, immunization poses a particular problem: every time a new strain of influenza A or B appears, the rapid production of large quantities of vaccine virus with the required antigenic characteristics, together with the need for routine tests of safety and efficacy, limits the amount of vaccine available.

Most national authorities immunize about 10 per cent of the population annually: these are the **'at-risk' group** who have a much increased chance of serious clinical complications after an attack of influenza, often caused by superinfecting bacteria such as pneumococci. There are two main categories of at-risk persons and it is most important that these individuals are vaccinated each year:

* the elderly (>65 years) or debilitated and those of any age with chronic heart, respiratory (asthmatics and chronic bronchitics), renal, or endocrine disease; and

* **people in closed institutions**, such as residential homes for the elderly, in which attack rates may be high.

It is also considered sensible to immunize groups in community service, such as healthcare staff, nurses and doctors, and police, who may need protection against wholesale sickness at times of major epidemics.

Inactivated vaccines are prepared from appropriate strains of influenza A and B grown in the chick embryo allantoic cavity (Chapter 37); the infected fluids are harvested, purified by ultracentrifugation, and inactivated with formalin. Two more modern vaccines are produced using cell culture techniques. Most of the vaccines are either subunit preparations containing purified HA and NA (Fig. 10.8) or so-called 'split' vaccines that have been extracted with ether and detergent to reduce the side-effects of whole-virus vaccines (Table 10.1). Apart from local erythema and soreness, sometimes with fever, these vaccines are generally very safe. Most governments have now set targets aimed at immunizing at least 70 per cent of the at risk group each year, because of the clear impact on hospitals of influenza in this group. Many new vaccines are being developed.

Live attenuated vaccines are made by reassorting genes of viruses possessing the required HA and NA antigens with various laboratory-derived mutants selected previously for inability to grow at 37°C or for ability to grow only at low temperatures, for example 25°C (cold-adapted mutants). Both mutants are of diminished virulence for humans.

The most recently developed cold-adapted vaccine, FluMist, is targeted in the USA at children. The concept here is to break the normal chain of infection within the family, from the child to the parents and grandparents. There is some evidence that in this situation the virus-induced mortality of the grandparents is reduced during the yearly influenza season.

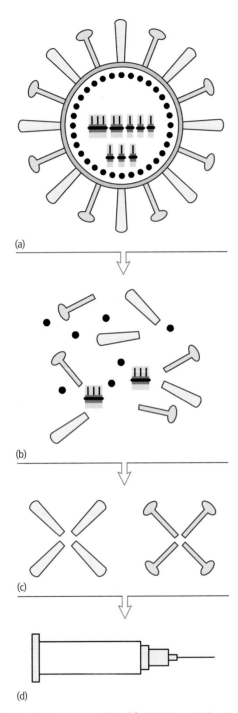

(a)

(b)

(c)

(d)

Fig. 10.8 Subunit influenza vaccine. **(a)** Virus is grown in eggs, purified, and concentrated. **(b)** Viral lipid is dissolved by detergent, releasing proteins and nucleic acid, which is removed. **(c)** HA and NA subunits are purified by ultracentrifugation. **(d)** Standardized quantities of HA and NA are incorporated into the final product (approximately 15 µg per dose).

Pandemic planning

Given the time span of 38 years since the last great world pandemic of influenza, WHO has requested all national governments to plan for the first global outbreak of the twenty-first century. The plan outlines strategy for vaccine and antiviral

Table 10.1 Inactivated influenza vaccines

Type	Remarks	Suitable for children
Whole virus	Good immunogen but may cause local and general reactions	No
'Split' vaccine	Whole virus extracted with ether	Yes
'Subunit' or 'surface' antigen	Purified HA and NA extracted with detergent; less liable to cause reactions	Yes

drugs. In reality this is a paper exercise until antivirals are stockpiled alongside experimental H1–16 vaccines. Given the overwhelming nature of previous pandemics and the speed of travel, these are important public health goals.

5 Reminders

- Influenza is primarily a short-lived infection of the upper respiratory tract; its severity is directly related to age. Complications include secondary bacterial infection and, rarely, **Reye's syndrome**. However, each year hundreds of thousands of deaths worldwide are attributed to influenza.

- Influenza is caused by the **orthomyxoviruses**, which contain segmented ssRNA genomes of negative polarity, 13 kb in size. They have **helical** symmetry.

- There are four genera, of which only two, the A and B viruses, are important in infections of humans. Influenza viruses are also prevalent in a number of mammalian and avian hosts and some can be transmitted between species.

- The **HA and NA antigens** are important in the infection of cells, and the corresponding antibodies to these spike- and mushroom-shaped proteins play a major role in preventing infection.

- **The genome has eight segments**, allowing reassortment of genes (**shift**). Shifted strains appear at long intervals and cause worldwide epidemics (pandemics) at long intervals. Virologists are planning for a new pandemic.

- By contrast, antigenic **drift**, due to minor mutations, affects both A and B viruses, is slowly progressive, and causes more frequent but localized outbreaks.

- The laboratory diagnosis, if needed, is made by isolation of the virus in chick embryos or cell cultures, or, more rapidly, by immunofluorescence staining or RT–PCR of nasopharyngeal washings.

- **Amantadine** and rimantadine are moderately effective in prophylaxis and therapy. Two new anti-NA drugs (oseltamivir and zanamivir) have shown prophylactic and therapeutic activity and are now being used in clinics throughout the world. They must be used as soon as an infection is apparent and certainly within 36 hours of the first symptoms. WHO recommends that these drugs are stockpiled in preparation for a global outbreak (pandemic). They can prevent 80 per cent of illness in the family when given early, or reduce the duration of illness by 1–2 days when administered within 36 hours of appearance of symptoms.

- *The main method of control is at present by means of inactivated virus vaccines, mainly consisting of the HA and NA proteins*, which are reformulated at intervals to match the prevalent strains. Supplies are limited, and are given as first priority to the 'at-risk' groups (about 15 per cent of the population). Influenza vaccines are 80 per cent effective.

Gastroenteritis viruses

1 Introduction

It is an odd fact that although the *Enteroviridae* replicate primarily in the gut, they do not cause gastroenteritis. Those that do are something of a rag-bag, which we can term **enteric viruses** to distinguish them from the enteroviruses. It is also curious that most of these agents cannot be propagated in cell cultures, which explains why some of them are poorly characterized.

Table 11.1 lists the viruses associated with D&V. Most of them were first recognized by EM of stool samples, a technique that is still the mainstay of diagnosis. For virologists, some at least of these viruses make up for their inability to grow in the laboratory by their elegant appearance under the EM.

These viruses are spread rapidly by the faecal–oral route, often because of failure to wash hands after defecation (Chapter 4, Fig. 4.4). There have been a number of explosive outbreaks on passenger ships, some of them severe enough to force cruises to be abandoned.

2 Rotaviruses

2.1 Properties of the viruses

Classification

These agents are members of the *Reoviridae*, 'reo' standing for respiratory enteric orphan; although they could be identified in the respiratory tract and gut, they were at first thought not to be associated with any disease, hence 'orphan'. The *Rotavirus* is a genus within the family; two others, *Orbivirus* and *Coltivirus*, will appear in Chapter 27.

Morphology

The shape of these viruses suggested their name (Latin *rota* = wheel). The capsid has a double shell and is 70 nm in diameter; some smaller, single-shelled particles may also be seen. In most of the virions a number of 'spokes' radiate from a central 'hub', although some appear empty by negative contrast staining. (Fig.11.1(a)). The cores appear to be icosahedral.

Moving from the inside towards the outside, the core is composed of the structural protein VP2 and the transcriptase (replicase) VP1. The inner icosahedral capsid is essentially the group specific antigen VP6, whereas the outer icosahedral capsid is VP7. Sixty spikes of the HA VP4 project outward.

Table 11.1 Viruses causing gastroenteritis

Virus	Approximate diameter of virion (nm)	Important morphological features	Genome
Rotavirus	70	A number of 'spokes' radiate from a central 'hub' (Latin *rota* = wheel)	Linear dsRNA, 18 kb, 11 segments
Adenovirus types 40, 41	80–110	Icosahedral; may have long fibres extending from the apices	Linear dsDNA, 36 kb. Inverted terminal repeats and a protein primer at each 5′ terminus
Calicivirus	35	32 cup-like indentations on surface (Latin *calix* = cup)	Linear positive sense ssRNA, 7.5 kb. Has a VPg protein at the 5′ terminus. The 3′ terminus has a poly(A) tail
Astrovirus	30	The arrangement of capsomeres gives the appearance of a five- or six-pointed star on the surface (Greek *astron* = star)	Linear positive-sense ssRNA, 7 kb. Has poly(A) tail at the 3′ terminus

Genome

The *Reoviridae* differ from all other RNA viruses in that their negative polarity segmented genomes are double-stranded. Furthermore, they are divided into 11 segments of varying size, coding for a similar number of structural and NS proteins (Fig. 11.2). The total size is 18 kbp. The electrophoretic pattern of the nucleic acid differs between strains (Fig. 11.3) and is used by some to define 'electropherotypes', which do not correspond with the serotypes but which may be useful for epidemiological studies.

Replication

Viruses bind to sialic acid receptors via the HA protein and enter cells by endocytosis or by direct entry through the plasma membrane. Degraded virions act as factory sites in the cell cytoplasm. The virion-associated transcriptase transcribes certain positive-stranded mRNAs coding for early viral enzymes that exit the factory sites via the hollow apices of the virus core. Negative RNA strands are then produced from the mRNA molecules and as a necessity of transcription dsRNA forms are made. The dsRNAs can then serve as templates for transcription of late mRNAs. Late mRNAs encode mainly virus structural proteins that trigger the self-assembly process. The infected cells lyse and release the accumulated new virions. Some members, such as rotavirus, employ a unique method of budding in the ER membrane of the cell.

Growth in cell culture

Unlike other reoviruses, rotaviruses can, if treated with trypsin, be propagated in primary monkey kidney cell cultures, but this method is not used for routine diagnosis.

2.2 Clinical and pathological aspects

Clinical features

Rotaviruses primarily infect the young of many species, including humans. **Babies under 2 years of age** are the main victims but there may also be outbreaks in the elderly, particularly those in institutions.

The incubation period is 2-4 days; the characteristic syndrome comprises **vomiting**, **diarrhoea**, and **fever**, but silent infections also occur. **Dehydration** must be dealt with promptly; it should be no problem in countries with adequate facilities, but causes untold numbers of infant deaths in the Third World.

Pathogenesis

Observations on infected animals show that rotaviruses attack the **columnar epithelium** at the apices of the villi of the **duodenum** and **upper ileum**; the loss of these cells results in malabsorption. Regeneration from the bases of the villi is normally rapid after the acute attack.

Immune response

Following infection, antibodies are demonstrable in the serum; tests for specific IgG are useful in epidemiological studies, which show that most adults have been infected at some time or another. IgA antibody produced in the gut is probably an important factor in the immune response, and there is also some cross-protection among the various serotypes.

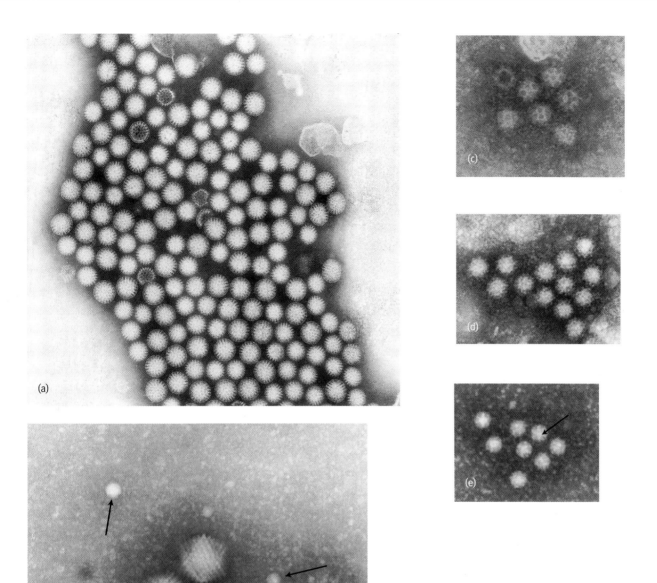

Fig. 11.1 Electron micrographs of gastroenteritis viruses found in stools of patients with diarrhoea. **(a) Rotavirus** (courtesy of Dr June Almeida). **(b) Adenovirus** from a child with diarrhoea. Note also the very small adeno-associated parvoviruses (arrowed). **(c) Caliciviruses** from faeces of a child with diarrhoea. Note the cup-like depressions on the surface. **(d) 'Small round structured virus'. (e) Astroviruses**. The six-pointed star pattern of the capsomeres is arrowed. (Parts **(b)** and **(e)** courtesy of Dr Ian Chrystie.) Scale bar = 50 nm.

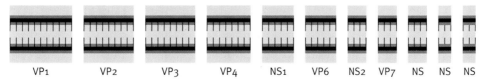

| VP1 | VP2 | VP3 | VP4 | NS1 | VP6 | NS2 | VP7 | NS | NS | NS |

Fig. 11.2 Rotavirus genome. The various structural proteins (VP) or non-structural (NS) proteins coded by each gene are labelled.

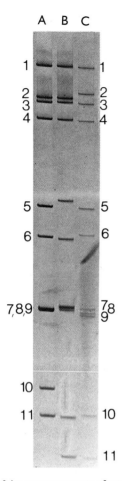

Fig. 11.3 Separation of the gene segments of rotavirus on a polyacrylamide gel. The 11 bands in each channel correspond with the individual genes of three different rotavirus (A–C).

Epidemiology

We tend to associate diarrhoea and vomiting (D&V) with the summer months, but in the northern hemisphere, rotavirus outbreaks typically occur in the winter. Spread is probably by the **faecal–oral route**; but the seasonal incidence suggests that respiratory infection cannot be ruled out. Outbreaks are common in institutions such as crèches and hospital-acquired infections are also fairly frequent. Unfortunately, the virus is relatively resistant to chemical disinfectants and spreads readily when hygiene is inadequate. In developing countries, infections with rotaviruses, along with other viruses and bacteria, are responsible for large numbers of infant deaths every year.

Transmission to infants from asymptomatic health care staff or relatives can occur; conversely, there is evidence that babies can infect adults in close contact with them. **Chronic rotavirus infection** can be troublesome in patients **with primary immunodeficiencies** (Chapter 32).

There are six serotypes (A–F) identified by antigenic differences in the capsid antigen VP6, but most human rotaviruses are members of group A.

The segmentation of the rotavirus genome permits reassortant strains to be made in the laboratory. As these viruses are widespread in nature and infect most if not all domestic and farm animals and birds, there is at least a theoretical possibility that infection of humans with mammalian or avian strains might take place, with the emergence of 'shifted' strains analogous to those of influenza A (Chapter 10); but so far, such hybrids have not been reported.

Rotavirus vaccine

There is no specific therapy for rotavirus infections, so that, especially in view of the problem they pose in developing countries, a vaccine would be a major benefit. During the last few years, promising results have been obtained with vaccines prepared by various methods. They include, alone or in combination:

- attenuated live vaccines;
- the use of animal strains, which cross-protect to a significant degree against human rotaviruses;
- the construction of attenuated reassortant strains with some genes from human and some from animal viruses, similar in principle to influenza vaccines (Chapter 10);
- the use of 'cocktail' vaccines containing several serotypes.

Reassortant and 'cocktail' vaccines have given encouraging results in field trials.

3 Adenoviruses

The properties of these viruses are described in Chapter 8.

Their relationship with respiratory and eye infections is well established, but their implication in diarrhoeal disease is often less clear. Like rotaviruses, their distinctive morphology makes them easy to spot in faecal specimens by EM (Fig. 11.1(b)), but again, their mere presence does not necessarily indicate that they are doing any harm. **Serotypes 40 and 41** are most commonly associated with acute diarrhoea in infants; other serotypes, that can readily be propagated from stool cultures, usually seem to be just passengers. These two serotypes differ from other adenoviruses in that they are 'fastidious', i.e. difficult to grow in cell cultures. Not uncommonly, adeno-associated parvoviruses (Chapter 13) can be seen in association with the adenoviruses (Fig. 11.1(b)). They do not seem to be pathogenic.

The clinical syndrome is similar to that caused by rotaviruses, except that the infants tend to be older; adenovirus gastroenteritis is sometimes complicated by **intussusception**.

4 Caliciviruses

4.1 Properties of the viruses

Classification

The members of the family *Caliciviridae* infect a very wide range of hosts, including mammals, birds, reptiles, and even fish. There are four genera, of which two, *Norovirus* (formerly 'Norwalk-like viruses') and *Sapporovirus* affect humans, causing outbreaks of gastroenteritis. Hepatitis E virus (HEV) is a calicivirus (see Chapter 23).

Morphology

The virion is 35 nm in diameter and has 32 cup-like indentations (Latin *calix* = cup), on the surface (Fig. 11.1(c)). Very similar viruses, mainly distinguished from the classical human caliciviruses (HuCV) by their amorphous surfaces (Fig. 11.1(d)) are known as 'small round structured viruses' (SRSV).

Genome

The positive sense ssRNA is 7.5 kb in size with a VPg protein at the 5′ terminus. The 3′ terminus has a poly(A) tail (Fig. 11.4).

Replication

The genomic mRNA is translated into a large polyprotein that is cleaved into structural and NS proteins. Separate subgenomic mRNAs code for the structural proteins. Replication occurs exclusively in the cytoplasm where self-assembly occurs. These viruses have not yet been cultivated in the laboratory.

4.2 Clinical and epidemiological aspects

A number of strains infect humans, mostly named after the places where they were first identified; the list includes the Norwalk, Hawaii, Taunton, and Snow Mountain viruses. The aetiological role of some of these viruses was proved by remarkably heroic volunteers, who developed gastroenteritis after drinking filtrates of faeces from patients.

There are several modes of transmission including the **faecal–oral route**, inhalation of **aerosols** from vomit and point source outbreaks from **contaminated food or water**. Shellfish are a frequent source of infection.

Caliciviruses cause outbreaks of vomiting, sometimes projectile, and diarrhoea. **The incubation period is 18–48 hours**, and the onset is often sudden. There may be abdominal pain and low-grade fever, but the stools do not contain blood or mucus.

SRSV and to a lesser extent HuCV are prevalent worldwide and are the major cause of outbreaks of D&V, many of which occur in closed institutions. SRSV infections tend to occur mainly in the winter, whereas HuCV epidemics are seen all the year round.

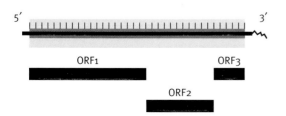

Fig. 11.4 Calicivirus genome and encoded proteins and open reading frames. ∿, poly(A) tail.

Diagnosis

EM using specific antisera (immunoelectron microscopy, IEM) remains a key method but RT–PCR kits are now available.

Management of outbreaks

Control is difficult because asymptomatic infection can occur and excretion of virus is prolonged for 1–2 weeks. However, virus-excreting food handlers can now be identified and removed from contact with food.

5 Astroviruses

5.1 Properties of the viruses

Classification

Like the *Caliciviridae*, the *Astroviridae* contains only one genus, *Astrovirus*, several species of which affect humans.

Morphology

By negative contrast EM, the surface of this 30 nm icosahedral virion has a curious five- or six-pointed star appearance (Greek *astron* = a star) (Fig. 11.1(e)). The capsid is composed of two or three structural proteins.

Genome

A linear, positive ssRNA molecule of ≈7 kb. The RNA has a poly(A) tract at the 3′ terminus and can act directly as mRNA.

Replication

The virus absorbs to a receptor and is internalized either by endocytosis or direct entry. Replication is entirely cytoplasmic. The RNA genome is replicated via a replicative intermediate dsRNA. In addition, a large subgenomic mRNA codes for a viral polyprotein, which is cleaved into capsid proteins. New virions self-assemble and may be seen as crystalline arrays in the cytoplasm, whence they are released by cell lysis.

These viruses can be cultivated in the laboratory in trypsin-treated human colon carcinoma or monkey kidney cells.

5.2 Clinical and epidemiological aspects

Astroviruses cause outbreaks of diarrhoea, predominantly in children. The modes of transmission resemble those of caliciviruses. **The incubation period is 3–4 days**. Vomiting is not a prominent feature. In temperate climates, there is a well-marked peak of incidence in the winter.

6 Laboratory diagnosis

We have already pointed out that detection of a micro-organism in a clinical specimen does not necessarily mean that it is causally related to the patient's signs and symptoms; enough has been said in this chapter to indicate that this is nowhere more obvious than in acute gastroenteritis. Under the EM, viruses, sometimes of more than one variety, can often be found in faecal specimens. Their association with disease is most probable in the case of rotaviruses, but as far as the others are concerned, epidemiological factors such as the presence of the same virus in a high proportion of people involved in the same outbreak must also be considered.

None of this makes the task of the virology laboratory any easier. There are two approaches to diagnosis:

- EM of faecal extract. This is sometimes called the **catch-all method**, because it is potentially capable of demonstrating all the viruses present in the specimen;
- Specific tests aimed at detecting a particular virus.

6.1 Electron microscopy

Some viruses commonly seen in stools, e.g. polio, other enteroviruses and some adenoviruses, can also be grown readily in cell cultures and thus identified; these are not associated with gastroenteritis. The viruses we are now hunting are all fastidious, growing poorly or not at all in the laboratory. All the viruses in Table 11.1 are, however, readily identified by their distinctive morphology.

A useful aid to the finding and identification of viruses in stool samples is **IEM**. A specific antiserum added before the specimen is mounted and stained will clump any virions of the same specificity, at one stroke making them easier to find and proving their identity. The method can be used for rota-, adeno- and enteroviruses.

6.2 Specific tests

Laboratories without EMs can utilize **ELISA tests** applied to stool samples; at present, tests for caliciviruses, astroviruses, rota- and adenoviruses are generally available. Specific antibodies can also be used to identify some fastidious viruses that undergo limited replication in cell cultures without inducing CPEs.

It should by now be apparent that attaching the right label to single cases of acute gastroenteritis is fraught with difficulties and that the best chance of success lies in the study of outbreaks in which the presence of a particular virus is a common factor. Such investigations demand the closest cooperation between physicians and laboratory staff; the haphazard collection and examination of specimens is useless.

7 Reminders

- Viruses of several families cause **D&V**. Identification of these agents is one of the few uses of EM in diagnosis.
- Transmission of these enteric viruses is mainly by the **faecal–oral route**, but spread by aerosols and ingestion of contaminated foods or water are also frequent.
- **Rotaviruses** have a complex double shell structure and a negative double-stranded and segmented RNA genome of 18 kbp. They are important causes of infantile diarrhoea; in the northern hemisphere, the incidence peaks in winter. Both infants and the elderly in institutions are particularly at risk. Correction of dehydration is an important element of treatment. Experimental vaccines are giving promising results.
- **Two serotypes (40 and 41)** of the **adenoviruses** cause acute diarrhoea in infants, intususseption is an occasional complication.
- **Caliciviruses**, ≈35 nm in diameter, have curious cup-like indentations on their surfaces. The positive sense ssRNA genome is 7.5 kb in size. These viruses, and the closely similar SRSVs are prevalent worldwide and are the most frequent cause of outbreaks of D&V.
- **Astroviruses** are 30 mm spherical virions with a five- or six-pointed star morphology. The genome is positive sense ssRNA, 7 kb in size. They cause outbreaks of diarrhoea, mainly in young children, with a peak prevalence in the winter.
- None of these viruses grow readily in routine cell cultures but all have morphological characteristics recognizable by EM. Other tests, particularly **ELISA**, are available for diagnosing some of these infections.

Rubella: postnatal infections

1 Introduction

Rubella is derived from the Latin *rubellus*, meaning 'reddish', and refers to the pink rash that is seen in most patients. Its popular name, German measles, probably derives from the fact that it was first described in Germany during the eighteenth century. Rubella is predominantly an infection of children, in whom it causes a mild febrile illness. Were this all, we should spend but little time on it; but, as a potent cause of fetal abnormality, rubella has a major claim on our attention. In this chapter we shall deal only with the virus itself and with postnatal infections; intrauterine infections are discussed in Chapter 31.

2 Properties of the virus

2.1 Classification

Rubella virus belongs to the family *Togaviridae*, which has two genera, *Alphavirus* and *Rubivirus*. The alphaviruses are mosquito-borne and infect a wide range of vertebrates. They are described in Chapter 27. Because it is the only togavirus that is not arthropod-borne, rubella has a genus all to itself, *Rubivirus*. This classification is supported by its lack of serological cross-reactions with other togaviruses.

2.2 Morphology, genome, and replication

These features (Fig. 12.1) are all very similar to those of the other togaviruses (Chapter 27). The genome, at ≈10 kb, is rather smaller. There is only one serotype, an important consideration both in the epidemiology of rubella and in the making of vaccines.

Rubella does not naturally infect species other than humans.

3 Clinical and pathological aspects

3.1 Clinical features

Rubella in children

The onset is marked by slight malaise, a small rise in temperature—usually to less than 38°C—and sometimes suffusion of the conjunctivae. Shotty enlargement of the **lymph nodes** in

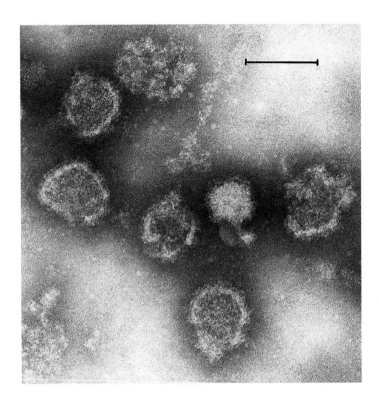

Fig. 12.1 Electron micrograph of rubella virus (courtesy of Dr David Hockley). Scale bar = 100 nm.

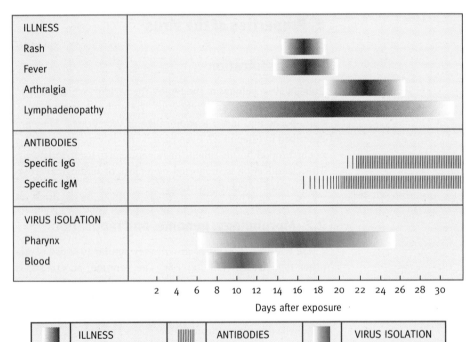

Fig. 12.2 The course of postnatal rubella. (Adapted, with permission, from Banatvala, J.E. and Best, J.M. (1984). In *Topley and Wilson's Principles of bacteriology, virology and immunity* (7th edn) (ed. G. Wilson, A.A. Miles, and M.T. Parker), Vol. 4, pp. 271–302. Edword Amold, London.)

the suboccipital region, behind the ears and in the neck and axillae is characteristic. The **rash** usually appears a day or two after the onset of symptoms, but is by no means a constant finding; its appearance is not diagnostic, as it may resemble those seen in other viral infections. It consists of small pinkish macules, rarely exceeding 3 mm in diameter, and usually more discrete and regular in appearance than the eruption of measles. The face and neck are first affected, followed by the trunk. Circumoral pallor is sometimes present, but is not diagnostic. Unlike the pronounced enanthem seen in measles, there may be some very small erythematous spots on the soft palate, but often the buccal mucosa appears normal. A purpuric rash has been described, but is rare.

The vast majority of patients get better within a few days. Postinfection **encephalitis** is rare, affecting one in several thousand patients, and the prognosis is generally good.

Rubella in adults

The main difference between rubella in children and in adults is that in the latter, **polyarthritis** is a not infrequent complication. It most often affects the hands and wrists, but may also involve the larger joints of the limbs. There may also be some myalgia. Rubella arthropathy predominantly affects postpubertal women. It usually clears up fairly quickly, but may persist for months or even years.

3.2 Epidemiology

Because rubella is of significance mainly in relation to fetal infection, an important epidemiological aspect is its prevalence in women of childbearing age. Rubella appears to be present in all countries, periods of endemicity alternating with epidemics at irregular intervals. Its distribution varies from country to country. Serological surveys (see Chapter 7) show that, in most populations, over 70 per cent of women have been infected, but in others, notably rural areas in some Third World countries, notably the Indian subcontinent, the figure is lower. This finding might explain the lower than average prevalence of rubella antibody in Asian women now living in London (see Chapter 7, Section 5.2).

Effective immunization programmes radically alter the prevalence, and where they are in force, rubella is now a rare infection.

3.3 Pathogenesis and pathology

The portal of entry is the respiratory tract; subsequent spread follows the pattern described in Chapter 4, Fig. 4.2. The incubation period is usually 14–16 days, but may range from 10 to 21 days. Because postnatal rubella is not a fatal illness, and animals cannot be infected, virtually nothing is known about its pathology. The pathology of fetal infections is described in Chapter 31 and may involve slowed growth rates of fetal cells infected by the virus and apoptosis induced by viral protein.

3.4 Immune response

Specific IgM antibody appears within a few days of the rash, and is followed soon after by IgG (Fig. 12.2). The titre of IgM increases rapidly, reaching a peak about 10 days after onset and thereafter declining to undetectable amounts over several weeks or months. The rapid appearance of specific IgM antibody is invaluable for diagnostic purposes. IgG antibody peaks at about the same time as IgM, and persists for many years, as does IgA antibody, which appears in the serum and nasopharyngeal secretions.

The cell-mediated response precedes the appearance of antibody by a few days, reaches a peak at about the same time, and is also detectable for many years.

3.5 Laboratory diagnosis

Because acute rubella is often difficult to diagnose on purely clinical grounds, laboratory diagnosis assumes considerable importance. Tests for rubella infection, past or present, can be considered under three headings:

- **screening tests** for rubella antibody, to ascertain the immune status of women of childbearing age;
- tests for acute infection in pregnancy;
- tests on infants for **congenital infection**.

We shall deal here only with the first category. Infections of the pregnant mother and fetus are discussed in Chapter 31.

Screening tests on women

In the UK and elsewhere, women attending antenatal clinics are routinely screened for rubella antibody. If the result is negative, immunization soon after the birth is advised in order to protect subsequent pregnancies. Screening is also advised for women of childbearing age at particular risk of infection, e.g. teachers and clinic and hospital staff in contact with children. Such tests should be done irrespective of a history of past infection or

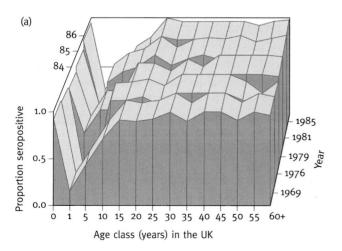
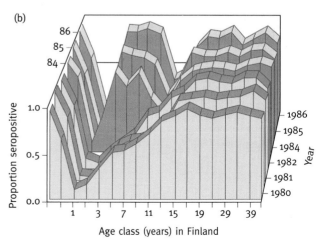

Fig. 12.3 The effects of different immunization policies on herd immunity to rubella. For explanation, see text. (Adapted with permission from Anderson, R.M. *et al.* (1990). *Lancet* **335**, 642.)

immunization, which may be unreliable. As many sera must be processed, the requirement is for a reliable test that can be done on a mass scale and that is not too labour-intensive. Some laboratories still **use single radial haemolysis** in which many sera can be tested simultaneously in a large gel plate containing both red cells sensitized with rubella antigen and complement. Plates are read after overnight incubation. ELISA tests for IgG antibody are now more commonly used. (See Chapter 36 for details of these tests.)

3.6 Control

Immunization

Rubella vaccine is the only one not given primarily for the benefit of the recipient, but to protect another, in this case, a fetus. As we shall see in Chapter 31, the risk of fetal malformation due to rubella acquired during the first trimester is very high.

Rubella vaccine

Rubella immunization was started in the USA during 1969 and in the UK a year later. Early immunization policies reduced the incidence of congenital rubella, but less so in the UK than in the USA. Figure 12.3a shows the antibody profiles by age group of people in a UK population during the period 1969–85, rubella immunization of teenage girls having been introduced in 1980. The antibody profiles are similar in pre- and postvaccination years. Figure 12.3b shows a similar analysis of a population in Finland which, in 1982, adopted a policy more like that of the USA, vaccine being given to both boys and girls aged 14 months and 6 years. Note the sharp increase in seropositivity in the younger age groups from 1984 onwards.

In 1988 a combined MMR vaccine was introduced into the UK, since when there has been much controversy concerning its safety. This issue is discussed in Chapter 37.

The policy is now, in outline, as follows.

- **Boys and girls aged 12–15 months.** First dose of MMR vaccine.
- **Boys and girls aged 3–5 years.** If no documentary evidence of previous vaccination, second dose of MMR before entering primary school (i.e. at same time as diphtheria–tetanus–polio booster).
- **School leavers** are offered MMR vaccine if they have not previously been immunized against rubella or measles.
- **Non-immune women**, before pregnancy or after delivery. Single rubella vaccine.

It is now accepted that the immunity resulting from vaccination, although not as solid as that following natural infection, is sufficiently durable to allow a programme of this type. Its aim is the eventual elimination of rubella, measles, and mumps from the UK. Now that the acceptance rate has reached 90 per cent, this goal is well within sight.

Contraindications to rubella vaccine

The main contraindications are those applying to other live vaccines, i.e. a febrile illness, allergy to one of the constituents (rare) and defective immunity. The important additional contraindication is **early pregnancy**; women are advised not to become pregnant a month before to a month after receiving rubella vaccine. That said, no instance of fetal damage has been recorded following inadvertent vaccination shortly before pregnancy or during the first trimester, although serological evidence of infection *in utero* has been obtained in a small proportion of the babies going to term. There is very little indication for terminating a pregnancy if rubella vaccine is given inadvertently.

Reinfections

Reinfections, both after second attacks of rubella and immunization, have been recorded and confirmed serologically. As far as is known, such episodes, if in early pregnancy, pose little or no risk to the fetus, probably because they are not accompanied by the viraemia characteristic of primary infections.

4 Reminders

- Rubella virus is an **enveloped ssRNA virus** belonging to the *Togaviridae*. It does not naturally infect species other than humans.
- Rubella (German measles) is a worldwide infection of childhood. It is spread by the **respiratory route** and causes a mild febrile illness with **lymphadenopathy** and **rash**. In older people, especially women, it is liable to cause **arthropathy**. It is important because **infection during early pregnancy damages the fetus** (Chapter 31).
- For this reason, efforts are made to prevent infection of women of childbearing age by:
  - **mass immunization** of the child population with MMR vaccine;
  - **serological screening** of certain categories of adult women and immunization of those without rubella antibody.

Parvoviruses

1 Introduction

It might be thought that viruses as a class represent the ultimate in parasitism, reliant as they are on their host cells to provide most of the machinery for replication. The parvoviruses, however, show a still further degree of dependence, as they can replicate only in the presence of another virus or of active DNA synthesis in rapidly dividing host cells. The reason lies in their minute size, for these are the smallest of all viruses (Latin *parvus* = small).

2 Properties of the viruses

2.1 Classification

The family *Parvoviridae* contains two subfamilies, the *Densovirinae*, which do not concern us as they infect only arthropods; and the *Parvovirinae*, in which there are three genera:

- *Parvovirus*, which takes its name from that of the family, and infects only animals and birds;
- *Dependovirus*, named for dependence on a helper virus, usually an adenovirus, but occasionally a herpesvirus, to assist in replication;
- *Erythrovirus*, which has only one member, known as B19, the only parvovirus causing significant disease in humans (Table 13.1).

Table 13.1 Parvoviruses infecting humans

Genus	Viruses	Diseases
Erythrovirus	B19	Erythema infectiosum Fetal infections Aplastic crises
Parvovirus	RAV-1*	Possibly implicated in rheumatoid arthritis
Dependovirus	Adeno-associated viruses (AAV) types 1–5	AAV-2 possibly implicated in fetal infections

* Classification in this genus is tentative.

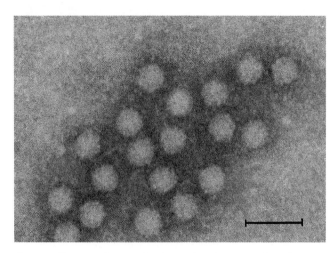

Fig. 13.1 Electron micrograph of parvovirus in serum. The virions are clumped together by antibody molecules. (Courtesy of Dr Ian Christie.) Scale bar = 50 nm.

2.2 Morphology

These are non-enveloped viruses, with icosahedral symmetry, about 22 nm in diameter (Fig. 13.1).

2.3 Genome

The *Parvoviridae* are the only DNA viruses with single-stranded nucleic acid. They were thought to be double-stranded until it was discovered that each virion contains either a positive or a negative-sense strand, a unique situation. A 'hairpin' loop at the end of each genome initiates replication of the complementary strand (Fig. 13.2). The ssDNA is about 5 kb long.

2.4 Polypeptides

The number of polypeptides that can be encoded by such a small genome is limited: there are only two or three structural and up to four NS proteins; this explains why parvoviruses are so dependent on external helper functions.

2.5 Replication

The virus attaches to a globoside or P antigen receptor, is endocytosed and migrates to the nucleus where replication of virus DNA and transcription of mRNA take place. Nine viral mRNA species and five viral proteins are detectable.

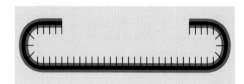

Fig. 13.2 Parvovirus genome.

The dependoviruses used to be called 'adeno-associated viruses' as they were seen by EM in association with enteric adenoviruses (Chapter 8). The genome becomes integrated into host-cell DNA and is active only when the cell becomes infected with a helper virus that can provide the enzymes essential for replication. The parvoviruses, on the other hand, replicate only in rapidly dividing host cells, in which S-phase functions provide the necessary help.

3 Clinical and pathological aspects

3.1 Clinical features

The parvoviruses infecting humans cause three main syndromes.

Erythema infectiosum

This 'infectious rash' is sometimes known as 'fifth disease', which is less of a mouthful. (The original classification of the exanthematous illnesses of childhood comprised six diseases: the other five are measles, rubella, scarlet fever, exanthem subitum, and Duke's disease, a rash of obscure aetiology.) A more picturesque name is 'slapped cheek syndrome ', which helps you to remember that, especially in children, the presenting feature is often **erythema over the malar areas**, followed within the next 4 days by a maculopapular rash on the trunk and limbs, which may persist for 2 or 3 weeks. Volunteer and field studies show the incubation period to be 13–18 days. There may be some fever and malaise in the early stages, and mild febrile illness without rash is common.

This is predominantly an infection of children but adults may also acquire it; in them, and **particularly in women**, the **joints** are much more likely to be involved. Those of the hand and fingers are most often affected, but there may also be arthropathy of the arms, legs, and spine. Arthralgia may persist for a few weeks.

Differential diagnosis

Erythema infectiosum may be diagnosed by the characteristic rash, especially during an epidemic, but differential diagnosis from other illnesses with fever and rashes is not always easy. The syndrome of fever, rash, and arthropathy may be clinically indistinguishable from rubella but it is essential to establish the correct diagnosis with absolute certainty in pregnancy; fortunately, laboratory tests can give the answer.

Meningitis and encephalitis following B19 infections have been described, but are very rare.

Fetal infection

B19 infection in pregnancy may result in fetal death; this topic is dealt with in Chapter 31.

Aplastic crisis

The need of parvoviruses for actively dividing cells in which to replicate is illustrated by their lytic effect on red cell precursors:

this is not clinically obvious in otherwise healthy people, but in those with a chronic haemolytic anaemia, e.g. sickle cell anaemia or thalassaemia, parvovirus infection may precipitate an **aplastic crisis** with very low haemoglobin and disappearance of circulating reticulocytes. This is because the virus replicates in and damages the rapidly dividing late normoblasts. Such events may be fatal if not treated rapidly by blood transfusion.

Persistent infection

Persistent infection with B19, associated with chronic anaemia, has been observed in a variety of conditions associated with immunodeficiency, including acute lymphocytic leukaemia, HIV infection, and therapeutic immunosuppression. Persistence may be aided by the continual appearance of new mutated strains.

3.2 Epidemiology

Infections with B19 occur worldwide, and tend to occur in cycles with peaks about every 5 years. Epidemics occur during late winter and early spring and mainly affect young school children. Spread is by the **respiratory route**: occasional transmissions by blood transfusion have been reported. In most areas, the prevalence of antibodies rises from ≈10 per cent in young children to over 80 per cent in the elderly.

3.3 Pathogenesis and pathology

After primary infection of the upper respiratory tract there is a viraemia lasting about a week. The dominant feature of infection is the high lytic activity of the virus in rapidly dividing cells, which accounts for its ravages both in fetal cells and in the adult haemopoietic system.

3.4 Immune response

Clearance of virus from the blood coincides with a sharp IgM antibody response, followed shortly by the appearance of IgG antibody. The rash and arthropathy in erythema infectiosum are probably mediated by immunological factors, including the deposition of immune complexes.

3.5 Laboratory diagnosis

These viruses cannot readily be grown in the laboratory, but can be found in the blood by **EM** during the viraemic stage. Virus DNA can also be identified by various tests, including the PCR and dot-blot hybridization. **Detection of IgM antibody by ELISA** indicates a current or recent infection, whereas the much more prolonged presence of IgG is a sign of past infection.

3.6 Control

There is at present no specific vaccine or antiviral therapy for parvovirus infections. Prophylaxis is directed mainly at prevention of spread to highly susceptible people, e.g. those with severe anaemias, and to laboratory staff who may be exposed to high concentrations of virus.

4 Reminders

- The *Parvoviridae* are the smallest viruses and the only ones containing **ssDNA**. Virions contain either positive or negative-sense strands. They need help from other viruses or from rapidly dividing host cells in order to replicate.

- The only parvovirus causing significant disease in humans is B19, the sole member of the genus *Erythrovirus*. It causes:
  - **erythema infectiosum**, a febrile illness with rash spread by the respiratory route, mainly in young children. Cure is spontaneous. In adults, especially women, there may be arthropathy;
  - **fetal infections** (see Chapter 31);
  - **aplastic crises** in people with pre-existing chronic haemolytic anaemia, e.g. thalassaemia or sickle cell disease, or who have immune deficiencies.

- The differential diagnosis of erythema infectiosum may be difficult clinically, but can be made by appropriate laboratory tests. In pregnancy, it is particularly important to distinguish it from rubella.

Poxviruses

1 Introduction

In a book of this size there is a great temptation to omit material that is no longer directly relevant to current practice; however, it would be unthinkable to discuss the poxviruses without an account, albeit briefly, of smallpox, the great success story in the fight against infectious disease and one that provides many valuable lessons. This epic provides at least three 'firsts': the first vaccine, the first disease to be totally eradicated by immunization, and the first virus infection against which chemotherapy was clinically effective. Although smallpox itself is now extinct, other poxviruses infect humans; and as we shall see in Chapter 37, one of them may be used in a rather surprising way to immunize against quite different diseases. Because of the threat of bioterrorism, some countries are stockpiling vaccinia vaccine against smallpox and safer vaccines are being developed to be held in a strategic reserve.

In many ways smallpox would be a poor choice for a biowarfare virus because of its relatively low infectivity and long incubation period, during which a population could be immunized. A more virulent or antigenically different virus could, in theory, be genetically engineered but only with great difficulty.

2 Properties of the viruses

2.1 Classification

The family *Poxviridae* contains two subfamilies: the *Chordopoxvirinae*, with eight genera infecting a wide range of mammals and birds; and the *Entomopoxvirinae*, with three genera that affect insects only. Most of these viruses do not infect humans. Others are pathogenic both for animals and humans and two, smallpox and molluscum, only for humans (Table 14.1). The genera are distinguished on the basis of morphology, genome structure, growth characteristics, and serological reactions; there is close serological relationship between the viruses within each genus and good cross-protection between genera.

2.2 Morphology

These are the largest viruses of all; the orthopoxviruses are brick-shaped, whereas orf and molluscum tend to be ovoid (Fig. 14.1). They measure about 230×270 nm and when suitably stained can just be seen with an ordinary light microscope.

Table 14.1 Poxviruses that infect humans

Genus	Virus	Primary host(s)	Clinical features in humans
Orthopoxvirus	Variola	Man	Smallpox
	Vaccinia	Man	Vesicular vaccination lesion
	Cowpox	Cattle, cats, rodents	Lesions on hands
	Monkeypox	Monkeys, squirrels	Resembles smallpox
Parapoxvirus	Pseudocowpox	Prairie dogs (USA), cattle	Localized nodular lesions ('milkers' nodes')
	Orf	Sheep, goats	Localized vesiculogranulomatous lesions
Yatapoxvirus	Tanapox	Monkeys	Vesicular skin lesions and febrile illness
Molluscipoxvirus	Molluscum	Man	Multiple small skin nodules

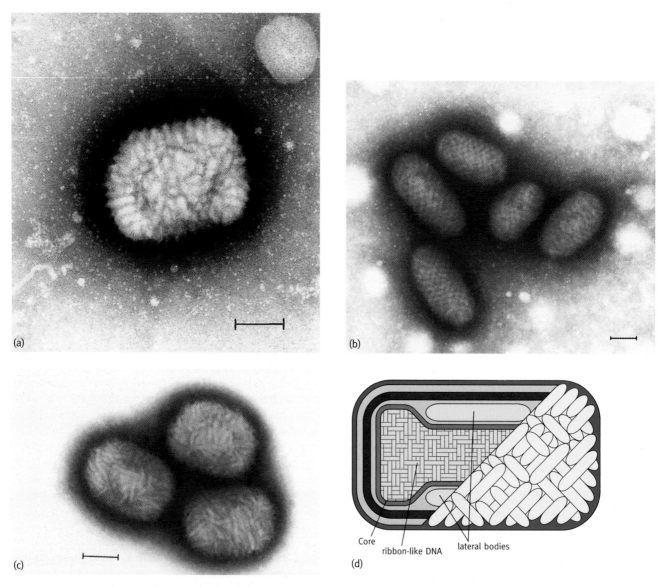

(a)

(b)

(c)

(d)

Core   ribbon-like DNA   lateral bodies

Fig. 14.1 Electron micrographs of poxvirus. **(a)** Vaccinia; **(b)** orf; **(c)** molluscum contagiosum; **(d)** model of poxvirus showing lateral bodies, ribbon-like DNA, and dumbbell core structure. Scale bar = 100 nm.

The poxviruses are neither icosahedral nor helical: their structure is referred to as **complex**. The outer membrane consists of a network of tubules and is sometimes surrounded by an envelope. Inside there is a dumbbell-shaped core structure and two accompanying lateral bodies, so named after their location in the virion.

2.3 Genome

*The nucleic acid is **dsDNA** ranging in size from 186 kbp (variola) to 220 kbp (cowpox). This large genome codes for more than 100 polypeptides, including a DNA-dependent RNA polymerase and other enzymes. Centrally located genes are conserved and are essential for virus replication, whereas genes near the two termini affect host range and virulence.*

2.4 Replication

Unlike most DNA viruses, the **poxviruses replicate only in the cytoplasm**, and can replicate in cells without a nucleus.

The virion enters the cell either by endocytosis or by a fusion event. The viral core enters the cytoplasm and acts as a scaffolding for subsequent replication events. Furthermore, the virus transports many essential enzymes such as viral transcriptase, transcription factors, capping and methylating enzymes and a poly(A) polymerase. Transcription of viral DNA is therefore initiated rapidly and approximately 100 early viral genes are activated, particularly genes coding for enzymes involved in viral DNA replication. Transcription of intermediate and late genes is initiated at the same time as DNA replication.

Certain viral gene products may interfere with the host response to infection and inhibit cytokine, chemokine, or complement production or confer resistance to IFN by interfering with IFN-induced antiviral proteins, cell signalling pathways, or apoptosis.

Virus assembly takes place in particular areas of the cytoplasm and immature viruses can be visualized quite easily. During maturation the virions move to the Golgi complex, where they are enveloped before being released by budding or by cell disruption. Some virions are enveloped and these may have some advantages, including speed of uptake by cells.

3 Clinical and pathological aspects of smallpox

3.1 Historical note

The Anglo-Saxon word 'pokkes' meant a pouch and refers to the characteristic vesicular lesions. The term 'small pox' was introduced during the sixteenth century to distinguish it from the 'great pox', or syphilis. The Latin term, *variola*, means a spot. It seems likely that smallpox has been with us for a very long time: the mummy of the Pharaoh Rameses V (1100 BC) bears lesions highly suggestive of this infection (Fig. 14.2) and there are many later accounts of its ravages. Indeed, smallpox was so wide-

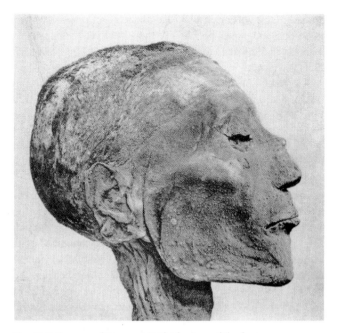

Fig. 14.2 Mummy of Rameses V. The lesions of the face are suggestive of smallpox. (Reproduced, with permission, from Dixon, C.W. (1962). *Smallpox*, J&A Churchill.)

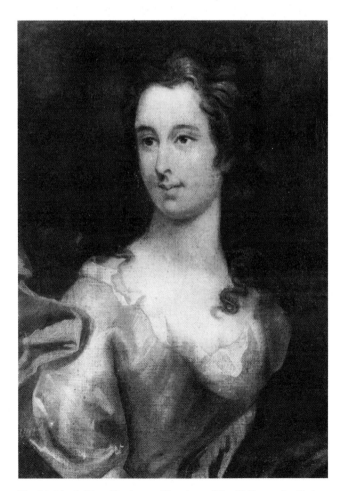

Fig. 14.3 Lady Mary Montague. (Courtesy of the Wellcome Institute Library, London.)

spread that it was often regarded as the norm rather than the exception and few people—if they survived—escaped its disfiguring scars. In India it was thought to be a divine visitation and even had its own goddess, Kakurani.

The observation that smallpox could be prevented by inoculation of healthy people with material from the lesions seems to have originated in China. From there an account of the practice (**variolation**) was sent by Joseph Lister to The Royal Society in 1700 and was followed by others from Turkey. Variolation caused a comparatively mild infection from which the subject usually recovered and effectively protected against the natural disease.

There now enters one of the most interesting characters in the story, Lady Mary Wortley Montague (Fig. 14.3). As wife of the British ambassador, this highly accomplished young woman saw variolation practised in Turkey and was so convinced of its safety and efficacy that in 1717 she had her own small son inoculated. Lady Mary had a vested interest in the subject because she herself had been scarred by the disease; on returning to England she used all her efforts and her many highly placed contacts to have the practice generally accepted. In the event, variolation enjoyed but a short vogue before being superseded by the safer method of vaccination.

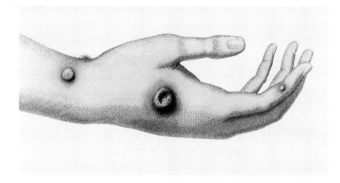

Fig. 14.5 Cowpox lesions on the arm of the milkmaid, Sarah Nelmes. Material from these lesions was used by Edward Jenner to vaccinate James Phipps. (Courtesy of the Wellcome Institute Library, London.)

The story of Edward Jenner's discovery in 1796 that inoculation with cowpox would prevent smallpox is well known; but it is not so widely appreciated that others had made similar observations, notably Benjamin Jesty, a Dorset farmer, who inoculated his own family. To Jenner, however, goes the credit for showing that, following the inoculation of young James Phipps with cowpox (Figs 14.4 and 14.5), deliberate inoculation with smallpox material failed to induce the disease.

The early vaccines were derived from cowpox (Latin *vacca* = cow) and propagated by arm-to-arm inoculation. During the twentieth century, other strains of poxvirus (vaccinia) that could be grown in quantity on the skins of calves and other animals were used.

With improved methods for preparing vaccine in bulk and for testing its safety and potency, vaccination was widely practised; nevertheless, wide regional differences in uptake ensured that the disease would continue to smoulder on, flaring at intervals into epidemics. In 1966, faced with this situation, WHO voted $2.5 million for an immunization campaign designed to eradicate smallpox completely within the next decade (Fig. 14.6). This vast enterprise is referred to again in Chapter 37, but needs a book to itself (see 'Further reading'). Its success may be judged by the fact that the last case of naturally acquired infection was recorded—in Somalia—in October 1977, only 10 months beyond the target date fixed 10 years previously.

3.2 Clinical aspects

It is very gratifying to be able to write this section in the past tense!

There were two main categories of smallpox, caused by slightly different viruses: **variola major** had a mortality of about 30 per cent whereas **variola minor**, or **alastrim**, killed less than 1 per cent of its victims. The incubation period was usually 10–12 days; a febrile illness of sudden onset lasting 3–4 days was followed by the appearance of a rash progressing from macules to papules, vesicles, and pustules (Fig. 14.7), which then formed crusts. Surviving patients were often left with unsightly scars or pockmarks. The distribution of the rash was **centrifugal**, i.e. it affected the extremities more than the

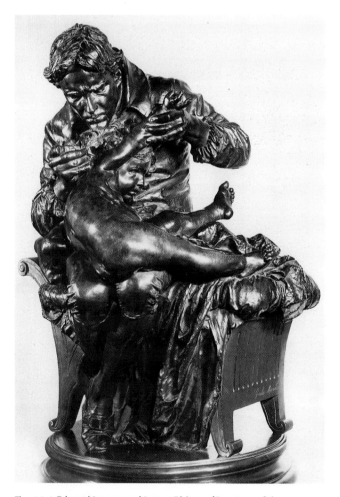

Fig. 14.4 Edward Jenner and James Phipps. (Courtesy of the Wellcome Institute Library, London.)

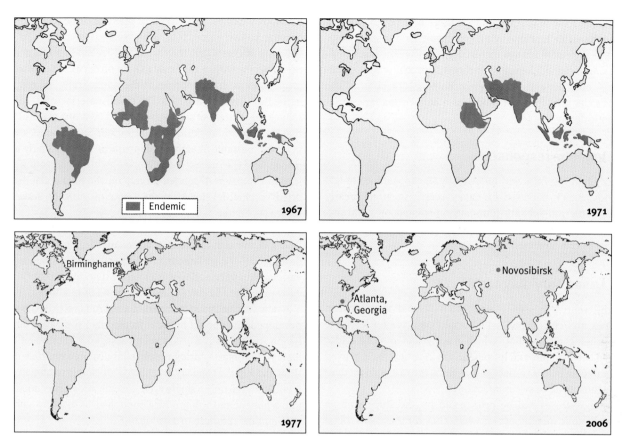

Fig. 14.6 The global eradication of smallpox by the World Health Organization. (Taken with permission from Fenner, F. *et al.* (1988). *Smallpox and its Eradication*, World Health Organization, Geneva.)

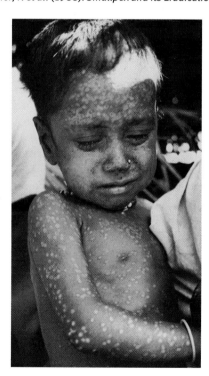

Fig. 14.7 Smallpox. This 2-year-old Bangladeshi girl was the last case of smallpox to be seen on the Asian subcontinent, and the last case in the world of variola major, the more severe form of the disease. (Photograph from World Health Organization.)

trunk, as opposed to the centripetal rash of chickenpox. Haemorrhagic and fulminating forms occurred, which were rapidly lethal. Modified smallpox with few lesions and comparatively little constitutional upset was sometimes seen in people who had been vaccinated some years previously.

3.3 Epidemiology

The main source of smallpox infection was the patient's upper respiratory tract in the early stages of the disease, but fomites such as bedding and clothing were also of some importance. The disease was mostly prevalent in the Eastern countries, the Indian subcontinent, and Latin America, both in endemic and epidemic form. Spread from country to country was facilitated by increases in the volume and speed of international travel; and, in the absence of universal vaccination, importations into Europe and North America occurred with some frequency well into the twentieth century. The last outbreak in the UK was 1962, due to imported smallpox; the last case, however, was a secondary infection from laboratory-acquired smallpox in the University of Birmingham in the UK in 1978.

3.4 Pathogenesis and pathology

The pattern was that of an acute generalized infection (see Chapter 4, Section 4.4). The lesions were caused by direct viral invasion and the vesicles contained large numbers of virions. Although variola is primarily a dermotropic virus, organs other than the skin were always involved, and in severe cases complications included keratitis, arthritis, bronchitis and pneumonitis, enteritis and encephalitis. Bacterial infection of the skin vesicles was frequent, and was a serious matter in pre-antibiotic days.

3.5 Immune response

An early IgM response was followed by the appearance of IgG antibody, which persisted for many years. An attack nearly always conferred lifelong immunity, mediated by neutralizing antibody. Recovery from infection was, however, largely effected by cell-mediated responses.

3.6 Laboratory diagnosis

The differential diagnosis most often needed was between smallpox and chickenpox, which could on occasion resemble each other clinically. **EM**, which readily and rapidly distinguished between pox and herpes virions in vesicle fluid, proved most valuable in this respect and remains the principal method for diagnosing all poxvirus infections.

Most poxviruses can be propagated on the chick embryo chorioallantoic membrane, on which they form circumscribed pocks, 2–3 mm in diameter, or in cell cultures. Molluscum has not so far been grown in the laboratory.

3.7 Control

Specific treatment

Methisazone, a thiosemicarbazone, would prevent or modify an attack if given during the incubation period; but soon after the discovery of this, the first effective antiviral compound, it was made redundant by the success of the vaccination campaign. New antivirals are now being developed in case the virus re-emerges. Marboran, a thio-semicarbazone, was used to treat some of the last smallpox infections three decades ago; a more modern drug, cidofovir (HPMPC) shows antiviral effects in animal models.

Immunization

Prophylaxis depended on vaccination, which not only induced immunity to subsequent exposure, but also protected if given early enough during the 12-day incubation period. The policy varied with time, place, and circumstances. In some countries, including the UK until 1948, vaccination of infants was—at least nominally—compulsory. Epidemics were contained by mass vaccination until the later stages of the world eradication programme, when this approach was replaced by selective vaccination of contacts.

Vaccinia and smallpox vaccine

We mentioned in the 'Historical note' (p. 113) that strains of poxviruses other than cowpox were developed for making smallpox vaccines. The origins of many of these strains, which became known as vaccinia, are obscure; but analysis of their genomes suggests that they are closely related and form a distinct species within the genus Orthopoxvirus. The virus was propagated in large quantities on the skins of calves, sheep, or—in the East—water buffaloes. The crude material was treated to reduce the content of skin bacteria, and kept in a glycerol solution at subzero temperatures until used. Such vaccines were, however, unstable at ambient temperatures, particularly in the tropics; and the success of the World Health Organization eradication campaign depended largely on the heat-stable freeze-dried vaccine developed at the Lister Institute of Preventive Medicine, Elstree.

Inoculation of a small quantity of vaccinia into the superficial layers of the skin resulted in a vesicular lesion that was well developed 7–9 days later and rapidly evoked cross-immunity to variola; thus vaccination was effective if performed during the early part of the 12-day incubation period of smallpox.

A new vaccine called 'more attenuated Ankara' (MVA) is being developed and should be safer to use than the earlier animal lymph strains. The virus has been passaged 500 times on chick embryo fibroblasts during which it has acquired multiple mutations and lost the capacity to replicate efficiently in human cells. It will undergo only a single cycle of replication once inoculated into a patient and will produce enough virus to allow a protective immune response to develop.

Survival of variola virus

Following tragic episodes of laboratory-acquired infection it was internationally agreed that samples of the virus should be held only in two maximum security laboratories, one in Atlanta, USA and the other in the Novosibirsk, Russia; furthermore, large stocks of vaccine are held in store for use in the unlikely event of a reappearance of the disease. Even so, in view of the depredations of smallpox, the herculean efforts needed to eradicate it from the planet and its possible use in biological warfare, the World Health Assembly recommended in 1996 that all remaining stocks of variola virus should be destroyed in June 1999. At the time of writing (April 2006) this decision has still not been implemented. The complete destruction of this virus is controversial, as, however dangerous, every living species embodies a unique fund of biological information and the obliteration of any one of them represents an irreplaceable loss to future generations. In this case, however, the complete nucleotide sequences of several smallpox viruses are known, and the viral DNA can be cloned into bacterial plasmids in such a way that it cannot be expressed, but still embodies the genetic information as a permanent record of one of the great viral plagues of mankind.

In view of the ability of poxviruses to survive for long periods in the dried state, it has been suggested that infective smallpox virus might still exist in preserved cadavers; this seems unlikely, but it is interesting that in 1986, Italian workers claimed to have serological and electron microscopic evidence of the virus in a Neapolitan mummy dating from the sixteenth century AD.

4 Other poxvirus infections

As we have seen, poxviruses are widespread in nature. Here, we shall briefly describe only those that infect humans.

4.1 Cowpox

Like most of the agents in this family, cowpox is, as its name implies, a zoonosis (Table 14.1); infection of humans is rare but may be seen in rural practices. Although recent evidence points to cats and rodents rather than bovines as the main reservoir of infection, most cases in humans seem to be acquired from cows with sores on their teats. The lesions usually present on the hands or face and resemble severe vaccinia infections.

Treatment with **anti-vaccinia immunoglobulin** may be helpful if given early.

4.2 Monkeypox

This orthopoxvirus zoonosis occurs in western and central Africa; it is of some concern because it causes an illness in humans very similar to smallpox, with a significant mortality rate. Importation into the USA of exotic pets from Africa, such as Gambian giant rats, is thought to be responsible for subsequent transmission of virus to other USA pet animals including prairie dogs. In 2003 there was an outbreak of monkeypox in several of the north-eastern states of the USA. As of July that year, 71 cases were reported to CDC: a number were severe but fortunately there were no deaths. The main clinical features were rash, fever, respiratory symptoms, and lymphadenopathy. Prairie dogs were an important source of infection, but elsewhere, squirrels seem to be the main reservoir, infection occurring mainly in children who can acquire it by playing with captive animals. Human-to-human transmission is more frequent than was at first thought, but control by vaccination is not difficult.

Monkeypox is the only poxvirus infection that might possibly call for prevention by vaccination, which, as mentioned above, is accomplished by inoculation of vaccinia virus into the skin. This procedure is normally very safe; however, recently, vaccination of relatively large numbers of people as a precaution against terrorist attacks revealed a previously unknown risk of cardiac myopathy in a small minority of patients.

Could monkeypox mutate to smallpox? The question was raised as soon as infections in humans were recognized; but fortunately the poxviruses, like others with DNA genomes, are genetically very stable, so that this dire possibility can, one hopes, be ignored.

4.3 Parapoxviruses

Pseudocowpox infects various species of cattle, whereas **orf** is found in sheep and goats in which it causes contagious pustular dermatitis; the viruses are very similar. In humans, lesions occur on the hands and face after contact with infected farm animals; the lesions of pseudocowpox are nodular ('milkers's nodes'), whereas those of orf are granulomatous. Parapoxvirus lesions are characteristically painless and resolve over a period of weeks without specific treatment.

4.4 Tanapox

This virus takes its name from the Tana River in Kenya, where it was first diagnosed. It is prevalent in monkeys in Kenya and Zaïre but, unlike monkeypox, appears to be spread by insect bites. There is usually only one vesicular lesion but its appearance is preceded by fever and quite severe malaise. Recovery is uneventful.

4.5 Molluscum contagiosum

Molluscum is the sole member of *the Molluscipoxvirus* genus; its study is not helped by our inability to grow it in the laboratory. **Molluscum contagiosum** affects only humans; it is a comparatively common skin condition, characterized by **multiple small (1–10 mm) nodular lesions** mostly on the trunk (Fig. 14.8). They become umbilicated and contain caseous material in which 'molluscum bodies' can be readily demonstrated. These are quite large (30 μm long) ovoid structures containing many

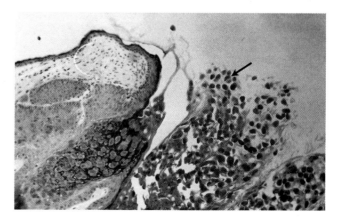

Fig. 14.8 Molluscum contagiosum. (courtesy of the Department of Dermatology, The Royal London Hospital, London).

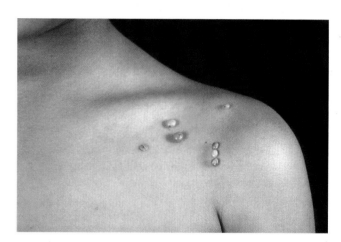

Fig. 14.9 Section of a molluscum contagiosum lesion of the skin. The small, ovoid molluscum bodies (arrowed) are packets of virus particles.

virions (Fig. 14.9). The diagnosis is usually obvious from the clinical appearance, but in case of doubt, a simple test is to identify the molluscum bodies in expressed material stained with Giemsa or Lugol's iodine. The virions themselves can readily be found by EM.

Transmission is by contamination of skin abrasions through contact; the infection can be sexually acquired. A molluscum lesion at the lid margin often results in severe **conjunctivitis** and **keratitis**, which resolve when the nodule is treated.

Disappearance of the lesions is often spontaneous, but can be helped along by cryotherapy, curettage, or treatment with caustic agents such as salicylic acid or phenol.

4.6 Ectromelia

Ectromelia, or mousepox, does not infect humans, but is mentioned here for two reasons. First, it provided the model for Dr Frank Fenner's research on the pathogenesis of acute viral infections in humans (Chapter 4); and second, it may become endemic—and very difficult to eradicate—in stocks of laboratory mice.

5 Reminders

- The Poxviridae are comparatively large, brick-shaped or ovoid viruses with a **complex** structure. Their genome is **dsDNA,** ranging in size from 186 kbp (variola) to 230 kbp (cowpox). **They replicate only in the cytoplasm** and transport into the cell transcriptases, capping and methylating enzymes and poly(A) polymerase.

- 100 early viral genes code for enzymes involved in DNA replication. Intermediate and late genes are transcribed at the onset of DNA replication and code for structural proteins and proteins, which may interfere with host response to infection.

- Most poxviruses cause zoonoses, but some are pathogenic for humans. Of these, smallpox was the most important until eradicated in 1977 by the WHO vaccination campaign. It was an acute generalized infection: the mortality of variola major was about 30 per cent and that of a milder form, variola minor or alastrim, less than 1 per cent.

- **Monkeypox** is a similar infection and occurs in West Africa; it is occasionally transmitted to humans, but person-to-person spread is rare and there was a recent outbreak in the USA linked to pet shops that had imported mammals from Africa, and prairie dogs.

- **Cowpox, pseudocowpox,** and **orf** affect farm animals and occasionally cause local lesions, which resolve spontaneously, on the fingers and faces of people coming in contact with them. Cowpox may be treated with anti-vaccinia serum.

- **Molluscum contagiosum** causes multiple small nodular lesions containing packets of virions known as molluscum bodies. A lesion at the lid margin may cause **conjunctivitis** and **keratitis**. The lesions may eventually disappear spontaneously, but can be treated by cryotherapy, curettage, or caustic chemicals.

- **EM** is the most important technique for diagnosing all poxvirus infections and units able to rapidly diagnose smallpox have been set up again to counter bioterrorism or natural emergence of monkey pox.

- A new generation of safer, more highly attenuated vaccines such as 'more attenuated Ankara' is being prepared in cell culture and can be stockpiled.

- Smallpox would be a poor choice as a bio-weapon, but the storage of vaccine just in case is a sensible public health strategy.

Papovaviruses

1 Introduction

In the last edition of this book, the family *Papovaviridae* was split into two genera, Papillomavirus and Polyomavirus, the latter containing cell vacuolating agents that are not associated with any disease. There are now two families, Papillomaviridae and Polyomaviridae, each containing only one genus, Papillomavirus and Polyomavirus respectively. These changes are of academic interest only as far as our readers are concerned.

The name of this family is yet another example of the acronyms so beloved by virologists; although Papova sounds like a Russian ballerina, its component syllables in fact help you to remember the characteristics of the viruses concerned.

pa = papillomaviruses

po = polyomaviruses

va = vacuolating agents.

The -oma components of these names immediately alert you to the fact that these agents have something to do with neoplasia (Greek *oma* = tumour) and indeed, the papillomaviruses have now displaced herpes simplex as the centre of attention in relation to cancers of the genital tract.

2 Properties of the viruses

2.1 Classification

The Family *Papovaviridae* consists of two genera, *Papillomavirus* and *Polyomavirus*; the vacuolating agents belong to the latter genus, but are distinguished from the other members by their lack of association with any known disease.

2.2 Morphology

The virions are **icosahedral** and have no envelopes. The papillomaviruses are about 55 nm in diameter (Fig. 15.1) and the polyomaviruses are slightly smaller, at about 45 nm.

2.3 Genomes

The polyomavirus genomes are circular supercoiled dsDNA, and code for a comparatively small number of polypeptides, some of which are, however, important in transforming normal cells to

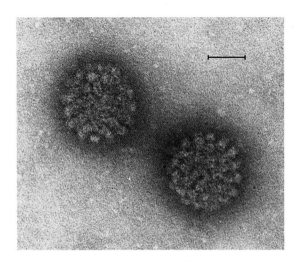

Fig. 15.1 Electron microscope of papillomaviruses. Scale bar = 50 nm.

the malignant state. The polyomaviruses particularly have compact regulatory regions and have a number of overlapping genes to compensate for the small size of the genome (see Fig. 2.7(c)).

The papillomavirus genome is 8 kbp in length with 8 ORF on one strand (Fig. 15.2). The early ORFs code for viral structural proteins. A long central region (1 kb in length) called the upstream regulatory region lies between the early and late ORFs that might determine human papillomavirus (HPV) tissue specificity. There are several internal transcription regulatory motifs including enhancers and silencers and these may act as cis-acting elements by binding to cellular and viral proteins that transregulate viral genome function. Transcription of viral genes results in many mRNAs because of multiple splicing patterns. Some mRNAs are translated as fusion proteins, whereas others are polycistronic. To give an example, early E1 (helicase) and E2 (transcript modular) proteins are involved in viral DNA replication, whereas E2 may also repress the activity of promotors by binding closely to them. E5 is a small protein that takes part in oncogenic events, perhaps by interacting with cellular growth factor receptors. The late ORF (L1 and L2) code for capsid proteins. L1 is the major capsid protein and L2 a minor capsid protein involved in DNA binding and encapsidation. Because of the multiple splicing patterns there are many more proteins than ORF.

2.4 Replication

Papillomavirus infection is initiated in dividing epidermal cells or basal layer cells of the skin. The viruses are very host and tissue specific and gene expression is linked to the differential state of the epithelial cell.

The polyomavirus binds to sialic containing glycoproteins and enters a cell by endocytosis and intracellular fusion, releasing virions to the perinuclear regions of the cell. Viral uncoating occurs in the nucleus. There are essentially two stages of viral replication. First, the mRNAs of the early viral proteins are transcribed from one DNA strand in a counter-clockwise direction. The mRNAs for late viral proteins are transcribed from the other strand in a clockwise direction. The first early proteins are the large and small T antigens, which bind to three sites on the viral genome, for example, binding

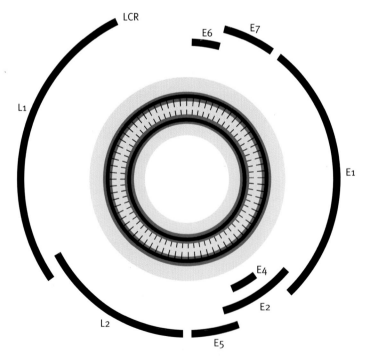

Fig. 15.2 Papillomavirus genome and encoded late proteins. Labelled late proteins are L1, L2 (capsid proteins), early proteins are E6, E7 (oncogenic proteins), E4, E5 and E1, E2 (DNA replication proteins). LCR is the long control region.

to one site stops binding of RNA polymerase and halts early transcription. Differential splicing occurs for late transcripts for VP1, VP2, and VP3 proteins. Finally, the large T antigen starts viral DNA replication. Replication begins with displacement of viral DNA histones. The supercoiled DNA is unwound. HPV DNA replication moves bidirectionally. The new viruses begin to assemble in the nucleus and are released by lysis of the cell. The 20–100 copies of the viral genome are detected per cell.

The oncogenic types 16 and 18 have two oncogenes (E6 and E7) that encode viral proteins; these interact with cellular gene products that normally have tumour suppressor activity.

3 Clinical and pathological aspects of papillomavirus infections

3.1 Clinical features

Papillomaviruses or their antigens have been detected in a wide range of mammals and in some birds. Because, for the reason just explained, they cannot be isolated and distinguished by serological tests, they **are classified on the basis of their degree of DNA homology**, i.e. on how closely their nucleotide sequences correspond: there must be less than 50% homology with any other type for a papillomavirus to be accepted as a new genotype. They cause disease only in skin and mucous mem-

branes, where they give rise to warty lesions. These are usually benign, but some may become malignant; there are distinct—but not invariable—associations between the type of HPV, the anatomical site involved, and the potential to cause malignant lesions. Table 15.1 gives examples of lesions caused by papillomaviruses and the types of virus most commonly associated with them; this list is not exhaustive and may vary somewhat according to the author.

Predominantly benign lesions

Cutaneous warts

The virus is transmitted from infected skin, either by direct contact or through fomites, and enters its new host through abrasions. Swimming pools and changing rooms are fertile sources of infection, and skin warts are most liable to affect the younger age groups.

   The common wart (verruca vulgaris, Fig. 15.3) has a characteristically roughened surface; the excrescences are usually a few millimetres in diameter and may occur in quite large numbers anywhere on the skin, but especially on the hands, knees, and feet. They usually cause no inconvenience, apart from the cosmetic aspect, but plantar warts on the soles of the feet are pressed inward by the weight of the body; they may be painful and call for more urgent treatment than those in other sites. **Flat warts (verrucae planae)**, as their name implies, are flatter and

Table 15.1 Lesions caused by human papillomaviruses (HPV)

Type of lesion	Site	HPV types*
Predominantly benign lesions		
Common warts	Skin, various sites	2,4
Plantar and palmar warts	Hands, feet	1,2,4
Butchers' warts	Hands	7
Flat warts	Skin, various sites	3
Genital warts (condylomata acuminate)	Cervix, various sites	6,11
Juvenile laryngeal papilloma	Larynx	6,11
Malignant or potentially malignant lesions		
Flat warts	Skin	**10**
Bowenoid papulosis	Vulva, penis	**16**
Pre-malignant and malignant intraepithelial	Cervix, penis	Many types, including 6, 11, **16**, **18**, 31, 39–45, 51–56
Neoplasia		
Carcinoma	Cervix, penis	**16**, **18**, 31, 33, 35, 39, 45, 51, 52, 56, 58, 59, 68, 73, 82
Papilloma/carcinoma	Larynx	**16**
Epidermodysplasia verruciformis	Skin, various sites	Many types including **5**, **8**, 9, **10**, 12, **14**, 15, 17, 19–29

* HPV types particularly liable to cause malignancies are printed in **bold**.

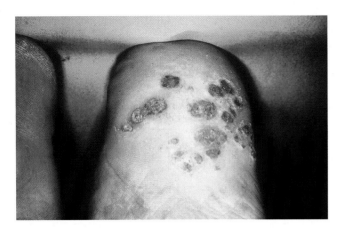

Fig. 15.3 Plantar warts.

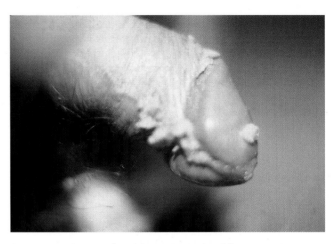

Fig. 15.4 Penile warts (condylomata acuminatea).

smoother than common warts; they also predominantly affect children. 'Butchers' warts', caused by HPV-7, are an occupational hazard. Why only this type affects butchers—and only butchers—is a mystery; there is certainly no relationship between it and any of the bovine papillomaviruses.

Genital warts

It is at this point, as we work down through Table 15.1, that we arrive at the somewhat blurred interface between the benign and malignant lesions caused by papillomaviruses.

As might be expected, genital warts are acquired by sexual contact: they are in fact one of the most common sexually transmitted diseases, and often occur in association with others, e.g. gonorrhoea or chlamydial infection. It follows that their highest incidence is the late teens and early adulthood. In 1996, papillomavirus infections were the most commonly diagnosed sexually transmitted viral diseases in the UK; nearly 54 000 first attacks were recorded, twice the number of first attacks of genital herpes simplex. In the USA 20 million persons are considered to be infected and the prevalence in the population is about 1% but could be 10 times higher in more sexually active groups.

Ordinary skin warts sometimes occur on the penis, but the most frequently seen lesions, both in men and women are **condylomata acuminata** (condyloma acuminatum, if, as rarely happens, there is only one of them). This Greco-Latin name means 'pointed lump', but sounds nicer. They are fleshy, moist, and vascular and may grow much larger than the common skin warts. By contrast with the latter, they may be pointed or filiform.

Condylomata acuminata may be seen at the following sites.

1. *In men*:
   - On the **penis**, affecting the area around the glans and prepuce more than the shaft (Fig. 15.4).
   - Within the **urethral meatus** and **urethra** itself.
   - Around the **anus** and within the **rectum**, particularly in homosexuals; in those practising receptive anal intercourse this site is more frequently affected than the penis.

It is unusual for condylomata acuminata to become malignant, but they occasionally progress to squamous cell carcinoma. This is particularly true of the comparatively rare giant condyloma, associated with HPV6 or HPV11, which forms huge masses of tissue on the penis or in the anoperineal area. The incidence of anal genital warts is increasing in the USA.

2. *In women*:
   - On the **vulva**.
   - Occasionally, in the vagina.
   - On the **cervix**. Here, the typical lesion is the flat, intraepithelial type, rather than the fleshy variety seen on the external genitalia. It is difficult to distinguish clinically between this lesion, caused by a papillomavirus, and other forms of cervical dysplasia.
   - Around the anus and on the perineum.

3. *In children* these lesions have been observed on the external genitalia of both male and female infants and children. Although they may be indicators of sexual abuse, it is dangerous to jump to this conclusion, as the infection may be transmitted from the mother during delivery, or even by close but innocent contact within the family.

Malignant or potentially malignant lesions

Bowenoid papulosis

This syndrome manifests as multiple papules on the penis or vulva; it is usually seen in young people, and although usually benign, may become malignant. It takes its name from Bowen's disease, which occurs in older people, is not associated with HPV, but with which there are histological resemblances.

Premalignant intraepithelial dysplasia

Irregularities in the histological pattern of the epithelium ('atypia') may occur on the penis, vulva (vulvar intraepithelial neoplasia, VIN), vagina (VAIN), or cervix (CIN). They are staged according to the degree of dysplasia and the most severe form (CIN 3 in the case of cervical lesions), which involves all layers of the stratified epithelium, has a high chance of progression to metastasizing carcinoma. It is now known that many of these lesions are associated with papillomaviruses. **HPV types 16** and **18** in particular are heavily implicated in the causation of carcinoma both of the **cervix** and of the **penis**.

Laryngeal infections with human papillomavirus

It is probably no accident that the types of HPV causing warts in the **juvenile larynx** are the same as those associated with genital warts, namely **HPV6 and 11**; they may well be transmitted during delivery and establish a persistent infection. Although they tend to recur after treatment, these papillomas do not become malignant in children; this is not, however, true of the **adult** variety, associated with **HPV16**, which may develop carcinomatous changes.

Epidermodysplasia verruciformis

This is a rare autosomal recessive disease associated with defects in T-cell function and numbers, but not with other varieties of immune deficiency. The multiple flat lesions may persist for years; they are associated with a wide range of HPV types and may become malignant, especially in areas of skin exposed to sunlight.

Immunosuppressed patients

Allograft recipients receiving immunosuppressive treatment are liable to develop squamous cell carcinomas of the skin; HPV5 has been demonstrated in the lesions of at least one such patient.

3.2 Epidemiology

As might be expected from the liability of genital warts to become malignant, most epidemiological studies have centred on them rather than on the comparatively trivial lesions seen elsewhere. The last few decades have seen a substantial rise in the numbers of genital HPV infections, and a corresponding increase in the prevalence of carcinomas of the cervix and penis. At least 90 per cent of cervical cancers are thought to be due to papillomavirus infections. Cervical cancer is the second most common cancer in women throughout the world and HPV is incriminated as a major cause. More than 80 types have been identified and classified as high, medium, or low risk.

The benign papillomavirus infections of the skin such as butchers' and plantar warts are acquired through breaks in the skin surface. **Swimming pools** are a fertile source of infection for the latter.

3.3 Pathogenesis and pathology

The papillomaviruses are something of a curiosity in that they can multiply only in **proliferating stratified squamous epithelium**, which cannot be grown as conventional cell cultures; the point of attack is often where one type of cell changes to another, e.g. the junction of the columnar epithelium of the cervical canal with the stratified squamous epithelium of the outer cervix. Study of these agents by the usual methods has therefore been considerably hampered; but this difficulty has a bonus,

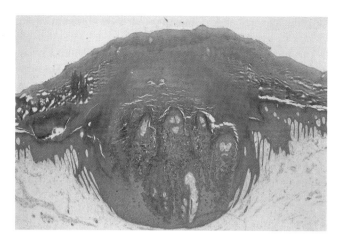

Fig. 15.5 Section of skin wart. Phloxine-tartrazine stain. The epidermis is hyperplasic. The epidermal cells, particularly those at the left in the body of the wart, contain many darkly stained inclusions.

because it pushed virologists into exploiting DNA technology for novel ways of detecting and classifying them; and this concentration upon the characteristics and functioning of the genome has taught us much about the mechanisms of oncogenesis.

A characteristic feature of the benign skin warts is **hyperkeratosis**, i.e. a massive proliferation of the keratinized layers of the dermis (Fig. 15.5). Particularly in plantar warts, there are deep extensions of the hypertrophic epidermis. Large, pale, vacuolated cells are present in the granular layer; these are more pronounced in plane warts than in verruca vulgaris. There are many eosinophilic cytoplasmic inclusions that are not of viral origin, but which consist of abnormally large keratohyalin granules. There are, however, **basophilic inclusions in the nuclei** of the epidermal cells in which typical papillomavirus virions can be seen by EM. HPV stimulates cell proliferation in the stratum spinosum by early expression of the immortality functions of E6 and E7 proteins. Late gene expression of L1 and

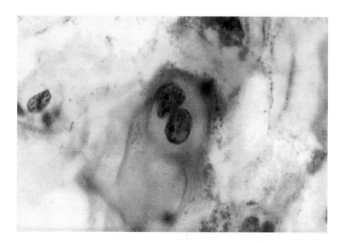

Fig. 15.6 Koilocyte in cervical scraping. The double nucleus, which is characteristic, is surrounded by an area of unstained cytoplasm. (Courtesy of Dr David Oriel.)

L2 proteins occur in the uppermost stratum corneum where virions are assembled and released.

The histology of condylomata acuminata is quite similar, except that hyperkeratosis is not a significant feature. The presence of vacuolated cells in cervical scrapings (Fig. 15.6) is diagnostically useful; they are known as **koilocytes** ('empty cells') because of their appearance in stained preparations, but the term is inappropriate as the apparently empty vacuoles contain enormous numbers of virions.

At this point, the histopathology of papillomavirus lesions merges into that of precancerous and cancerous changes, which is beyond the scope of this book.

3.4 Immune response

The failure to culture papillomaviruses has greatly hindered our ability to unravel the immune reactions to infection. This is a pity, because the little that we do know poses tantalizing suggestions that the immunology of papillomavirus infections may have some unique characteristics. Why, for example, may cutaneous warts persist for years and then suddenly disappear for no obvious reason? What is the relationship between the immune response and oncogenesis? What are the respective roles of CMI and antibody? We know from immunofluorescence studies that both IgM and IgG antibodies may appear, particularly in those with regressing warts; but not all those with antibody have warts and not all warty individuals have antibody. On the other hand, CMI may be equally or more important, as regressing lesions contain many macrophages and lymphocytes, of both T-suppressor (CD8+) and T-helper (CD4+) subclasses. Circumstantial evidence of the importance of the immune responses is provided by patients with epidermodysplasia verruciformis, who have an inborn defect of immunity, and by the high prevalence of warts in immunosuppressed patients.

There is an association between histocompatibility (HLA) type and the development of cervical carcinoma. The mechanisms by which papilloma and other viruses give rise to malignant tumours are dealt with in Chapter 6.

3.5 Laboratory diagnosis

The presence of warty lesions is usually so obvious to the eye, aided when necessary by a magnifying glass, colposcope, or urethroscope, that laboratory methods are largely redundant except for determining, if possible, whether a given lesion is benign or malignant. At colposcopy, lesions in the vagina (or rectum) are rendered more visible by painting the area with 5 per cent acetic acid. The histological appearances are characteristic, and Papanicolaou staining of smears may reveal characteristic features, notably the presence of koilocytes. The presence of HPV—but not its type—can be verified by an antiserum against disrupted bovine papillomavirus particles. For typing HPVs within lesions, recourse must be had to DNA hybridization techniques, e.g. Southern blot, PCR, and hybridization *in situ*.

3.6 Control

Treatment

Skin warts may need treatment on cosmetic grounds, or, in the case of plantar warts, because of pain and disability on walking. They may be removed by treatment with **podophyllin**, extracted from the roots of the American mandrake, or by **freezing** with liquid nitrogen. It is a curious but quite well authenticated observation that common skin warts can sometimes be made to disappear by suggestion. There are a variety of methods of dealing with cervical lesions, including **freezing, electrodiathermy**, and **cone biopsy**. Recurrent laryngeal warts may be removed surgically, but must never be treated with irradiation, as this induces malignant change. Injection of **IFN** directly into the lesions has met with limited success, but by no means in all patients so treated.

Immunization

Controlled clinical trial of a vaccine directed against HPV16 and 18 has yielded promising results and it may well be that such a vaccine will make a useful contribution to control of these carcinogenic serotypes.

Other measures

Warts, especially on the feet, are readily acquired in **swimming pools and changing rooms**, where adequate hygienic measures should be maintained. Measures for preventing genital warts are similar to those for other sexually transmitted diseases.

4 Clinical and pathological aspects of polyomavirus infections

Poly-oma means what it sounds like—'many tumours'. In 1951, Ludwik Gross, in the USA, injected tissues from mice suffering from a naturally occurring leukaemia into newborn mice; unexpectedly, they did not develop leukaemia but malignant tumours of the salivary glands (see Chapter 6). After a number of passages in the laboratory, the agent was able to cause various types of tumour, which accounts for its name. This property was very noticeable when it was injected into other species of animal. Polyomaviruses naturally infect various animals and birds; when spread is vertical, i.e. from mother to offspring, infection is life-long, but without tumour formation. (The leukaemia affecting the mice from which polyomavirus was first isolated proved to be due to concurrent infection with a different agent, a retrovirus.)

Here, then, we have other papovaviruses with oncogenic potential; but in terms of their ability to cause disease in humans they bear no resemblance whatsoever to HPV. Another important difference is their ability to grow and induce CPEs in cultured cells, notably those from embryo mice.

4.1 Clinical features

Only two polyomaviruses cause significant disease in humans, and then but rarely, although antibodies to them are present in a high proportion of sera.

JC virus and progressive multifocal leucoencephalopathy

First described in 1958, this syndrome is characterized by hemiparesis, disturbances of speech and vision, dementia, and a relentless progression to death within a few months. It is noteworthy that progressive multifocal leucoencephalopathy (PML), which is quite rare, often occurs in **elderly** patients already suffering from disease of the **reticuloendothelial system**; the first three to be described suffered from chronic lymphatic leukaemia or Hodgkin's disease. The lesions in the brain comprise multiple areas of **demyelination, abnormal oligodendrocytes**, and, in the later stages, pronounced **astrocytosis**. The name of the syndrome derives from these clinical and pathological features.

A few years later, virions with the morphology of polyomavirus were found in the nuclei of affected glial cells; and in 1971, a virus, termed JC after the initials of the patient, was isolated from PML in cultures of human fetal glial cells. This virus is widespread in humans, in whom it causes persistent infection, primarily in the urinary tract, until stirred into more dangerous activity by immunosuppression. It is almost unheard of in immunologically normal people.

PML was a comparatively rare disease until, quite recently, it came to greater prominence as a presenting feature or complication of AIDS, which is not surprising in these severely immunocompromised patients.

BK virus: another persistent agent

In the same year as the detection of JC virus, a similar agent, termed BK, was isolated from the urine of an immunosuppressed renal transplant patient in London. This virus grows in human fibroblasts and monkey kidney (VERO) cells and has now been isolated from the urine of many immunocompromised patients. Although its physical characteristics are very similar to those of JC virus, its pathogenicity for humans is quite different.

Vacuolating agents

During the 1950s, the widespread use of monkey kidney cells for isolating polioviruses and preparing vaccine brought to light many viruses that caused inapparent infections; not until the cells were explanted into culture vessels did CPEs become obvious. These agents were termed 'simian viruses' (SV). One of them, that induced a vacuolated, or foamy, appearance in the cytoplasm, was termed SV40. This agent proved to be a polyomavirus, and like other members of the genus was oncogenic, this time for hamsters. It did not, however, seem to cause disease in the monkeys from which it was isolated; and it would probably have remained of academic interest but for the fact that it proved comparatively resistant to formalin, which was used to inactivate the polio vaccine widely used at that time. Unfortunately, many thousands of doses had been issued before the discovery of SV40, and there was a real worry that some of the inoculated children would develop tumours in later life. Luckily, intensive follow-ups have revealed no evidence of any such effects; but the scare created by this episode did much to improve the testing of biological products to ensure that they contain no extraneous viruses.

4.2 Epidemiology

As determined by tests for antibody, the prevalence of BK in the general population is also high; like wild mice, people seem to become infected with polyomaviruses early in life without suffering obvious ill effects. Normal people do not excrete BK virus unless they are immunocompromised or pregnant, in both of which cases the virus is liable to reactivate. Even when it does, however, overt disease is rare, the main exception being small numbers of cases of ureteric stenosis in renal transplant recipients and of acute haemorrhagic urethritis or cystitis. BK virus does not appear to cause PML.

4.3 Pathogenesis and pathology

Primary infections are asymptomatic and nothing is known about the portal of entry; the presence of virus in the urinary tract gives a clue to at least one site where BK virus may lurk after the primary infection, but apart from this, little is known of its pathogenicity.

In the brains of patients with PML, there are areas of **demyelination**, and basophilic inclusions can be found in the oligodendroglia.

There is virtually no evidence that either virus causes tumours in humans.

4.4 Immune response

By contrast with papillomaviruses, polyoma agents induce a good **antibody response**, but little is known about the role of CMI. In view of the persistent nature of these infections, it seems that immune mechanisms serve only to keep the viruses at bay, without actually eradicating them.

4.5 Laboratory diagnosis

Antibody is measurable by a haemagglutination-inhibition test employing human group O erythrocytes; however, as latent infection is so widespread, such tests are of limited value.

The clinical diagnosis of PML can be confirmed at autopsy by the characteristic histological appearances. Isolation of JC virus is difficult and can be done only in a very few specialized laboratories. Papovavirus virions, often in crystalline arrays, can be found by EM in ultrathin sections of oligodendrocyte nuclei.

Isolation of BK infections by cultural methods is slow; a faster diagnosis may be made by staining exfoliated cells in the urine for viral antigen by immunofluorescence or immunoperoxidase methods.

4.6 Control

Treatment and prevention

Limited success has been claimed for cytarabine in the treatment of PML, but for practical purposes the prognosis is dire. Other than this, there is no treatment for polyomavirus infections. We can however, end this chapter on an optimistic note, as at the time of writing clinical trial of a vaccine against the oncogenic strains 16 and 18 suggests that it is highly effective.

5 Reminders

- There are two families of papovavirus:
  - Papillomaviridae, with one genus, Papillomavirus
  - Polyomaviridae, also with one genus, Polyomavirus
- HPVs replicate only in **proliferating epithelium** and thus cannot be grown in conventional cell cultures.
- HPV cause warts in **skin** and **mucous membranes**, which are usually benign but may become malignant, especially in the genital tract. Certain types of HPV, notably **16** and **18**, are strongly implicated in the causation of cancer of the genital tract, notably **carcinoma of the cervix**.
- HPV are particularly liable to cause malignant disease in **immunocompromised patients.**
- HPV infection is now the most common **sexually transmitted disease** in the UK.
- **Polyomaviruses** are widespread in humans and animals, causing **persistent but silent infections of the urinary tract**. They are, however, oncogenic if injected into newborn animals or into other species.
- The two best characterized human polyomaviruses are JC and BK
  - **JC virus** causes **PML,** a fatal demyelinating disease of the CNS, usually seen in later life and particularly affecting those with disease of the reticuloendothelial system.
  - **BK virus** also reactivates in **immunocompromised patients,** but rarely causes overt disease.
- Another polyomavirus, SV40, causes persistent but inapparent infection of the kidneys of some monkeys, and is liable to be present in cultures prepared from them.
- The preparation of a successful vaccine against HPVs 16 and 18 now appears to be a possibility.

Chapter 16

Poliomyelitis and other picornavirus infections

The family *Picornaviridae* is one of the largest in numerical terms to be considered in this book and contains some of the smallest viruses, of which poliovirus is the most important. Poliomyelitis was one of the first diseases to be recorded; an Egyptian tomb carving of the Nineteenth Dynasty shows the dead man to have had a foot-drop deformity typical of paralytic poliomyelitis (Fig. 16.1). A world polio eradication campaign should result in this virus becoming extinct by 2006.

The extraordinarily wide range of diseases caused by different members of the family is summarized in Table 16.1. The syndromes include asymptomatic infection, which, fortunately, is by far the most common, disease of the CNS, febrile illness with rash, conjunctivitis, herpangina, infections involving the muscles and heart, and hepatitis. Probably no other family of viruses causes such a diversity of illnesses.

1 Properties of the viruses

1.1 Classification

The family *Picornaviridae* contains six genera (Table 16.1). Its name derives from the small size of these viruses (*pico* = small) and their RNA genome. Picornaviruses are found in several mammalian species, but we shall describe only those that infect humans. They are acid-resistant, which enables them to survive passage through the stomach. They replicate in the small intestine, can readily be isolated from faeces and are spread by the faecal–oral route. Gastroenteritis is, however, not a major feature of picornavirus infections.

Poliovirus was the first of the genus—indeed, of the whole family—to be isolated. This accomplishment by Enders, Weller, and Robins in 1948 earned them a Nobel Prize, because it was the first occasion on which a neurotropic virus was grown in non-neural tissue, in this instance derived from monkey kidney.

Soon after the isolation of the polioviruses, similar viruses were discovered that paralysed infant mice. On the basis of the pathological changes in mice, two groups were defined, termed Coxsackieviruses A and B after the town Coxsackie, New York, where they were first isolated. (Note that by convention we write 'coxsackieviruses A', rather than 'Coxsackie A virus'.)

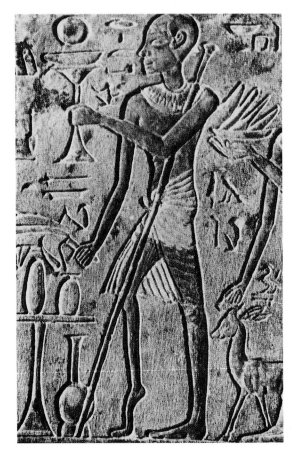

Fig. 16.1 Egyptian tomb carving of the Nineteenth Dynasty. The 'foot-drop' deformity is characteristic of residual paralysis due to poliomyelitis, shortly a disease to be confined to history.

Table 16.1 The *Picornaviridae*

Genus	Main syndromes
Enterovirus	Infections of the central nervous system, heart, skeletal muscles, skin, and mucous membranes
Hepatovirus	Hepatitis A
Rhinovirus	Common colds
Aphthovirus	Foot and mouth disease of cattle (rarely in humans)
Cardiovirus	Encephalitits and myocarditis
Parechovirus	Diarrhoea

In the late 1950s, with the increasing use of mammalian tissue cultures, faecal samples yielded yet more viruses of the same sort, but which did not at first appear pathogenic for animals or humans. Such viruses are called echoviruses, a term derived from enteric *c*ytopathogenic *h*uman *o*rphan viruses—orphan because they seemed to be viruses that lacked a disease. Many of the orphans now have parent diseases.

Table 16.2 Picornaviruses that infect humans

Group	No. of serotypes
Poliovirus	3
Coxsackie A	23
Coxsackie B	6
Echovirus	32
Enterovirus	5*

* Numbered 68–72.

The terminology of these agents is indeed somewhat confusing. To summarize, the genus *Enterovirus* comprises all the viruses shown in Table 16.2, of which five serotypes are also called enteroviruses to distinguish them from the echo- and coxsackieviruses. To make life even more difficult, the whole genus is often referred to colloquially as 'enteroviruses'. In this chapter, it should be clear from the context exactly what we mean when we use this term.

So many enteroviruses are now known that those newly identified are referred to by numbers (which are *not* related to the number of serotypes) (Table 16.2). Enterovirus 72, the cause of hepatitis A, is dealt with in Chapter 35.

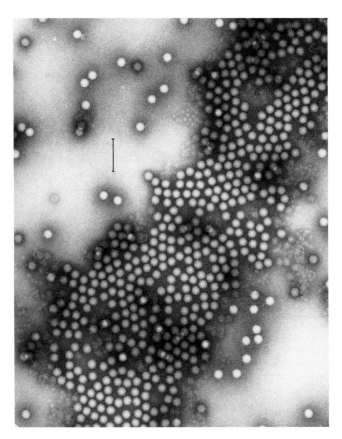

Fig. 16.2 Electron micrograph of a cluster of picornaviruses (poliovirus). (Courtesy of Dr David Hockley.) Scale bar = 100 nm.

1.2 Morphology

Picornaviruses are only 18–30 nm in diameter and icosahedral, with a regular protein capsid composed of 60 protomers each containing a single copy of four structural proteins called VP1, VP2, VP3, and VP4; there is no envelope (Fig. 16.2).

Some remarkable studies have been performed with polio- and rhinoviruses using X-ray crystallography. These analyses have helped to pinpoint functional areas in the virion, the most interesting being the 'canyon' or cleft where the cell receptor-binding site is located. There is great interest in this saucer-shaped depression as a target for antiviral drugs, particularly against rhinoviruses. Immunogenic sites are present on the exposed external parts of the capsid. These antigenic areas are binding sites for neutralizing antibody and are a key feature in the immunogenicity of poliomyelitis vaccines.

1.3 Genome and polypeptides

Picornaviruses are positive-strand RNA viruses and the genome of 7.5 kb is thus infective for cells. The genome RNA has a covalently attached protein termed VPg at the 5' end; it is polyadenylated at the 3' end and can act directly as the viral messenger. There is a single large ORF for translation into one very large polyprotein. The polyprotein is cleaved into intermediates P1, P2, and P3; polypeptide P1 undergoes further cleavage to give the four viral capsid proteins (VP1, VP2, VP3, and VP4). About 20 other proteins are derived from the polyprotein, thus enhancing the information base of the genome (Fig. 16.3). P2 codes for three NS proteins including a protease, whereas P4 codes for four proteins including the RNA replicase. The protein coding region is flanked by a 750 nucleotide long 5' untranslated region and a 3' untranslated region ending in a poly(A) tail.

1.4 Replication

Poliovirus and the other members of the family, with the exception of echoviruses, attach to the cellular adhesion protein ICAM-1. The echoviruses attach to the integrin VLA 2. Replication of viral RNA starts within 1 hour of infection of a cell and as is typical for a positive strand RNA virus, is initiated by the newly synthesized virus-coded RNA replicase. The parental positive-sense RNA strand is transcribed into a negative-sense strand which serves repeatedly as a template for transcription into progeny positive-sense RNA strands (Fig. 16.4). The dsRNA, termed a replicative intermediate, has only a fleeting

existence. Assembly of viral RNA nucleic acid and structural proteins takes place in the cytoplasm. Translation of cellular mRNAs is effectively shut down by these viruses because the viral protease inactivates the cellular cap binding complex termed αIF-4F, which is needed for binding of cellular mRNAs to ribosomes. This complex is not required for polio mRNAs. The cell normally dies, and after a viral replication period of 4 hours and about a million virus particles are released by cell death and lysis.

2 Clinical and pathological aspects

2.1 Poliomyelitis

This term is derived from the Greek *polios* (grey) and *muelos* (marrow), and refers to the propensity of the virus to attack the grey matter of the spinal cord. The shortened form 'polio' is often used to indicate the paralytic form of the disease. From 2005 the world should have seen the last case of clinical polio.

Clinical features

The incubation period is usually 7–14 days, with extremes of 2–35 days. The course is variable; there may be inapparent infection; a minor illness with malaise, fever, and sore throat; or a major illness heralded by a meningitic phase. Each of these, except the major illness, may resolve without sequelae.

The minor illness is due to viraemia. As well as the non-specific signs mentioned, there may be a personality change, especially in young children. In those progressing to the major illness there may be a few days of apparent well-being before the onset of the meningitic phase, giving a biphasic presentation.

The major illness may occur with or without preceding symptoms; the onset is abrupt, with headache, fever, vomiting, and neck stiffness. The meningitic phase often concludes in a week. However, in a minority of persons, about 1%, paralysis sets in. Its extent ranges from part of a single muscle to virtually every skeletal muscle, in which case severe impairment of respiration may demand the use of artificial ventilation. Paralysis is of the lower motor neuron type with flaccidity of affected muscles. In bulbar poliomyelitis involvement of cranial nerves results in paralysis of the pharynx, again bringing difficulty with respiration.

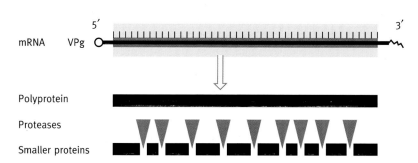

Fig. 16.3 Proteolytic cleavage of poliovirus polyprotein to yield structural proteins. The viral mRNA encodes a single large polyprotein, which is then cut by proteases at precise positions to produce a number of smaller proteins with different functions.

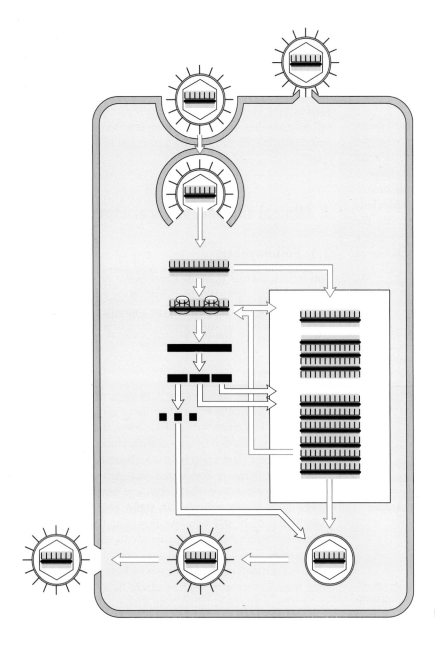

Fig. 16.4 **Replication cycle of poliovirus (see text).**

When there is paralysis, its full extent is apparent within 72 hours of the first signs, although a firm prognosis cannot be made for about a month, by which time most reversible neuronal damage will have disappeared and the residual permanent damage can be assessed (Fig. 16.5). Fortunately, there is often great improvement during this anxious waiting period. In bulbar polio the outlook is good if the patient is still alive by the tenth day or so, as the pharyngeal muscles then begin to show signs of recovery.

Pathogenesis

Poliovirus may be acquired by the respiratory route, but the faecal–oral mode of transmission is much the more important. The virus replicates in the lymphoid tissue of the pharynx and gut, including Peyer's patches. A viraemic phase is followed by extension to the CNS, within which the virus spreads along axons. Lytic infection of neurons, with secondary degeneration of axons, is the primary cause of paralysis. Typically, the anterior horn cells of the spinal cord are the worst affected, which accounts for the lower motor neuron type of limb paralysis. The virus does not replicate within the muscles themselves. In severe cases, various centres within the bulb and brain may be attacked, with respiratory paralysis sometimes leading to death. More transient damage results from inflammatory infiltration in the CNS. Pregnancy increases the incidence of paralysis as does intramuscular injection—e.g. of other vaccines or antibiotics.

Pathology

The most remarkable feature is the high selectivity of the virus for the nervous tissue. In addition to the lytic destruction of neurons there is an inflammatory reaction, an initial poly-

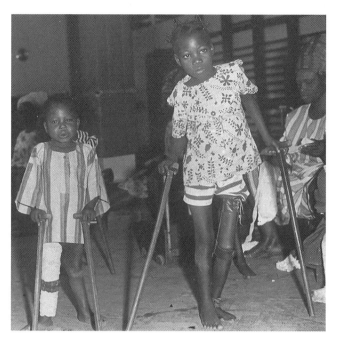

Fig. 16.5 Children crippled by poliomyelitis. Hopefully this will now become a disease of the past.

morphonuclear response giving way to lymphocytes. There is perivascular infiltration with lymphocytes ('cuffing') characteristic of inflammatory reaction in the CNS, microglial proliferation, and oedema. Inflammatory foci in lymphoid tissue are also present.

Experimental observations suggest that the virus is often disseminated throughout the CNS to a much greater degree than is suggested by the clinical signs.

Immune response

Infection induces antibodies with complement-fixing and neutralizing activities and they may be used retrospectively for laboratory confirmation at polio infection. There is the usual early specific IgM response, rapidly followed by a much longer-lasting production of specific IgG. Neutralizing antibodies—IgG in the blood and IgA at mucous surfaces—are important in protecting against reinfection. However, antibody against one of the three serotypes does not in general protect against the others, although there may be some cross-protection between types 1 and 2.

Epidemiology

Before the advent of immunization, outbreaks in temperate countries tended to occur in the summer; there is, however, no marked seasonal variation in tropical areas.

The mode of spread of poliovirus by the faecal–oral route (see Fig. 4.4) tells us immediately that this disease is likely to be have its highest prevalence in areas where hygiene is defective. The virus may be excreted for 2–3 weeks in faeces. Transmission is also favoured by the ability of this and other enteroviruses to survive for some weeks in water and sewage. Like other infec-

tions that flourish under these conditions, poliomyelitis is likely to be acquired early in life. In Chapter 7, we showed how the pattern of infection varies in communities according to their socio-economic status. In deprived areas, especially in the subtropics and tropics, most children—after a 6-month period of grace conferred by maternal antibody—have been infected by all three serotypes by the age of 5 years or so (the 'Cairo model', Chapter 7). This is the endemic pattern. By contrast, the average age of acquisition in more affluent communities (the 'Miami model') was, in the days before mass immunization, much later; this meant that an epidemic situation was created in which, every few years, outbreaks occurred among the accumulated reservoir of susceptibles in the population. The advent of mass immunization in such countries introduced the vaccine era, in which the behaviour of poliomyelitis again changed: the disease has now been virtually abolished in most regions of the world and in 2006 should be totally eradicated.

Viruses of increased neurovirulence, 1 case per 2.5 million cases of vaccine, have been recorded and these viruses can circulate silently leading to polio outbreaks. Therefore only inactivated poliomyelitis vaccine (IPV) will be used after polio has been eradicated.

Polio vaccine

Although for the foreseeable future the world is suffering its last cases of polio the vaccination campaign will continue using the inactivated polio vaccine.

Inactivated vaccine

By the mid-1950s, Jonas Salk's group in the USA had demonstrated that a poliovirus suspension from the supernatant fluid of infected monkey kidney cell cultures, treated with formalin to destroy its infectivity, induced immunity in susceptible persons. This IPV contains the three serotypes and is given as three injections at monthly intervals. The modern vaccine uses Vero cells, a continuous line of monkey kidney cells, as a substrate.

Live attenuated vaccine

While Salk's researches were still in progress, Albert Sabin and co-workers were using a different approach; they were trying to attenuate highly virulent polioviruses by repeated subcultures (passages) of virus in monkey kidney cells.

These attenuated strains were used to prepare live vaccine, which was given by mouth (oral polio vaccine, or OPV). This too was given in three doses at monthly intervals, but the reason is quite different from that on which the similar schedule for IPV is based. The first dose of the latter induces the classical primary immune response to a non-replicating antigen, followed by enhanced (secondary) responses to the second and third doses (Chapter 5). By contrast, the virus in the attenuated vaccine replicates in the lymphoid tissue of the gut; when the first dose is given, only one of the three serotypes (say type 2) secures a foothold to the exclusion of the others, and induces immunity to type 2 strains only. At the next dose, either type 1 or type 3 wins; similarly, the third dose provides immunity against whichever of the three stereotypes is left.

Table 16.3 Comparison of inactivated and attenuated (oral) poliomyelitis vaccines (IPV and OPV)

	IPV	OPV
Stimulates IgG antibody in blood	Yes	Yes
Stimulates IgG antibody, hence local immunity, in gut	No	Yes
Duration of immunity	Medium	Long
Cost	High	Low
Route of administration	Injection	Oral
Skilled staff needed	Yes	No
Inadequate response in some tropical countries	No	Yes
Involuntary transmission to susceptibles within the community	No	Yes
Possible mutation to neurovirulence	No	Yes, but very rare
Contraindicated in immunodeficiency states or pregnancy	No	Yes

The global polio eradication campaign

Most countries have eradicated polio using live attenuated vaccines. However, the type III vaccine, can, albeit rarely, cause poliomyelitis in vaccinees. So for the final months of the eradication strategy killed vaccine will mostly be used.

Finally, there is a word of caution about the post polio era: vaccination will have to be continued for some years until the world can be declared 'polio free'.

The WHO set out to eradicate polio in 1988 (Fig. 16.6(a)) when the disease was endemic in 125 countries and some 350 000 children were paralysed. By 2002 polio was reported in only a handful of countries (Fig. 16.6(b)). In 2004 only 32 cases had been confirmed in the whole world. However, children will continue to be vaccinated because of the fear that polio could re-emerge from undisclosed laboratory samples or from immunosuppressed persons who can continue to excrete polio for a lifetime. Also WHO plans to have an emergency stockpile of 75 million doses of oral vaccine.

The huge efforts made in every country of the world to eradicate polio should never be underestimated. This year vaccinator volunteers will deliver two drops of OPV to 105 million children twice during the year. Up to 100 million children will receive an extra two or three doses to be sure. In one month in 2004 the Indian government set up 640 000 vaccine booths and send 1 million mobile vaccinations teams to visit 191 million houses. In Uttar Pradesh alone there are 500 000 babies born each month and 80 per cent of Indian cases are concentrated here. In some villages parents will not allow their children to be vaccinated. Most countries experienced social and religious problems during the global eradication of smallpox. European countries, including the UK, have recently changed their vaccine and all children will now receive IPV because, in the final analysis, polio cannot be eradicated by a live vaccine where in one vaccinee per million the vaccine virus genetically mutates and reverts to virulence.

Is total eradication possible?

In theory, yes. However, the target year set by WHO in 1988 was 2004, but that year has come and gone with the disease still endemic in several countries, namely Sudan, Nigeria, Niger, Egypt, Pakistan, India, and Afghanistan. It is unfortunate to say the least that the campaign is impeded by propaganda directed against the vaccine in a number of areas.

2.2 Infections caused by enteroviruses other than polioviruses

At least 65 HEV types are diluted and five species HEV-1 to D and polio, but we will continue with the older subdivision.

Table 16.4 lists the diseases caused by these agents; there is much overlap between the syndromes caused by the various groups and it may help you to remember them better if we classify them in terms of the body systems affected rather than of the virus groups involved.

Most textbooks list the serotypes predominantly involved in each syndrome, but there is no need to memorize them in such detail; we shall merely indicate the broad relationships. Table 16.4, therefore, gives only a rough idea of the quantitative involvement of the viruses in the various syndromes. The 'plus' scores compare the frequencies of occurrence **only within the same row**, and not overall.

Central nervous system

Like their relatives, the polioviruses, the enteroviruses give rise to CNS infections, which may, on occasion, closely mimic poliomyelitis; paralytic disease is, however, less common than with poliovirus infections. Enterovirus 71 is a prominent cause of CNS infections, including encephalitis. (See also Chapter 30.)

Heart

Acute myocarditis and pericarditis are caused particularly by Coxsackie B viruses. They occur both in children and adults, and are sometimes fatal.

Skeletal muscle

Epidemic pleurodynia (or myalgia) is also mostly caused by Coxsackie B viruses. This syndrome is sometimes called Bornholm disease, after the island on which the first well described outbreak occurred. It is characterized by fever and severe pain in the chest and, if the diaphragm is involved, in the abdomen. Symptoms last from a few days to 2 weeks, and resolve without ill effects; relapses are, however, fairly common. Virus is thought to invade the muscle itself.

A mysterious syndrome, known variously as **myalgic encephalomyelitis (ME), postviral disease syndrome,** or Royal Free disease (after the London hospital in which there was a large outbreak) is still the subject of much controversy. It affects women more often than men; in the Royal Free Hospital out-

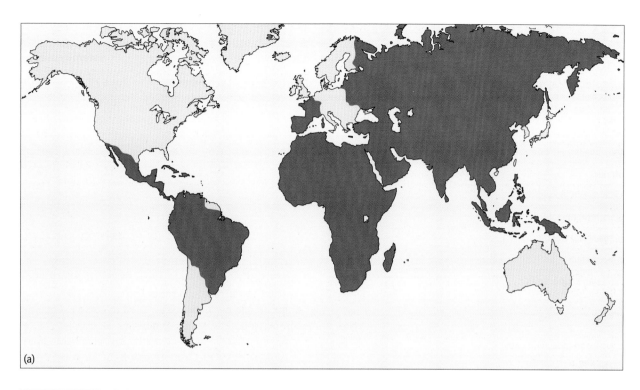

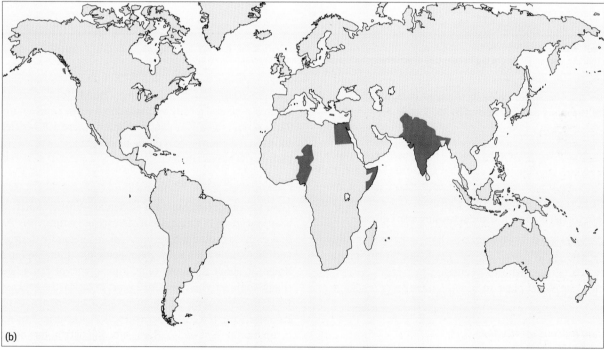

Fig. 16.6 **(a)** Distribution of polio virus in 1988. **(b)** Distribution of polio virus in 2002.

break in 1955, female nurses were predominantly affected. ME patients have few if any physical signs, but many symptoms , of which the most prominent are fatigue following even minor physical activity and depressive psychological illness. ME, which may persist for years and resist all forms of treatment, has been dismissed in the past as psychological in origin. Nevertheless, there is mounting serological evidence that ME is associ-

ated with Coxsackievirus B4 infections; and there is evidence that enteroviral VP1 antigen (Section 2.3), either free or complexed with antibody, is present in the sera of a significant proportion of ME patients. Recently, enteroviral RNA sequences were detected by the PCR (see Chapter 36) in muscle biopsies from a significant proportion of patients with this syndrome. The use of such techniques for detecting viral antigens may help

Table 16.4 Syndromes caused by coxsackieviruses, echoviruses, and enteroviruses 70 and 71

System affected/syndrome	Coxsackieviruses A[†]	Coxsackieviruses B	Echoviruses[‡]	Enteroviruses[†] Type 70	Type 71
Central nervous system					
Meningitis	+	+	+		+
Paralytic disease	+	+	+		+
Encephalitis	+	++	++		++
Myalgic encephalomyelitis		+			
Heart/skeletal muscle	+	++	+		
Gastrointestinal tract			++		
Respiratory tract	++	++	+		
Skin, mucous membranes					
Rashes	+		+		
Herpangina	++				
Hand, foot, and mouth disease	++	+			++
Conjunctiva	+*			++	
Pancreas		+			
	+	++	+		

* A variant of Coxsackievirus A24.
[†] Note that the + scores compare the frequencies of occurrence only within the same row and not overall.

to solve the puzzle presented by the syndrome, which is all too real for the many people affected by it.

Gastrointestinal tract

Although echoviruses may be isolated from cases of diarrhoea it is not always possible to be sure that they are the cause; they may be simply passengers. In this connection their name—enteric cytopathic human orphan viruses—is a reminder that they often exist in the gut without causing overt disease.

Respiratory tract

Both Coxsackie A and B viruses are sometimes implicated in mild upper or lower respiratory tract infections; but, as with gastrointestinal illnesses mentioned in the previous paragraph, it is not always easy to prove an aetiological relationship.

Skin and mucous membranes

Enteroviral infections of these tissues are caused almost by Coxsackie A viruses. **Rashes** may accompany infections of other systems. **Herpangina** as its name suggests, is painful infection of the pharynx with herpes-like features. It mainly afflicts young children. The onset of fever and sore throat is sudden, and accompanied by difficulty in swallowing. In a typical case there are vesicles on the soft palate, fauces, uvula, and posterior wall of the pharynx. They are usually smaller than herpetic vesicles and are further distinguished from them by being confined to the **posterior** part of the buccal cavity, whereas herpes primarily affects the anterior parts of the mouth. The infection resolves

spontaneously within a few days. **Hand, foot, and mouth disease** is caused mostly by Coxsackie A viruses and enterovirus 71. It occurs mainly in young children; there are vesicles and ulcers in the anterior part of the mouth, followed by a vesicular rash on the hands and feet.

Conjunctiva

The most important causes of epidemic acute conjunctivitis are a variant strain of Coxsackie A24 virus and enterovirus 70. The first of these caused a large outbreak in Singapore during 1970 and there have been subsequent epidemics there and in Hong Kong. At about the same time, a pandemic of acute haemorrhagic conjunctivitis raged for 2 years in Africa, the Far East, and India, involving some 10 million people. This was a more serious infection than the A24 type, and was characterized by a short incubation period of 1–2 days, subconjunctival haemorrhage, severe pain in the eyes, photophobia, and sometimes by keratitis. A small proportion of patients suffered from polio-like infections of the CNS. Apart from this complication, recovery was usually complete. During 1981, the disease reappeared in the East, and this time also affected large areas of Latin America, North America, and Canada.

Pancreas

There is evidence, still mostly circumstantial, linking infections with Coxsackie B viruses—especially B4—to acute-onset, insulin-dependent diabetes mellitus (IDDM) in young children.

There is experimental evidence that Coxsackie B4 virus can destroy beta cells in the islets of Langerhans, but the pathogenesis is still not clear; it may be that the viral infection precipitates rather than initiates the diabetes.

Perinatal infections

Neonatal infections with Coxsackie B virus serotypes and echoviruses may occur in outbreaks, severe cases of the former being associated with myocarditis and of the latter with hepatitis. Infections of the newborn carry an appreciable mortality rate, and every effort should be made to prevent spread via aerosols or unwashed hands.

Pathogenesis of enterovirus infections

Enteroviruses are mainly transmitted either by the respiratory or the faecal–oral route. Those causing conjunctivitis are spread by eye secretions, probably via soiled clothing, handkerchiefs, etc., or contaminated hands. Infections of the mucosae of the upper respiratory tract, conjunctiva, and gut result from direct viral invasion, whereas the pathogenesis of generalized infections, e.g. those involving the CNS, heart, or muscles, has a viraemic phase and is similar to that of poliomyelitis (Section 2.1); it follows the pattern of acute infection described in Chapter 4, section 4.4. Destruction of tissue is in the main due to direct lysis of cells, but some damage may be caused by immunopathological mechanisms, especially in the case of coxsackievirus infections.

The susceptibility of patients with primary immunodeficiencies to enterovirus infections is referred to in Chapter 32. Even in those with no obvious defects in immunity, some infections, notably those due to Coxsackie B viruses, seem to be **persistent**. This finding may explain their implication in conditions such as ME, and possibly in some cases of chronic heart disease.

Paralysis caused by novel recombinant viruses

Recent outbreaks of poliomyelitis in the island of Hispaniola were shown to be caused by a novel virus with genes of polio type 1 and another enterovirus. The non-poliovirus contributed to the NS proteins.

Immune response to enterovirus infections

Specific IgM, IgG, and IgA antibodies are formed, the latter particularly in mucosal infections. In generalized infections with a viraemic phase, circulating IgM and IgG antibodies are particularly important in recovery from infection; IgG antibody confers long-term protection against reinfection with the same serotype, and may also provide some immunity against closely related serotypes.

Epidemiology of enterovirus infections

In view of the many types of infection and the multiplicity of viruses involved, it is not possible here to provide more than some important general points about the behaviour of these infections.

- Most enteroviruses survive well in moist or wet environments, and are thus readily transmitted via the faecal–oral route, as described for polioviruses, and are therefore most prevalent in hot countries and during the summer months.

- The transmission of infections acquired by the respiratory or conjunctival routes is facilitated by overcrowding.

- Most infections are subclinical.

- Enterovirus infections occur predominantly in children; some, particularly those of the CNS, affect boys more often, or more severely, than girls.

- Epidemics of some—but not all—enteroviruses occur periodically.

2.3 Laboratory diagnosis

Warning!

Because these viruses—with the exception of polio—are so widespread, particularly in children, it is essential to bear in mind that isolation of a particular agent does not necessarily prove its casual relationship with the patient's illness; all the findings—clinical, virological, and serological—must be taken into account. The exception is when virus is isolated from the cerebrospinal fluid (CSF); this is strong evidence of association with a CNS infection.

Specimens

As a routine, throat swabs, faeces, and serum and CSF are collected during the acute phase. As excretion of virus may be intermittent, it is prudent to take further samples of faeces if the first is negative. Samples should also be taken from vesicular lesions, if present, as the fluid contains virus.

Virus isolation

Human or monkey cells must be used as only primate cells possess the specific receptors for human enteroviruses. All these viruses cause a somewhat similar CPE within 2–3 days of inoculation; it consists of rounding up of cells and eventually, complete destruction of the monolayer. It is necessary to identify the virus concerned by neutralization tests. In view of the many viruses involved, this is best done by using several pools of reference sera, each containing antibodies to some viruses but not others. By noting which pools do or do not neutralize infectivity, it is possible to identify the virus in the specimen. Such tests can be done only in specialist laboratories.

If a coxsackievirus infection is suspected, clinical specimens or infected cell cultures are inoculated into newborn mice, in which Coxsackie A and B viruses induce flaccid and spastic paralysis respectively. This is the only virus diagnostic test still employing animals; it will certainly be superseded by tests *in vitro*.

Detection of antibody

A rising titre of antibody in paired sera taken early in infection and 10–14 days later is good evidence of infection, but such tests are of little value in practice, both because of the time involved and the many possible antibodies. They are now being superseded by IgM antibody capture ELISA tests (see Chapter 36); again these are limited by the number of viruses and their corresponding antibodies, but may be useful when infection with a specific virus, e.g. a Coxsackie B, is suspected.

Detection of viral genome

Detection of viral genome in tissues and isolates can be effected by hybridization or PCR. Further information on diagnostic methods will be found in Chapter 36.

3 Control measures

None of the enteroviruses, including poliovirus, is susceptible to chemotherapy and there are no vaccines, except of course for poliomyelitis. Control therefore depends on hygienic measures, particularly those aimed at reducing the risk of spread by the faecal–oral route. These include not only the proper management of food, water supplies, and sewage, but also individual measures such as hand washing and correct disposal or disinfection of potentially contaminated materials.

4 Reminders

- The family *Picornaviridae* comprises five genera of small RNA viruses, of which three, *Enterovirus*, *Rhinovirus* (Chapter 8), and *Hepatovirus* (Chapter 23) frequently infect humans.

- The picornaviruses are **icosahedral**, about 25 nm in diameter, non-enveloped and have a **positive-sense RNA genome** 7.5 kb in size with a covalently attached protein (vpg) at the 5′ end. The genome extends its information base by coding for a long polyprotein which is subsequently cleaved into 20 viral proteins.

- Polioviruses can specifically shut down cellular mRNA translation by a viral protease that inactivates the cellular cap binding complex αIF-4F. The virus is therefore cytocidal for cells including neuronal cells.

- The *Enterovirus* genus comprises the three polioviruses, Coxsackie A and B viruses, echoviruses, and enteroviruses. Those infecting humans replicate only in primate cells. They cause a wide range of illnesses, including poliomyelitis, other infections of the CNS, and infections of the heart, skeletal muscles, liver (Chapter 16), skin, and mucous membranes, including the conjunctiva.

- Enteroviruses are transmitted predominantly by the **faecal–oral route**, but sometimes via the respiratory tract; conjunctival infections are spread by contact with infective secretions.

- In infections of the respiratory tract, gut, and conjunctiva the viruses invade the mucous membranes directly. In infections of other organs, e.g. CNS and heart, there is a viraemic phase followed by dispersion of virus to the target organs.

- Enteroviruses are ubiquitous and **many infections are inapparent**; they affect children more often than adults and are most prevalent in areas where hygiene is poor, or where there is overcrowding.

- Laboratory diagnosis involves **isolation of virus** from faeces, throat swabs, CSF, or vesicle fluid. Identification requires **neutralization tests** or, in the case of coxsackieviruses, inoculation of newborn mice. IgM antibody capture tests of the ELISA type may also be useful. **Specific viral RNA** can be identified by hybridization or PCR tests. Prevention of poliomyelitis is accomplished by immunization with **IPV** or live **attenuated OPV**. Both are highly effective, but OPV has a number of advantages, including ease of administration and low cost. However, IPV may be most important during the final stages of the WHO plan to eradicate polio.

- There is no specific antiviral therapy for enterovirus infections and no vaccine other than polio vaccine. Prevention thus depends on **hygienic measures**, particularly those designed to block faecal–oral spread.

Chapter 17

The herpesviruses: general properties

A herpetologist is not a virologist who specializes in herpes infections; he or she is in fact an expert on reptiles (Greek, *herpeton*). The name herpes seems to have become attached long ago to this group of viruses because of a rather fanciful idea of the creeping nature of the lesions caused by some of them. The name is, however, appropriate in a more modern context, because these viruses are excellent examples of 'creepers' (Chapter 4).

The herpesviruses form a large and most important group of infective agents, and affect many species both of warm- and cold-blooded animals. In humans they cause a wide range of syndromes, varying from trivial mucocutaneous lesions to life-threatening infections; they may also be implicated in certain cancers. An important property of all herpesviruses is their ability to cause latent infections that may subsequently become reactivated. They occupy a great deal of medical time both in the clinic and in the laboratory and thus merit detailed attention.

1 Classification

The family *Herpesviridae* contains several members that affect humans (Table 17.1); none, except for herpesvirus B, naturally infects other animals. The subfamily designations are rarely used and for convenience we shall refer to these viruses by their abbreviations. The morphology of all herpes viruses is similar and distinctive. Although they share a number of antigens, they can be distinguished by differences in their genomes and by serological tests. HSV-1 and HSV-2 have most in common, particularly in terms of biological activities, but differ sufficiently to be classed separately. Of the remaining subfamilies, they most closely resemble VZV. We shall first consider the general properties of the group and then in separate sections describe the biological activities of the viruses.

Although biological features such as latency, cytopathic changes, and reproductive cycle are still important features of herpes classification, in the future comparative analysis of nucleotide sequences and identification of gene clusters, gene order, and arrangements of sequences for genome packaging will be of more importance.

2 Morphology

The virions are **icosahedral**, built up of 162 tubular capsomeres surrounding a core of DNA. The core is surrounded by a tegu-

Table 17.1 Members of the family *Herpesviridae* that infect humans

Subfamily	Colloquial name and abbreviation	Numerical designation
Alphaherpesvirinae	Herpes simplex type 1 (HSV-1)	HHV-1*
	Herpes simplex type 2 (HSV-2)	HHV-2
	Varicella-zoster (VZV)	HHV-3
	Herpesvirus B (or herpes simiae virus)	–
Betaherpesvirinae	Cytomegalovirus (CMV)	HHV-5
	Human herpesvirus 6 (HHV-6)	HHV-6
	Human herpesvirus 7 (HHV-7)	HHV-7
Gammaherpesvirinae	Epstein–Barr virus (EBV)	HHV-4
	Kaposi's sarcoma-associated herpesvirus (KSHV)	HHV-8

* HHV = human herpesvirus.

ment and outermost there is a large baggy **envelope** (Fig. 17.1); unenveloped particles may also be present. The diameter of the naked particle is about 100 nm and of the complete enveloped virion 120–200 nm.

3 Genome

The dsDNA is **linear,** with molecular weights varying from 125 to 229 kbp, according to the subfamily. The genome is

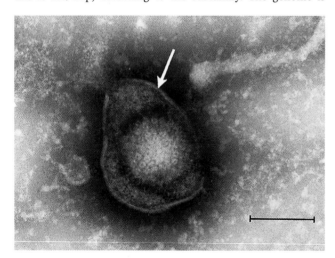

Fig 17.1 Electron micrograph of HSV. The baggy appearance of the outer envelope (arrowed) is characteristic, but is an artefact arising during preparation of a specimen. (Courtesy of Dr David Hockley.) Scale bar = 100 nm.

infectious. The genomes of the subfamilies differ remarkably in their organization; those of HSV-1 and HSV-2 resemble each other most closely. However, it is obvious that the α, β, and γ herpesviruses have evolved from a common ancestor.

Herpes simplex is the prototype virus of the family and the genome has been completely sequenced. It has 152 kbp, containing 80 genes. Each gene is expressed from its own promotor. There are many overlapping reading frames. The HSV-1 genome has two covalently joined sections termed the **unique long** *and* **unique short** *regions. Each is bounded by inverted repeats, which allow structural rearrangements of the unique regions and hence* **the HSV-1 genome exists as a mixture of four isomers,** *which are functionally equivalent to each other. All herpes genomes have repeated sequences and this introduces another variation in genome size in the family.*

Herpes simplex has 80 tightly packed genes orientated in either direction; most have a protein coding function.

It is assumed that, although most genes are required for growth in humans, only half of them are utilized when the virus replicates in cell culture. Other members of the same subfamily share most of the genes, which have similar layouts. For example, there are only five genes in VZV that do not have counterparts in HSV-1.

As expected, comparison of the genomes in the three subfamilies reveals more variation, but even so, nearly half of the genes are conserved.

Extra genes are found in two of the subfamilies and may represent captured cellular genes, whereas some other genes present in the prototype virus HSV-1 may be missing: thus the β herpesviruses do not have a TK gene.

Between the subfamilies, there is variation in the genes encoding the virion surface glycoproteins. Whereas gB, gH, gL, and gM are present in all HHVs, VZV does not have three proteins possessed by HSV-1; CMV, however, has a vast array of glycoprotein genes.

4 Polypeptides

The large genome codes for 80–100 polypeptides, many of which are NS proteins, including a DNA polymerase that is essential for replication. HSV-1, HSV-2, and VZV code for a phosphorylating enzyme, a **TK** essential for the activation of certain antiviral drugs (Chapter 38). Structural proteins are present in the nucleocapsid, the tegument, and the lipid envelope.

5 Antigens

As might be expected from the many polypeptides contained in these viruses, antigenic analysis and the study of serological cross-reactions are difficult. Conventional tests such as neutralization and complement fixation identify the subfamilies. HSV-1 and HSV-2 can be distinguished by cross-absorptions, but the use of **monoclonal antibodies** or **restriction endonuclease analysis** of viral DNA are more efficient. In the diagnostic laboratory, the antigens of EBV have received most attention as their pattern can give useful information about the stage of infection.

6 Replication

The docking protein of the most studied member of the family, HSV-1, is the glycoprotein C, which attaches to cellular proteoglycans. Other viral glycoproteins (B, D, and H) then become involved in a complex fusion process of the viral lipid envelope with the plasma membrane. The viral capsid is transported to a nuclear pore, at which point the linear DNA is released and enters the nucleus of the cell where most events of transcription, viral DNA replication and capsid assembly occur. The virus induces a shutdown of host protein and nucleic acid synthesis.

Initially there is a burst of transcription activity from early viral genes whereas slightly later, after initiation of viral DNA replication, intermediate and late genes are transcribed. Not unexpectedly the whole process is carefully controlled. Transcription of the immediate early α mRNAs is stimulated by a viral tegument protein and once transferred to the cytoplasm, translation into α proteins commences. These α proteins are, on the whole, *trans*-acting regulatory proteins, which control the expression of later β and γ genes.

The β proteins are predominantly enzymes such as **TK, DNA polymerase**, and **helicase**, which are required for viral DNA replication. The late γ mRNAs are triggered after viral DNA replication and code for **structural proteins**.

New viral DNA is synthesized by a rolling circle mechanism and the appropriate cleaved fragments are packaged into nucleocapsids, migrate to the nuclear membrane and associate there with both viral tegument proteins and envelope proteins. **Budding** takes place through the nuclear membrane and enveloped viruses congregate in the endoplasmic reticulum before they are released from the cell.

7 Reminders

- The family *Herpesviridae* contains three subfamilies: the *Alphaherpesvirinae*, *Betaherpesvirinae*, and *Gammaherpesvirinae*, distinguished by their different genome structures and biological properties.

- Herpesviruses have four concentric layers, an outer envelope, a tegument, an **icosahedral** nucleocapsid and an inner core; they are 120–200 nm in diameter.

- Their genomes are **dsDNA**; they vary in size from 125 to 229 kbp and encode 80–100 polypeptides. HSV-1, HSV-2, and VZV code for **TK**, which helps to mediate the action of certain antiviral drugs. The unique viral DNA polymerase is a target for antiviral drugs.

- Viral replication is entirely **nuclear** and is strictly controlled with α, β, and γ genes coding for corresponding proteins. The α proteins are *trans*-acting regulatory proteins, whereas β proteins are enzymes such as DNA polymerases; the γ proteins are structural.

- The viruses of the three subfamilies cause diverse clinical syndromes, ranging from minor cutaneous lesions to life-threatening illnesses. They can all cause latent infections.

Chapter 18

The alphaherpesviruses: herpes simplex and varicella-zoster

1 Herpes simplex viruses

1.1 Clinical aspects

The HSVs, HSV-1 and HSV-2, have many features in common but can be distinguished by laboratory tests. There is no sharp demarcation between the syndromes caused by the two viruses. All of them may be caused by either virus, but as a general rule, HSV-1 primarily affects the upper part of the body, whereas HSV-2 is more usually, but not exclusively, the cause of genital infections.

HSV infections can be established in many species of animal, which facilitates research on them.

Terminology

Primary infection refers to the first infection with either HSV. As there is little cross-protection between HSV-1 and HSV-2 it is possible to be infected later with the other variety; to distinguish it from a primary infection in a completely non-immune person, such an episode is known as an **initial infection**.

The term **reactivation** properly applies to production of infective virus by a latently infected cell. If clinically apparent disease results, it is termed a recurrence or **recrudescence**.

Oropharyngeal infection

The primary infection with HSV is often acquired in infancy or early childhood from close contact with an older person, often as the result of a kiss. In many instances the infection is asymptomatic, but it may present as **acute gingivostomatitis** (Fig. 18.1): vesicles on the gums and oral mucosa break down to form ulcers. By contrast with Coxsackie infections (Chapter 16) in which the vesicles appear on the hard palate and fauces, herpetic lesions affect the anterior part of the mouth, often with involvement of the lips and circumoral skin. The child is febrile, uncomfortable and has difficulty in feeding. The time from onset to healing is about 2 weeks.

In later life, recurrences manifest around the mouth, commonly at the lip margin (Fig. 18.2), as a cluster of vesicles heralded some hours previously by an itching sensation. They are milder, more localized and of shorter duration than the primary

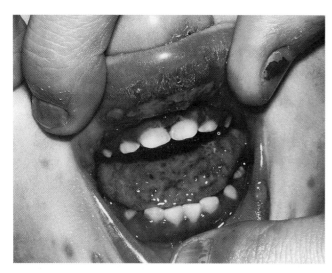

Fig. 18.1 Herpetic gingivostomatitis in a child. Note the vesicles around the mouth and on the tongue and the intensely inflamed gingivae. (Courtesy of the late Dr W. Marshall.)

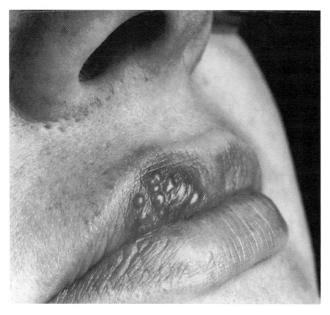

Fig. 18.2 Recurrent herpes simplex.

or initial infection; the lesions, which at first contain a clear watery fluid, crust over and heal within a few days. With the passage of years, recurrences tend to become less frequent and often cease altogether.

Dermal infections

Primary infections of the skin are not uncommon in healthcare staff whose hands come into contact with oral secretions. Many people shed HSV infections in respiratory secretions and saliva, so that for example, nurses, particularly those looking after tracheostomy patients, and dentists are at risk of **herpetic whitlow**, a lesion on a finger, which is very painful but heals without treatment. The temptation to open such lesions must be resisted as the interior contains not pus but necrotic material and inci-

sion will make matters worse. Such infections can of course be prevented by wearing gloves.

Sportsmen, e.g. wrestlers, may acquire skin lesions ('herpes gladiatorum') from contact with another competitor, or from contaminated mats or other articles.

People with eczema are particularly liable to acquire skin infection with HSV, an unpleasant and occasionally fatal condition known as **eczema herpeticum**.

Genital infections

These have in recent years attracted much attention in Western countries, where publicity about them in the 'media' has contributed to the realization that gonorrhoea and syphilis are not the only sexually transmitted diseases. Nevertheless, their existence has been known for many years.

Because most people have been infected with HSV-1 early in life, genital infection is more often acquired as an initial episode than as a true primary infection. In the male it presents as a crop of vesicles on the **penis**; lesions may also occur within the meatus causing dysuria. **Herpetic proctitis** is sometimes seen in homosexuals. In the female, the lesions are on the **labia, vulva**, and **perineum**, sometimes extending to the inner surface of the thighs (Fig. 18.3). **Cervicitis** with vesicular lesions also occurs. **Inguinal lymphadenopathy** is pronounced in both sexes and there is often some fever and malaise. Not infrequently, particularly in male homosexuals, there is also an attack of **meningitis**. Recurrences of infections with HSV-2 are likely to be more frequent and severe than those due to HSV-1. They are the cause of much sexual disability and mental distress.

In children, herpetic vulvovaginitis may indicate sexual abuse, but needless to say, other causes of infection, such as auto-inoculation from an oral lesion, must also be considered.

There has been much discussion about the relationship of HSV infection of the cervix and cervical carcinoma. There is

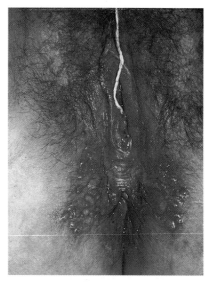

Fig. 18.3 Genital herpes. (Photography courtesy of the late Dr David Oriel.)

certainly a correlation between the incidence of both conditions, but it is by no means certain that HSV is the primary cause, although some workers claim to have identified HSV DNA sequences in carcinoma cells. Many other factors such as promiscuity, smoking and infections with other microorganisms, in particular papillomaviruses (Chapter 15) may, however, be implicated and the role of HSV, if any, awaits clarification.

Ophthalmic infections

Herpetic keratoconjunctivitis is a comparatively frequent infection, nearly always caused by HSV-1. It is often characterized by **dendritic ulcers**, so called because of their branching appearance. The corneal stroma may also be affected (disciform keratitis), and **iridocyclitis** is a serious complication. Recurrent attacks of keratitis or keratoconjunctivitis, if untreated, may also cause considerable damage to the eye, with corneal scarring and loss of vision.

Meningitis and encephalitis

We mentioned earlier that meningitis occasionally complicates genital tract infections. By itself it is a benign condition; but HSV encephalitis is a serious, life-threatening illness with a high rate of neurological sequelae after recovery from the acute infection. It may occur at any age and is usually caused by HSV-1; there may be concurrent signs of herpes elsewhere, but more often than not it strikes without warning. The onset is often insidious with malaise and fever lasting a few days, followed by headache and changes in behaviour. Clouding of consciousness proceeding to coma is a bad prognostic sign. Untreated, the mortality is about 70 per cent with a high rate of neurological sequelae, including mental defect, in survivors.

Infections of the newborn

These are almost always caused by HSV-2 during passage through an infected birth canal. They are described in Chapter 31.

Infection in the immunodeficient host

This is discussed in Chapter 32. HSV infections, sometimes severe and persistent, are common in patients whose cellular immunity has been impaired by malignant disease or cytotoxic therapy. They are also frequent in patients with AIDS, who may suffer from severe perianal infections.

1.2 Pathogenesis

Skin and mucous membranes are the portals of entry in which the virus also multiplies, causing lysis of cells and formation of **vesicles**. In mucous membranes these soon rupture to form shallow ulcers, but in skin they remain intact for several days before crusting over and healing. The clear fluid within the vesicles contains large numbers of virions. In scrapings or sections of vesicles there are cells containing **eosinophilic intranuclear inclusion bodies** (Chapter 4), characteristically surrounded by a clear halo (see Fig. 32.7) they represent sites of replication ('virus factories').

Local replication is followed by spread to the regional lymph nodes and then by viraemia, which is of little significance unless there is haematogenous spread to the CNS, causing meningitis or even encephalitis (Chapter 30). Such events are, however, comparatively rare; the nervous system is involved by a more subtle mechanism that is central to the pathogenesis of HSV infection.

Soon after replication is under way in the skin or a mucous membrane, virions travel to the **root ganglia** via the sensory

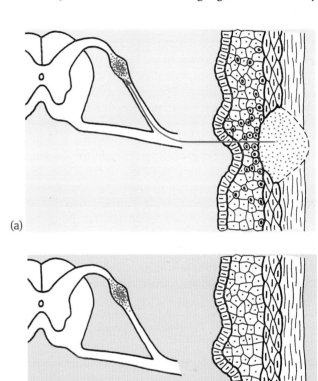

(a)

(b)

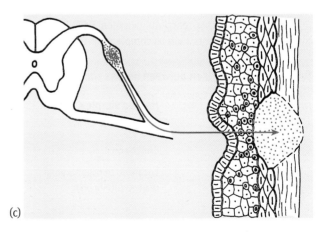

(c)

Fig. 18.4 Latency and recurrence in herpes simplex infections. From the primary lesion, the virus **(a)** travels up the sensory nerves to the dorsal root ganglion, and **(b)** becomes latent; **(c)** when reactivated, it returns to the skin by the same route and gives rise to a recurrent lesion.

nerves supplying the area (Fig. 18.4). Primary infections of the orofacial and genital areas involve respectively the **trigeminal** and **lumbosacral** dorsal root ganglia. The virus then becomes latent in the ganglia in a way that is not fully understood. We know that the viral DNA, normally a linear molecule, is integrated into neurones in the form of a circular episome, but many other aspects of latency are not as yet understood. It is a curious fact that latent virus can be reactivated by removing a ganglion from a latently infected animal and incubating it in culture medium for several days.

Whatever the mechanism, once HSV has established itself in a ganglion *in vivo*, **reactivations** are liable to take place at intervals of weeks or months thereafter. Such attacks may be triggered by a variety of stimuli. The popular terms 'cold sores', or in the USA, 'fever blisters' illustrate their association with colds and other febrile illnesses; sunlight, menstruation, and therapeutic irradiation are other well-known factors, as is surgical interference with the trigeminal nerve. Again, the mechanism is not clear, but it seems likely that the host cell is stimulated to produce infective virions that pass down the sensory axons to replicate once again in dermal cells, with the production of vesicles at or near the site of the original infection. It may be that those nerve cells in which virus is reactivated become lysed in the process; if so, it is plausible that the gradual destruction of the whole pool of latently infected cells, possibly in combination with the immune response, accounts for the fading away of recurrences.

1.3 Immune response

IgM, IgG, and IgA antibodies are produced and seroconversion following a true primary infection is diagnostically useful. IgG antibody persists for many years but does not prevent reactivations, the virus presumably being protected from neutralization within the 'immunologically privileged' site of the nervous system. The antibody response to recurrences is variable, often undetectable by routine methods, and thus of no diagnostic value.

Because of the cross-reactions between HSV-1 and HSV-2, routine serological tests such as complement fixation and neu-tralization do not distinguish between them. Nevertheless, although infection with one of these viruses usually protects against reinfection with the same variety, it often fails to confer immunity against the other; thus people who have had, say, an HSV-1 infection of the mouth are not fully protected against subsequent genital infection with HSV-2.

The importance of **CMI** in controlling the course of infection is amply illustrated by the tendency of HSV infections to become generalized in some patients with defects in their T-cell response (Chapter 32, Section 1.3).

1.4 Epidemiology

Most people are infected by the time they are adults. The virus is usually acquired in infancy or childhood but there is, at least in some communities, a second peak at adolescence when opportunities for spread are renewed by sexual activity. Primary infections after the age of 30 are rare. Once acquired, HSV is carried throughout life as a latent infection. There are recurrences in about half of those infected, but asymptomatic shedding of virus in oral and genital secretions takes place both in them and in those without clinical signs.

Table 18.1 summarizes the differences between the clinical features of herpes simplex, varicella, and zoster infections.

1.5 Laboratory diagnosis

The clinical appearances of mucocutaneous herpes are usually distinctive enough to make laboratory tests unnecessary. They are, however, useful in genital and eye infections, in distinguishing between generalized herpes and varicella-zoster in an immunodeficient patient, and in herpetic meningo-encephalitis; the latter topic is dealt with in Chapter 30.

Serological tests are by and large of limited value, especially in diagnosing recurrences. When they are used, complement fixation remains the standard technique in many laboratories, but is now being replaced by more sensitive assays such as ELISA. Weak cross-reactions with varicella-zoster are a possible source of error.

Table 18.1 Comparison between herpes simplex and varicella-zoster infections

	Herpes simplex	Varicella	Zoster
Transmission	Contact	Aerosol	Recurrence of latent infection
Age of acquisition	Childhood	Childhood	Adolescence/adulthood
Areas mainly affected	Localized to oropharynx, skin, genitalia, eye	Generalized: oropharynx and skin	Usually a trigeminal, cervical, thoracic, or lumbosacral dermotome. Usually unilateral
Reactivations	Frequent	Once only (as zoster) or never	Second attacks rare
Congenital infections	Intrapartum. Relatively infrequent. May be localized or generalized	Acquired *in utero*. Rare. Fetus usually dies	None

Detection of virus

Detection of virus rather than of antibody is thus usually the method of choice. In most instances, the distinction between HSV-1 and HSV-2 is academic and there is no need to do the more sophisticated tests needed for identification at this level.

Virus isolation

Scrapings or swabs from active lesions are inoculated into a suitable cell culture—human diploid lines are highly susceptible—and observed for CPE. Foci of enlarged cells, some of which are multinucleate, appear within 72 hours. HSV-2 usually causes more 'ballooning' of the cells than HSV-1 and an experienced observer can often make an accurate guess as to the type of virus. The identity of any doubtful appearances can be established by serial passage, or, much more quickly, by **immunofluorescence staining** or **EM**.

It must be remembered that by itself, isolation of HSV from body fluids such as saliva or genital secretions does not prove that it is causing disease, as many apparently normal people shed virus intermittently.

Giant cells and inclusions

Stained smears made from vigorous scrapings of the base of an active lesion often reveal multinucleate cells containing intranuclear inclusions. These appearances may also be observed in sections of biopsy or necropsy material. Such techniques are, however, rarely used nowadays, although they may still be useful in laboratories with limited facilities.

Electron microscopy

If vesicles with clear fluid are present this method is fast and reliable. It is not recommended if there is secondary infection or if crusting has taken place. A drop of fluid is taken by opening the top of a vesicle with a needle or, preferably, a scalpel point, spreading it on an ordinary microscope slide and allowing it to dry. In the laboratory the material is taken up in distilled water for negative staining and EM. The fluid contains numerous virions that are easy to recognize, so that a diagnosis can often be made with a drop only 2 or 3 mm in diameter within an hour of collecting the specimen.

Immunofluorescence

Monoclonal antibodies against both HSV-1 and HSV-2 are now available; these are conjugated with a fluorescent label and used to stain vesicle fluid; by this method, the virions appear in the ultraviolet microscope as bright yellow–green particles. The method has the advantage of immediately distinguishing between the two HSVs, but like EM, demands properly collected specimens taken from suitable lesions.

Polymerase chain reaction

This is useful for detecting viral DNA in CSF when herpetic infection of the CNS is suspected.

1.6 Immunization

There is as yet no vaccine against HSV-1 or HSV-2, and indeed, it is difficult to see how such a vaccine could be effective against latent infections with recurrences. There may be some scope for immunization against HSV-2 before adolescence, but the expense and risk associated with such a vaccine probably makes it a non-starter, especially now that effective chemotherapy is available.

1.7 Treatment

ACV is the drug of choice for treating and, in some situations, preventing HSV infections. Intravenous, oral, and topical preparations are available. The mode of action is described in Chapter 38. In practice, the following general points are important.

As with all antiviral therapy, ACV must be given early to be fully effective. It should not be used indiscriminately for trivial infections. In the eye, topical applications are relatively effective. ACV may, however, be indicated for infections in immunodeficient patients that would not otherwise need treatment. ACV-resistant mutants are rare, and in general are isolated only from patients with immunodeficiencies.

ACV is excreted in the urine and the dosage must be reduced in patients with impaired renal function.

Treatment of specific syndromes

Mucocutaneous herpes

Except for severe genital tract infections, primary and recurrent mucocutaneous herpes simplex does not normally need specific treatment. Facial lesions should be kept dry with boric acid or methylated spirit. Long-term continuous oral prophylaxis is very effective in preventing severe recurrent genital herpes but is also very expensive.

Ophthalmic infections

These are treatable with topical applications of ACV. Steroids are strongly contraindicated.

Encephalitis

A double-blind trial in Scandinavia clearly showed that ACV is superior to vidarabine, both for preventing sequelae and diminishing mortality. Early treatment is particularly important in this condition.

Infections in pregnancy

It seems logical to treat a genital infection occurring late in pregnancy in order to protect the baby at birth. As data are still being collected about the safety of this procedure, it is not as yet officially recommended, but there have been no untoward effects on either mother or baby in the cases so far reported.

Immunodeficiency

New infections in severely immunodeficient patients may be prevented by oral administration. Severe and generalized infections need intravenous treatment, the recommended dosage being 5 mg/kg body weight every 8 hours. There is usually no point in continuing treatment beyond 5 days.

2 Varicella-zoster virus

By contrast with the HSVs there is only one varicella-zoster agent, named after the two main syndromes that it causes: **varicella**, or chickenpox, and **herpes zoster**, popularly known as shingles (or hives in the USA). There are similarities with HSV infections in terms of lesions, pathogenesis, and pathology.

2.1 Clinical aspects

Varicella (chickenpox)

Chickenpox is a common childhood infection. The **incubation period** is about 2 weeks but may vary by several days each side of this figure. In children, the rash is usually the first sign, associated with a mild feverish illness. Adults usually suffer much more constitutional upset. The rash is characteristically **centripetal**, i.e. more pronounced on the trunk than on the limbs. It first appears as flat **macules**, which rapidly become raised into **papules**; these are succeeded by **vesicles**, which finally form crusts **that** are shed from the skin (Fig. 18.5). The rash

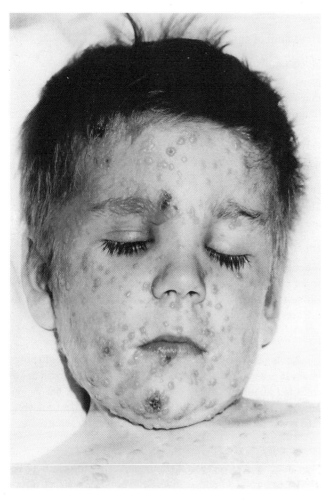

Fig. 18.5 Chickenpox rash. The lesions are mostly at the vesicular stage; the darker ones have started to form crusts. (Courtesy of the late Dr W. Marshall.)

appears in successive crops, so that all stages of the eruption can be seen at the same time. Recovery is usually uneventful.

Complications

Bacterial infection of the vesicular fluid leading to pustule formation may occur. In patients with thrombocytopenia the rash may become haemorrhagic and there may be bleeding from body orifices. Postinfection **encephalitis** may occur, particularly in immunodeficient patients (Chapter 32).

The complications most to be feared are **varicella pneumonitis** and generalized varicella, which again mainly affect immunocompromised patients. **Leukaemic children** are at particular risk of pneumonitis, which is often fatal. The term 'generalized varicella' is tautologous, but is used to imply clinically apparent involvement of the viscera, joints, and CNS.

Congenital and neonatal infections

These are described in Chapter 31.

Herpes zoster

'Zoster' is derived from the Latin word for a belt or girdle and refers to the characteristic distribution of the rash when a thoracic dermatome is involved. The attack is heralded by hyperaesthesia and sometimes by pain in the affected area, followed within a day or so by a crop of typical herpetic vesicles that eventually crust over and heal in the usual way.

Complications

- **Postherpetic pain** in the affected area is frequent, particularly in the elderly. It usually ceases within a month, but may persist for years. If severe, its resistance to treatment can make life a misery for a minority of patients.

- **Ophthalmic zoster** is a potentially serious complication, when as often happens, the ophthalmic branch of the trigeminal nerve is affected. Both superficial and deep structures of the eye may be involved.

- **Generalized zoster** is similar to generalized varicella, but is distinguished clinically by the presence of vesicles distributed along a dermatome in addition to the more general rash. Encephalitis is a rare complication of herpes zoster.

2.2 Pathogenesis

Varicella is acquired by the **respiratory route**. Because there is no animal model, the pathogenesis has not been verified experimentally, but probably follows the pattern of other acute childhood fevers (Chapter 4). Dissemination of virus in the bloodstream is followed by a rash, at first macular, but rapidly developing into papules followed by vesicles similar to those caused by HSV and like them, containing many virions. The lesions become crusted and separate as scabs within 10 days of onset; contrary to early ideas, the scabs are virtually without infectivity.

In some patients the virus becomes **latent** in a dorsal root ganglion. This event is analogous to what happens in HSV infections, but, as one might expect in such a generalized infection, VZV may affect any sensory nerve, those most commonly involved being the thoracic, trigeminal, cervical, and lumbosacral; it is rare for more than one of these to be involved. Unlike HSV, VZV infects only humans, so that research on latent infections is very limited. Unfortunately, latent VZV in cadavers cannot be reactivated by the incubation method described for HSV. Nevertheless, viral DNA can be detected in the sensory ganglia, and this technique has yielded some information on the distribution of latent virus.

In humans, VZV can reactivate, causing an attack of herpes zoster with a characteristic distribution of vesicular lesions along the affected dermatome. Almost invariably, there is only one such episode in a lifetime. Even less is known about the trigger mechanism than in the case of HSV infections, but it is noteworthy that many attacks of zoster occur in the elderly, in whom immunity is waning, and in **immunocompromised patients**.

2.3 Immune response

The antibody response to chickenpox is more clear-cut than in HSV infections. IgM antibody appears within the first week and persists for about 3 months; IgG antibody is detectable for many years. A subsequent attack of zoster results in renewed production of IgM antibody. The role of the humoral response in immunity is not clear, but as in HSV infections, intact T-cell responses are most important in controlling recovery from infection.

2.4 Epidemiology

In temperate climates, chickenpox is primarily a disease of young children, but at least two reports show that the age of onset in the Indian subcontinent is much higher, adults being mainly affected with correspondingly more severe infections. The reason for this is not clear.

As herpes zoster is a reactivation of a latent infection it cannot—or should not—be 'caught' in the same way as varicella. The qualification is necessary because there are reports suggesting that zoster can be acquired by contact with other cases; but this seems inherently unlikely and the evidence is circumstantial. By contrast, **varicella can be readily acquired from patients with an active zoster infection**. This can present a problem in wards containing immunodeficient patients who are liable to develop zoster if they have previously had chickenpox, or who are unduly susceptible to VZV infection if they have not. Furthermore, spread from patients to non-immune nursing staff occurs readily. Management of such situations includes adequate isolation of patients with VZV infections, who ideally should be attended only by staff with antibody to the virus.

2.5 Laboratory diagnosis

When laboratory confirmation is needed, it depends on techniques similar to those used for HSV. As we have seen, serological tests are more informative than with HSV, although the results may be blurred by cross-reactions with these viruses. Detection of IgM by radioimmunoassay (RIA) is useful for diagnosing current or recent infection.

Direct demonstration of the virus by isolation in cell cultures can be a slow business because the CPE may take up to 3 weeks to become apparent. Under the EM, the virions appear identical to those of HSV; immunofluorescence tests on infected cell cultures will, however, distinguish between these agents.

2.6 Active immunization

A **live attenuated VZV vaccine** is available for preventing chickenpox in immunodeficient children, e.g. those with leukaemia. It is licensed in some countries, but not as yet in the UK, where it is available only on a named patient basis (see also Chapter 37).

2.7 Passive immunization

Although there are no really well-controlled trials, **immunoglobulin** prepared from the sera of blood donors with high titres of antibody to VZV seems to be of some use in preventing or modifying severe disease in immunodeficient patients who come into contact with chickenpox or herpes zoster. This preparation, **zoster immune globulin** (**ZIG**), must be given as soon as possible, and certainly within 4 days of contact. It is of no value for treating established infection.

2.8 Treatment

Chickenpox in the immunocompetent child does not require antiviral therapy. Calamine lotion containing 1 per cent phenol is useful for preventing itching. In immunocompromised patients there is always the danger of generalization and varicella pneumonia, for which ACV is useful both for prevention and treatment.

ACV is used to treat severe VZV infections. *In vitro* it is about 20 times less active against this virus than against HSV, but is still effective clinically: for intravenous use, twice the usual dose is given, i.e. 10 mg/kg every 8 hours. Two compounds with a similar mode of action, **famciclovir** and **valaciclovir**, are also available.

ACV in high dosage can be given during the prodromal stage in an attempt to modify the severity of the infection, but seems to have little or no effect in reducing the incidence of postherpetic pain.

3 Herpesvirus B

This alphaherpesvirus is not usually considered as a HHV as it normally infects only macaque monkeys, hence its alternative name, *herpesvirus simiae* (not to be confused with *herpesvirus saimiri*, which infects squirrel monkeys). Such infections are silent, or at worst cause vesicular lesions in the mouth and skin. Humans exposed to saliva, e.g. by being bitten, are liable to contract severe **encephalomyelitis**, which is almost always fatal. There have been several such cases in laboratory staff handling apparently normal monkeys.

4 Reminders

4.1 Herpes simplex infections

- **Primary** infections with HSV-1 usually affect the oropharynx or facial skin, and infections with HSV-2, the genitalia. The lesions are **vesicles**, which contain much infective virus.

- During the primary infection, virus travels up the sensory nerves supplying the affected area and becomes **latent** in the dorsal root ganglia. **Reactivation** of latent virus may result in **recurrences** at intervals, with renewed formation of vesicles in the skin or mucous membrane.

- HSVs are also liable to cause **ophthalmic infections, meningitis**, and **encephalitis**.

- Severe infections, sometimes widespread, may be caused in **neonates**, who acquire the infection at birth, and in patients suffering from **immunodeficiencies**.

- Methods used in the laboratory diagnosis include virus isolation, **EM** and detection of antigen by **immunofluorescence**.

- **ACV** is the drug of choice for all herpes simplex infections.

4.2 Varicella-zoster infections

- **Varicella** (chickenpox) is a common childhood infection acquired by **the respiratory route**. The **incubation period** is about 2 weeks.

- It causes a generalized **rash**, progressing from macules to papules and then to **vesicles**, similar to those of herpes simplex.

- Recovery is usually uneventful, except in **immunocompromised** patients, e.g. leukaemic children, who may develop severe **pneumonitis**.

- **Herpes zoster** (shingles) results from reactivation of latent virus in dorsal root ganglia and appears as a crop of vesicles on one or more of the dermatomes of the trunk, or, if the trigeminal ganglion is affected, on the head. Postherpetic pain in the affected area may be troublesome, especially in the elderly. Like varicella, zoster may become generalized in immunocompromised patients.

- Herpes zoster is infective for non-immune contacts, in whom it may cause chickenpox.

- The clinical diagnosis may be confirmed by finding **specific IgM antibody** or by demonstrating virus in vesicle fluid by **EM** or **immunofluorescence**.

- **Passive immunization** of susceptible contacts may be effected with **ZIG**. **An attenuated live vaccine** shows promise for protecting immunodeficient children.

- **ACV** is used for treating severe varicella or herpes zoster in immunodeficient and other patients.

Chapter 19

The betaherpesviruses: cytomegalovirus and human herpesviruses 6 and 7

1 Cytomegalovirus

The name means 'large cell virus' and derives from the swollen cells containing large intranuclear inclusions that characterize these infections.

1.1 Clinical aspects

At first encounter, CMV infections are confusing because they vary so much in terms of age groups affected, mode of acquisition, and clinical presentation. A good aid to memory is to classify them by the ages predominantly affected, as this factor strongly influences the type of disease likely to be encountered. CMV can be a problem even before the cradle and certainly to the grave.

CMV is transmissible to the **fetus** via the placenta, and is an important cause of neonatal morbidity and mortality (Chapter 31).

Normal infants can acquire infection from **colostrum** or **breast milk**; maternal antibody does not seem to confer protection. Such infections are usually asymptomatic.

Young children readily become infected, again without overt disease, when they enter crèches or play schools, in which the environment is liable to become contaminated by virus shed in **urine** and **saliva**.

The next wave of infection occurs at **adolescence and early adulthood**, when infection is spread by **kissing and sexual intercourse**. At this age, CMV sometimes causes a syndrome like the infectious mononucleosis resulting from infection with EBV, another herpesvirus (Chapter 20). CMV causes a febrile illness with splenomegaly, impaired liver function—sometimes with jaundice—and the appearance of abnormal lymphocytes in the blood; the pharyngitis and lymphadenopathy characterizing EBV infection are, however, absent. A similar illness occasionally follows blood transfusion, the risk being increased when large volumes are used. CMV is found so constantly in promiscuous male homosexuals that before the discovery of HIV it was considered as a possible cause of AIDS.

Transplant recipients

The last of our categories is not age-related. The source of infection can be

- **exogenous**, deriving from the donor's tissues or from blood transfusions given in support of surgery, or
- **endogenous**, i.e. reactivation of an existing infection in the recipient.

Both types of infection, and particularly the second, are facilitated by the associated immunosuppressive treatment. Primary infections are the most dangerous and may result in glomerulonephritis with rejection of a transplanted kidney or in CMV infection of the lungs. This is **an interstitial pneumonitis** with oedema and pronounced cellular infiltration. The mortality is about 20 per cent in bone marrow recipients but only 1–2 per cent in kidney transplant patients. Reactivations are less serious than primary infections and may result in nothing worse than a febrile illness. For further discussion of CMV infections in renal and bone marrow transplantation, see Chapter 32.

Although rare, cases of CMV encephalitis have been reported in apparently immunocompetent adults.

1.2 Pathogenesis

The pathogenesis of the herpesvirus infections so far described is reasonably straightforward; CMV presents more difficult problems. Infection is acquired by various routes, and lasts for life. How this happens is not clear; it may well involve a combination of true **latency**, with integration of viral genome into leucocytes, and **chronic infection** with production of infective virions. The finding of CMV inclusions in renal and salivary cells of people without clinical disease is good evidence for the latter mechanism. Throughout life, there is **intermittent shedding of virus in body fluids**, including saliva, urine, cervical secretion, semen, and breast milk, giving ample opportunities for transmission; transfused blood may also be a source of infection. In most people, the infection is silent, but in overt disease almost any organ is liable to be damaged. As with other herpesviruses, **reactivations** are an important feature of pathogenesis, and to complicate matters further, **reinfections** with other strains are also possible.

CMV infection is particularly serious in **AIDS patients** because of their lack of CD4+ cells.

1.3 Immune response

Primary infections, but not reactivations, induce **IgM antibody**, which is therefore useful diagnostically. As might be imagined from the persistence of infection, IgG antibodies are present throughout life. The importance of CMI is again emphasized by the tendency to reactivation in immunosuppressed patients.

1.4 Epidemiology

The propensity of CMV to be reactivated intermittently and shed in urine and other body fluids, even in the absence of overt illness, makes it a very successful parasite. As might be expected, the opportunities for acquiring CMV are greatest under conditions of poverty, overcrowding, and poor hygiene. In one sense this is an advantage, because infection is acquired early in life when it is usually symptomless. Conversely, the average age of acquisition is greater in communities with high living standards and the outcomes, in terms of the more severe primary infections, are correspondingly worse; this is particularly true of first infections during pregnancy.

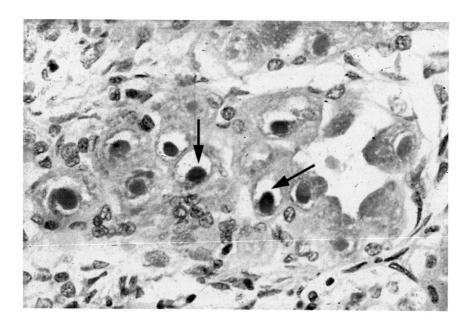

Fig. 19.1 'Owls' eye' intranuclear inclusions of cytomegalovirus, arrowed.

1.5 Laboratory diagnosis

Serological methods

Tests for IgM antibody are best done by RIA after absorbing out rheumatoid factor, which is liable to give false positive results. They can be used on cord blood to test for infection acquired *in utero* and for diagnosing current or recent primary infections in immunocompetent adults. IgM antibody is not induced by recurrent infection or in immunodeficient patients.

Tests for **IgG antibody** include complement fixation, ELISA, the latter being the more sensitive. Such tests are useful for identifying potentially infective blood or tissue donors and for epidemiological surveys.

Detection of virus

CMV can be isolated from urine, saliva and the **buffy coat of heparinized blood**. This virus can be propagated only in human fibroblasts, in which it gives rise to foci of swollen multinucleate cells with characteristic intranuclear inclusions. Such changes may take up to 4 weeks to appear, but infection can be diagnosed as early as 24 hours after inoculation by **immunofluorescent staining with monoclonal antibody.**

In histological sections, CMV can be identified by the characteristic enlarged cells containing **'owl's eye' inclusions** (Fig. 19.1). Like other herpesvirus inclusions these are intranuclear, but are more basophilic than those of HSV and VZV. These cytomegalic cells are present in the epithelial or endothelial cells of most viscera. They can also be found in the salivary glands of about 10 per cent of infants dying of unrelated causes. In the kidney, they are seen in the convoluted tubules but not in the glomeruli: the affected cells are shed into the urine, in which they can sometimes be found after centrifugation.

Immunofluorescence with monoclonal antibody can also be used to detect virus in tissue sections, but its main value is in staining bronchoalveolar washings for the diagnosis of CMV pneumonitis.

Viral DNA is detectable in blood and other body fluids by PCR and hybridization methods (Chapter 36).

1.6 Active immunization

A vaccine prepared from the Towne strain of CMV has appeared to protect renal allograft recipients against infection, but failed to induce an adequate antibody response in normal women exposed to young children in group care.

1.7 Passive immunization

There is some evidence that the administration of high titre anti-CMV immunoglobulin protects immunosuppressed patients against CMV pneumonitis.

1.8 Treatment

Because CMV lacks the TK possessed by HSV and VZV, ACV is inactive. Ganciclovir, a similar compound, is however phosphor-ylated by a different enzyme and is used with some success in treating immunosuppressed patients, including those with AIDS. Unfortunately, it is relatively toxic and its bioavailability is poor, so that a satisfactory treatment for CMV must await further advances in chemotherapy (see also Chapter 38).

2 Human herpesviruses types 6 and 7

The comparatively recent identification of these viruses supports the speculation that, despite all the diagnostic advances in the last few decades, there are still others waiting to be discovered.

2.1 Human herpesvirus 6

Isolation

This agent was first isolated in 1986 from blood leucocytes of six patients suffering from lymphomas or acute lymphocytic leukaemia. It induces CPE with inclusion bodies in human B lymphocytes and is morphologically similar to other herpesviruses, but varies in several biological characteristics. HHV-6 was at first thought to be associated with AIDS, but was later established as the cause of a febrile illness of children, **exanthem subitum**, or **roseola**; on the basis of its distinctive genome structure and other characteristics it was assigned to a new genus, *Roseolovirus,* within the subfamily *Betaherpesvirinae*. There are two groups, A and B, defined by differences in serological reactions and genetic composition.

Clinical features

Both names of this illness refer to the **rash**, and 'subitum' reminds us of its sudden onset. These designations are not really appropriate, as the rash appears in only ≈30 per cent of cases, although it is of course the feature causing most parental alarm. It usually follows the febrile stage, and is macular or maculopapular, most evident on the trunk. The cervical lymph nodes, and sometimes the spleen, are enlarged.

Convulsions are not uncommon soon after onset, suggesting some involvement of the CNS; nevertheless, complete recovery is the rule. Treatment is symptomatic.

In normal adults, infection with HHV-6 may cause an illness resembling infectious mononucleosis. In immunocompromised patients, however, it may be severe, involving various organs, including the bone marrow.

Epidemiology

The virus is widely disseminated, and is shed in body fluids, including blood.

The prevalence of antibody in infants is biphasic: most are seropositive at birth, having acquired it transplacentally. Most of this maternal antibody disappears by 6 months of age, after which the seroprevalence rate increases as a result of silent infections, so that by the second year of life nearly all children in developed countries are again seropositive.

Laboratory diagnosis

This is unnecessary except in the case of a suspected infection in an immunosuppressed patient, when virus can be isolated in cell culture, or detected by tests with monoclonal antibodies. Such tests are made primarily to exclude other causes of fever.

2.2 Human herpesvirus 7

This one was isolated from CD4+ T cells taken from a healthy person. Like HHV-6, it is widespread and most people have antibody by late childhood. It too may cause an illness resembling infectious mononucleosis, but the results of primary infections are not as clear as those caused by HHV-6. Some cases of exanthem subitum have been associated with HHV-7, and a possible association with pityriasis rosea, a transient inflammatory rash, has also been reported.

Laboratory diagnosis follows the methods used for HHV-6.

3 Reminders

- CMV may be acquired at any age and gives rise to **persistent** infections, during which virus is shed intermittently in **urine** and other body fluids.

- In infancy or childhood, transmission is facilitated by poor hygienic conditions; these infections are **silent**, but those acquired later, usually through **sexual activity**, may cause an illness like infectious mononucleosis.

- **Transplant recipients** are at particular risk, either from virus transmitted from **donor tissues** or **blood transfusion**, or from reactivation of a persistent infection. In these cases, **immunosuppression** is an important factor in increasing the severity of the illness. Primary infection may result in a dangerous **interstitial pneumonitis**.

- Diagnosis of **primary** infections depends on demonstrating specific **IgM antibody**, or, by immunofluorescence, viral antigen in human fibroblast cultures inoculated with **urine**, saliva, or **buffy coat** of heparinized blood. In histological sections of kidney, **intranuclear 'owl's eye' inclusions** can be seen in the convoluted tubules.

- As CMV does not code for TK, ACV has little or no therapeutic effect. However, **ganciclovir**, a similar compound, is phosphorylated by a different enzyme and, although toxic to bone marrow, may be useful in treatment.

- **HHV-6 and -7** are both lymphotropic agents. HHV-6 causes **roseola (erythema subitum)** a mild febrile illness with rash occurring in young children. The primary illness in normal adults resembles infectious mononucleosis, but may be severe in immunocompromised patients, involving major body systems. HHV-7 also causes an illness such as glandular fever, but its clinical features are still not fully identified.

Chapter 20

The gammaherpesviruses: Epstein–Barr virus and Kaposi's sarcoma-associated herpesvirus

1 Epstein–Barr virus

EBV is in some respects the most sinister herpesvirus, for its association with malignant disease is now well established. In 1958, Burkitt described a tumour in African children that occurred in areas with a high prevalence of malaria. He thought that it might be caused by an infectious agent spread by mosquitoes. The mosquito theory was wrong, but 6 years later Epstein and his colleagues discovered a herpesvirus in cultures of the tumour cells. In 1966, American workers showed the association of this virus both with infectious mononucleosis (glandular fever) and with another form of cancer, nasopharyngeal carcinoma, occurring mostly in southern China. In addition to its association with these three syndromes, EBV causes B-cell lymphomas in immunodeficient patients (Table 20.1). Some species of monkey can be infected experimentally.

There are two types of the virus, A and B (also known as types 1 and 2), with differing biological characteristics. Worldwide, type A is predominant, but type B appears to have a particularly

Table 20.1 Epstein–Barr virus infections

Syndrome	Age group mainly affected	Remarks
Infectious mononucleosis	Adolescents, young adults	Worldwide distribution
Burkitt's lymphoma (BL)	Children 4–12 years	Endemic in sub-Saharan Africa and New Guinea
Nasopharyngeal carcinoma	Adults 20–50 years	Endemic in southern China
B-cell lymphoma	Children and adults	Occurs in some primary and acquired immunodeficiencies

high prevalence in equatorial Africa and in immunocompromised patients, including those with AIDS. However, there is as yet no firm evidence that the two types differ in terms of pathogenicity or oncogenicity. Both types may coexist in the same person.

EBV differs considerably from the other herpesviruses in two important respects; these are now described before the clinical features.

1.1 Viral antigens

EBV induces more than 80 virus-specified antigens in B lymphocytes, some of which are encoded by 'latent genes', i.e. are expressed in cells latently infected. The first of these to appear are viral nuclear antigens (Epstein–Barr (virus) nuclear antigen (**EBNA**)), which, as their name implies, are found in the nuclei of infected cells. Other important antigens are

- **LYDMA** (lymphocyte-detected membrane antigen), the target for cytotoxic T cells.
- **EA** (early antigen), involved in viral DNA replication.
- **VCA** (viral capsid antigen), a structural protein complex.

In addition, there are several glycoproteins, mostly associated with the cell membrane and hence with infectivity. The major antigen of this sort is **gp340/220**, which induces neutralizing antibody.

1.2 Immortalization of host cells

In vivo, the full lytic cycle of virus replication takes place in differentiating squamous epithelium, from which the virus is shed. When B cells are exposed to EBV *in vitro*, however, a proportion of them develop a latent infection, characterized by circularization of the viral genome. These cells can multiply indefinitely, a condition known as **immortalization**, and give rise to a **lymphoid cell line**. This process has obvious implications for the oncogenic potential of the virus (Chapter 6). Similar events take place *in vivo* so that, once infected, a person carries B cells containing EBV genome throughout life. There are six EBNAs, three of which are involved in maintaining the immortalized state. A few cells in such lines possess a plasma cell antigen, PC1, which, together with the presence of VCA, marks those cells that are due to undergo a lytic infection, an activity triggered by cell differentiation.

1.3 Clinical syndromes

EBV induces no CPE like those caused by other herpesviruses, although its ability to cause inflammatory disease shows its capacity for directly or indirectly damaging cells *in vivo*.

Infectious mononucleosis

Clinical aspects

Like CMV, EBV is shed intermittently by a substantial proportion of the population. Infectious virus is generated in the **pharynx**, probably in lymphoid tissue, and appears in the saliva. Thus,

like CMV mononucleosis, glandular fever is a 'kissing disease' and the peak incidence is in **adolescents and young adults**. The incubation period is a month or more. There is fever, **pharyngitis**, and **enlargement of the lymph nodes**, first in the neck and later elsewhere. In most patients the spleen is palpable and there is some **liver dysfunction**, occasionally with frank jaundice. There may be a transient macular rash; it is a peculiarity of the disease that patients given **ampicillin** develop a more severe rash due to the formation by transformed B cells of antibody to this antibiotic.

Complications are relatively uncommon. They include Guillain–Barré syndrome or other signs of CNS involvement and rarely, rupture of the spleen. Complete recovery within 3 weeks is the rule but convalescence is sometimes lengthy, with prolonged lassitude and loss of well-being.

Epidemiology

In poor communities, EBV, like CMV, is acquired early in life when it causes mainly inapparent infections (Fig. 20.1). Unlike CMV, however, the initial infection confers lifelong immunity to subsequent encounters. Infectious mononucleosis is thus most frequent in the developed countries where the infection is acquired later in life, with a peak incidence at 16–18 years.

Laboratory diagnosis

Virus isolation, depending as it does on the transformation of lymphocyte cultures, is impracticable; diagnosis in the routine laboratory is based on the haematological findings and on serological tests.

The feature that gives infectious mononucleosis its name is the **raised leucocyte count** (20×10^9 per litre, 50 per cent of which are lymphocytes). Up to 20 per cent of the lymphocytes are atypical in appearance, with bulky cytoplasm and irregular nuclei. These are not, as you might suppose, infected B cells, but

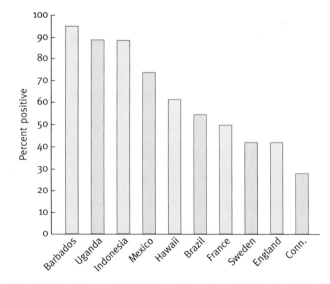

Fig. 20.1 Prevalence of EBV viral capsid antigen (VCA) antibody by age 4–6 years in 10 different population groups. (Reproduced with permission from Oxford, J.S. and Oberg, B. (1985). In: *Conquest of Viral Diseases*. Elsevier, Oxford.)

T cells reacting against viral antigens expressed on the B cells and capable of killing the latter.

Heterophil antibodies

B cells transformed by EBV undergo polyclonal expansion, i.e. they produce antibodies with a number of specificities (Greek *hetero* = different). Oddly, one is directed against ampicillin (see 'Clinical aspects', above). Others agglutinate sheep or horse red cells and are the basis for the Paul-Bunnell test. This is done by absorbing the patient's serum with guinea-pig kidney tissue to remove any irrelevant heterophil antibodies of the Forssman type, and then mixing it with the test erythrocytes. In a true positive test, the agglutinating ability can be removed by absorption with ox red cells. In its original form the **Paul-Bunnell test** is cumbersome, and has been replaced in many laboratories by a slide agglutination test ('**Monospot**') based on the same principle. These tests are negative in CMV mononucleosis.

Specific antibodies

Tests of the Paul-Bunnell type may give false negative results in young children. In specialized laboratories, tests for specific EBV antibodies can be undertaken. Selected cell populations expressing the required antigens are stained with the patient's serum by the indirect method. IgM antibody to VCA indicates a current or recent infection, whereas IgG antibody to this antigen is evidence of past infection. These tests are, however, technically demanding and are not in routine use.

Burkitt's lymphoma

This highly malignant neoplasm (see Fig. 4.1(c)) occurs mainly in **African children** living in the belt where malaria is hyperendemic, roughly speaking between the Tropics of Capricorn and Cancer (Fig. 20.2(a)). The peak incidence is in children 6–7 years old. There is another focus in **Papua New Guinea** and sporadic cases occur elsewhere. It presents as a tumour, usually of the jaw, less often of the orbit and other sites. Untreated, it is nearly always fatal within a few months, but is very responsive to **cyclophosphamide**, which if given early enough, may effect a cure.

EBV genome in circular episomal form can be demonstrated in the tumour cells of most cases of African and New Guinea BL, but not usually in those of the sporadic cases seen elsewhere. All children with African BL possess antibodies to the virus, and there is thus a strong association between the virus infection and the tumour (see also Chapter 6). Falciparum malaria is an important co-factor; its similar geographical distribution is striking, and there is some evidence that its ability to cause immunosuppression interferes with the control by cytotoxic T cells of tumour development; but this is not as yet proven.

Patients in the earlier stages of AIDS are also liable to develop BL.

Nasopharyngeal carcinoma

People in **southern China**, or who originate from there, are subject to an undifferentiated and invasive form of nasopharyngeal cancer, usually presenting as enlarged cervical lymph nodes to which the tumour has metastasized. It is the most common form of cancer in that area, with an incidence of 0.1 per cent of the population (Fig. 20.2(b)). It mainly affects people **20–50 years old**, males preponderating. This neoplasm is also associated with EBV, the evidence being similar to that for BL. In this instance, however, epithelial cells rather than lymphocytes are involved, and the epidemiology is quite different. Not only is the age of onset much later, but there is no association with malaria. Other co-factors appear to operate, one being an **association with certain HLA haplotypes**. It has also been suggested that dietary habits may play a part, in particular a high consumption of **nitrosamines** in salted foods. These tumours are relatively inaccessible to surgery or chemotherapy. Even after irradiation, the prognosis is poor.

B-cell lymphoma

Probably as a result of failure of T-cell control, those with primary or acquired immune deficiencies, including organ graft recipients and AIDS patients are liable to develop B-cell lymphomas associated with EBV infection.

Oral hairy leucoplakia

EBV is often detectable in these lesions, which appear as white roughened patches on the buccal mucosa and the sides of the tongue and are seen in male homosexuals who are HIV-positive, with or without signs of AIDS.

Other syndromes

EBV has been linked with T-cell lymphomas and Hodgkin's disease, but causal relationships are not fully established. There is recent evidence of a relationship between high titres of antibody to EBV and multiple sclerosis.

For a general discussion of the complex association of virus infections with malignant disease, see Chapter 6.

1.4 Immunization and treatment

Immunization

An EBV vaccine might confer enormous benefits in protecting against BL and nasopharyngeal carcinoma. An experimental subunit vaccine made from one of the viral envelope glycoproteins, gp340 (Section 1.1) has given promising results in Tamarind monkeys; nevertheless, the application of an EBV vaccine on a mass scale is still a long way off.

Antiviral therapy

Like CMV, EBV does not code for TK; and although ACV in high doses has been claimed to have some therapeutic value in EBV-related neoplasms, and in oral hairy leucoplakia, the effect is only palliative.

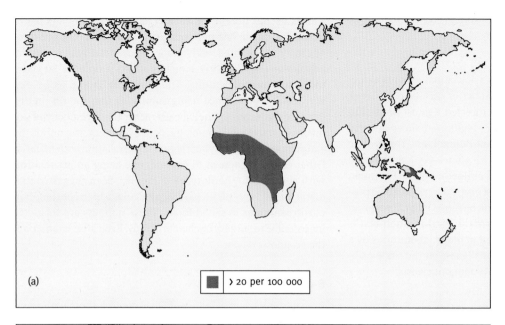

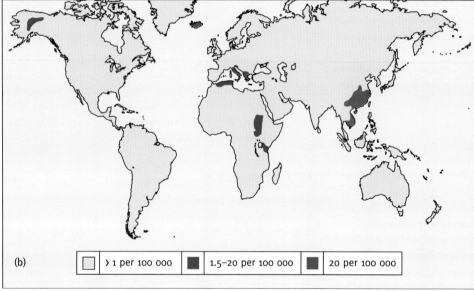

Fig 20.2 Geographical distributions of **(a)** Burkitt's lymphoma, and **(b)** nasopharyngeal carcinoma. (Redrawn, with permission, from Zuckerman, A.J., Banatvala, J.E., and Pattison, J.R. (1987), *Principles and Practice of Clinical Virology*. John Wiley & Sons, Chichester.)

2 Kaposi's sarcoma-associated herpesvirus (human herpesvirus 8)

The tumour described by Kaposi appears to arise from **endothelial cells** at multiple sites in the dermis. An indolent form used to be the main presentation, mostly in elderly men of Jewish or Italian origin, but a much more aggressive form is now prevalent, mainly in the USA and Africa, where it is a characteristic feature of **AIDS**. The lesions occur mainly in the **skin**, **lymph nodes**, and **gastrointestinal tract**. HHV-8 was first detected in the form of its DNA, and causes lytic infection in a B-cell lymphoma line. Diagnosis depends mainly on detection of viral DNA by PCR.

There is some evidence linking HHV-8 with multiple myeloma.

3 Reminders

- Like CMV, EBV is acquired early in poorer countries and later in more affluent communities. It causes **persistent infection of B lymphocytes**, in which it induces various virus-specific antigens, some of which mediate latency, and others, notably glycoproteins, infectivity.

- **Infectious mononucleosis** (glandular fever) has a peak incidence in adolescents and young adults, in whom it is spread by sexual activity, including kissing. The physical signs include **fever**, **pharyngitis**, and **enlargement of the lymph nodes and spleen**.

- Laboratory diagnosis depends on (1) the **raised leucocyte count** and **atypical T lymphocytes** in the blood film, and

(2) the presence of **heterophil (Forsmann) antibodies** detectable by the Paul-Bunnell or '**Monospot**' haemagglutination tests.

- **BL** is a malignant tumour occurring mostly in **Africa**; endemic malaria is a co-factor. It affects **young children** and is strongly associated with EBV infection, the viral genome being demonstrable in the tumour cells. This association may not hold true for areas other than Africa and Papua New Guinea.

- **Nasopharyngeal carcinoma** is associated with EBV infection. It occurs mainly in southern China and in people originating from there. The incidence is highest in the 20–50-year age group, males predominating. Cofactors may include particular **HLA haplotypes** and consumption of **nitrosamines** in salted foods.

- EBV is also associated with various forms of **lymphoma**, and with **oral hairy leucoplakia**, a condition often seen in HIV-infected homosexuals.

- DNA sequences of **Kaposi's sarcoma-associated virus (HHV-8)** have been detected in tissue from the tumour. It now seems fairly certain that this virus is causally associated with Kaposi's sarcoma.

- As with CMV, ACV is in general of no value in treating acute EBV infections; it may, however, have a palliative effect in oral hairy leucoplakia and in some tumours.

Introduction to the hepatitis viruses

It is paradoxical that the liver, a site of massive viral replication in the acute infectious fevers, nearly always escapes serious damage during such episodes. This is because the viruses concerned multiply in the Kuppfer cells of the reticuloendothelial system; however, the main targets of the true hepatitis viruses to be discussed in this chapter (Table 21.1) are the hepatocytes themselves. Nevertheless, liver damage may also be caused by other viruses, which for completeness are listed in Table 21.2. One of them, YF virus, also has the liver as its main target organ, but differs in several important respects from the other infections described here. It is arthropod-borne, and is dealt with in Chapter 27.

In the days when syphilis was treated with Ehrlich's 'magic bullet', arsphenamine, patients sometimes became jaundiced, an effect put down to a toxic effect of the drug on the liver. We now know that the cause was a virus spread from one person to another by inadequately sterilized needles. Later, it became apparent that there were at least two forms of transmissible hepatitis. One type seemed to be acquired by the oral route and was labelled 'infectious' or 'catarrhal' hepatitis. The other, known as 'serum hepatitis', was spread by injections, blood transfusions, and sexual contact. The first type had an incubation period of about 2–6 weeks, whereas that of the second was longer, 2–5 months. Neither form was infective for the usual laboratory animals or culture systems and there was confusion about their true nature until experimental inoculations of humans distinguished between the infective agents now known, respectively, as the hepatitis A virus (HAV) and HBV.

Table 21.1 The hepatitis viruses

Virus	Classification	Main route of transmission	Chapter
HAV	*Picornaviridae*	Enteric	16
HEV	*Caliciviridae*		23
HBV	*Hepadnaviridae*	Parenteral	22
HDV	Deltavirus		22
HCV	*Flaviviridae*	Parenteral	24
GBV-A, B, C	Flavi-like viruses		24

Table 21.2 Viruses causing hepatitis as part of a general infection

Virus	Remarks
Epstein–Barr virus	
Cytomegalovirus, generalized herpes simplex	Especially in congenital infections
Rubella	Congenital form
Mumps	Rare
ECHO viruses	Rare
Yellow fever	Generalized infection; liver is main target organ

Several viruses cause hepatitis as part of a general infection, but the primary target cells of the 'true' hepatitis viruses are the hepatocytes. Except for HAV, none has been propagated in quantity in the laboratory, but all are infective for chimpanzees.

1 Hepatitis A

The form of hepatitis with the shorter incubation period, originally termed 'catarrhal' or 'infectious' hepatitis, differed from hepatitis B not only in severity, but in being transmitted by the enteric route. HAV proved to be an RNA virus, a member of the *Picornaviridae* (Chapter 16). As such, virologists were already familiar with its main characteristics. Diagnosis by conventional serological tests was easy enough; the main problem was that, unlike other picornaviruses, it could not readily be propagated in the usual cell cultures. Control originally depended on hygienic measures and on passive immunization with immunoglobulin, but the latter conferred only short-term protection. Later, an inactivated vaccine was produced that confers much longer protection.

2 Hepatitis B and deltavirus

Of the two infections, HBV was the more dangerous on account of its tendency to become chronic, sometimes giving rise to cirrhosis of the liver, or worse still, liver cancer. Occasionally, fulminant cases died rapidly from massive liver failure. HAV on the other hand was a transient infection with little or nothing in the way of long-term effects or mortality. For this reason, interest was at first focused mainly on HBV, which proved to be a hitherto unknown type of DNA virus with several unusual features, including its genomic structure and mode of replication. Because it could be transmitted in very small amounts of blood or body fluids it posed a particular threat in hospitals, blood transfusion centres, and renal dialysis units. Worse still, in highly epidemic areas with many carriers, HBV could be acquired by infants during or after birth, and its ability to spread by sexual contact created yet more public health problems. These dangers prompted intense research on methods of laboratory diagnosis and the development of a vaccine. Both lines of investigation were successful, so that we now have highly effective means of controlling hepatitis B; the problem is to apply them, particularly in developing countries where carrier rates are highest.

Another novel feature of HBV was the discovery of an associated agent, delta virus, or HDV. This proved to be a very small RNA virus, more properly termed a satellite, as it depends on HBV to provide its envelope protein. HDV may be transmitted along with HBV, or as a superinfection, and tends to cause exacerbations of the liver disease.

3 Hepatitis C

This virus, like HBV, is transmitted by exposure to blood and body fluids, and is very liable to cause chronic infections, sometimes terminating in cirrhosis of the liver or HCC. It is described in more detail in Chapter 24.

4 Other hepatitis viruses

When laboratory tests for HAV and HBV became available, it became clear that some cases of hepatitis fell into neither category. They, together with hepatitis C, were at first referred to by the clumsy term 'non-A, non-B' (NANB) agents. They resembled the known infections in being spread either by the parenteral or enteric routes, but were even more difficult to identify in the laboratory. Nevertheless, intensive application of molecular methods resulted in the identification of yet more hepatitis viruses.

Hepatitis E (HEV) resembles HAV in being primarily spread by ingestion, but proved to be a calicivirus (Chapter 11).

The 'Reminders' for the various hepatitis viruses will be found in the appropriate chapters.

The blood-borne hepatitis viruses B and delta

Although the worldwide incidence of hepatitis A must run into millions, as a cause of serious disease and death this infection pales almost into insignificance beside hepatitis B. Like HAV, the causal agent of hepatitis B cannot be readily propagated in laboratory systems. The first clue to its nature was obtained in 1964 by Blumberg, who, during a survey quite unconnected with hepatitis, found that an antibody in serum from a haemophiliac precipitated with an antigen in the blood of an Australian aborigine. The antigen, originally termed 'Australia antigen', proved to be a component of the elusive HBV.

1 Properties of hepatitis B virus

Perhaps in no other virus infection is a knowledge of the causal agent and immune responses so important for understanding the clinical and epidemiological aspects and the principles of laboratory diagnosis. Hepatitis B is rather complicated, but a little concentrated study here will serve you well when you meet the infection in practice.

1.1 Classification

The family name is *Hepadnaviridae* (HEPAtitis DNA viruses). There are two genera, *Orthohepadnavirus* and *Avihepadnavirus*, which respectively affect certain mammals (woodchucks and squirrels) and birds (Peking ducks).

1.2 Morphology

EM of the blood of acute and some chronic cases of hepatitis B reveals many particles differing in shape (Fig. 22.1(a)). One type is 42 nm in diameter, and double-shelled; this is the complete virion (Fig. 22.1(b)), sometimes called the Dane particle after its discoverer. The others are spheres or tubules 20–22 nm in diameter; they consist only of excess surface antigen, i.e. the glycoprotein forming the outer layer of the double-shelled Dane particle. The core of the latter is an icosahedral nucleocapsid containing:

- the DNA genome;
- a DNA-dependent DNA polymerase involved in replication;
- hepatitis B core antigen (HBcAg);
- hepatitis B e antigen (HBeAg).

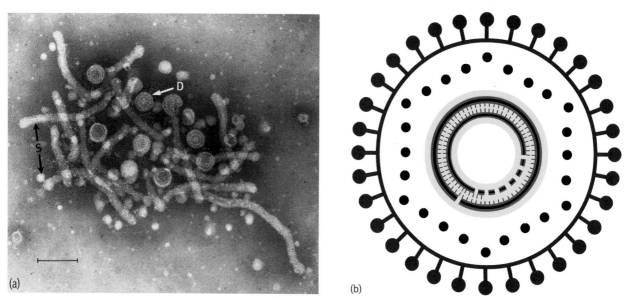

Fig. 22.1 **(a)** Electron micrograph of hepatitis B virus. D, Dane particles; S, filaments and spheres of HBsAg. (Courtesy of Dr David Hockley.) Scale bar = 100 nm. **(b)** Model of the Dane particle of HBV.

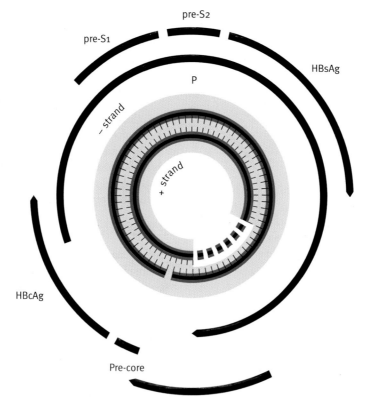

Fig. 22.2 Hepatitis B genome and encoded proteins. Labelled proteins are HBsAg (surface antigen), HBcAg (core antigen), P (polymerase), pre-S1 and pre-S2 core proteins.

1.3 Genome

The genome is extremely compact and consists of circular dsDNA some 32 kbp in size (Fig. 22.2). There are four overlapping ORFs. Its conformation is unique in that for most of its length the DNA is double-stranded but one strand ('short') has a gap about 700 nucleotides in length. The 'long' strand has a nick near the 5′ end. The virus can code 50 per cent more protein than would be expected from the genome size.

1.4 Replication

The virus attaches to a hepatocyte using the virion S protein and enters by endocytosis. The virus nucleocapsid moves to the nucleus where transcription takes place. The minus strand is transcribed to give mRNAs plus a 3.4 kb RNA transcript called the pregenome. The pregenome and the shorter mRNAs move to the cytoplasm and are translated. The mode of replication of the genome is unusual and entails a reverse transcription of the DNA from an RNA intermediate. The RNA is digested away and a plus DNA strand is transcribed.

The replication strategy is unique for a DNA virus, using an RNA intermediate and a reverse transcription step. The RT with its lack of proof reading leads to relatively high mutation rates but the extremely small genome size prevents a large degree of genetic variability. Most variation occurs in the pre S region, which is important for virus attachment and entry.

The newly synthesized virus cores congregate in the cytoplasm, associate with viral DNA and bud through the endoplasmic reticulum at areas already containing S antigens. The new enveloped viruses emerge without cell lysis.

1.5 Antigens and antibodies

The core itself has its own antigenic specificity, referred to as HBcAg. The surface antigen is named HBsAg and is in fact the one originally found in the blood of the aborigine; for this reason it was at first referred to as 'Australia antigen', but this term is no longer used.

HBV markers

The main antigens **HBsAg**, **HBcAg**, and **HBeAg** each induce corresponding antibodies (Table 22.1) With the exception of

Table 22.1 Serological markers of hepatitis B infection

Marker	Remarks	Present in Antigens
HBsAg	Surface antigen, not infective	Acute and chronic infections, including antigenaemia
HBeAg	Found in core of virion. Presence in blood indicates infectivity	Acute and chronic hepatitis
Viral DNA polymerase	As for HBeAg, above	As for HBeAg, above
Antibodies		
Anti-HBs	Indicates recovery; protects against reinfection	Convalescence
Anti-HBe	Presence indicates little or no infectivity	Convalescence
Anti-HBc	In IgM form, indicates recent infection	The first antibody to appear. Persists in IgG form for life

N.B. HBcAg, the core antigen, is not readily detectable in blood and is not used as a marker.

Table 22.2 Infectivity of HBV carriers

Degree of infectivity	Markers				
	Antigens		Antibodies		
	HBsAg	HBeAg	Anti-HBs	Anti-HBe	Anti-HBc
High	+	+	–	–	+
Intermediate	+	–	–	+	+
Low	+	–	+	+	+

HBcAg, all these antigens and antibodies, together with the viral DNA polymerase, can be detected in the blood at various times after infection and are referred to as 'markers', because their presence or absence in an individual patient mark the course of the disease and also give a good idea of the degree of infectivity for others (Table 22.2). HBcAg is readily detectable only in the hepatocyte nuclei.

Hepatitis B virus subtypes and genotypes

As well as the main antigens already mentioned, HBcAg, HBeAg, and HBsAg, the surface antigen is endowed with serological specificities that enable us to define subtypes of the virus (Fig. 22.3). There is a group-specific antigenic determinant, *a*, associated with various combinations of subtype determinants *d*, *y*, *w*, and *r*. These combinations are themselves grouped into six or more genotypes (A–F), which are useful epidemiologically as their geographical distributions differ. Thus genotypes B and C are prevalent in the Far East, whereas E occurs more often in sub-Saharan Africa. In combination with HBV DNA sequencing they may also be helpful in deciding whether a particular carrier—e.g. a surgeon or dentist—is the source of infection of another person. The finding of identical subtypes would not of course confirm the possibility, but differing subtypes would rule it out.

Genetic analysis has revealed seven genotypes of the virus showing about 8 per cent nucleotide sequence divergence and there is increasing evidence that the clinical picture, long-term progression, and even response to drug therapy may relate to the genotype.

2 Clinical and pathological aspects of hepatitis B virus infections

2.1 Clinical features

Patterns of infection are variable and are influenced by age, sex, and the state of the immune system. It is now thought that the genotype of the virus also contributes. We shall start with acute infections acquired well after infancy and then consider the special problems posed by perinatal infection.

Postnatal infections

The incubation period is usually within the range 60–80 days. Acute infection may be **subclinical**, especially in young children

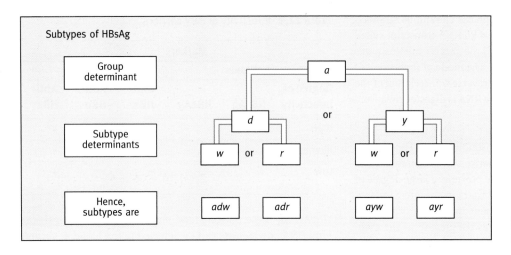

Fig. 22.3 The antigenic subtypes of HBsAg.

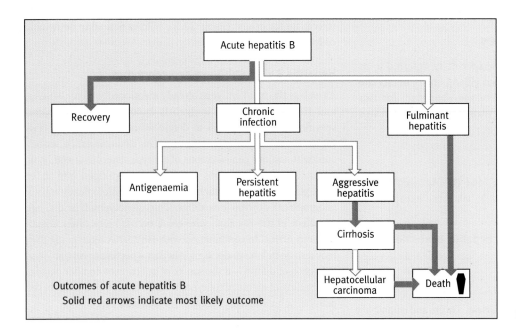

Fig. 22.4 Clinical outcomes of hepatitis B infection.

or in those with impaired immunity. Typically, however, there is a **prodromal phase** similar to that of hepatitis A, but sometimes marked by a transient rash and arthropathy, probably due to virus/antibody interaction. This is followed by overt **jaundice**, after which 90 per cent of patients recover uneventfully within a month or so. In others, however, the outcome may be chronic infection or even rapid death (Fig. 22.4).

Figure 22.5(a) shows the course of a typical acute infection in an immunocompetent adult. Even before the appearance of jaundice there is a rise in **serum transaminases** and **HBsAg** is detectable in the serum, followed soon afterwards by **HBeAg** and **DNA polymerase** (not shown). **Anti-HBc** is the first antibody to appear. The next is **anti-HBe**, a good prognostic sign as its production heralds the disappearance of HBeAg and thus of infectivity. Although HBsAg is the first antigen to appear, **anti-HBs** is the last antibody to do so; its arrival indicates complete recovery and immunity to reinfection.

At the other end of the spectrum (Fig. 22.4) one patient in a thousand, usually a female, develops fulminant **hepatitis** and dies within 10 days in hepatic coma; this is the result of an abnormally active destruction of infected hepatocytes by cytotoxic T lymphocytes.

We are now left with the 10 per cent or so of patients who do not come into either of these categories, but who become **chronic carriers**. This diagnosis is made when the serological profile has not reverted to the normal postrecovery pattern within 6 months of onset. There are three varieties.

In **chronic antigenaemia** the patient fails to form anti-HBs and the appearance of anti-HBe may be delayed (Fig. 22.5(b)). Although HBsAg persists in the blood for many years, liver function is normal, the patient is well and is of little or no danger to others. This picture is often seen in those with impaired immunity. The serological pattern is similar in chronic persistent hepatitis, in which however there is a mild degree of liver damage.

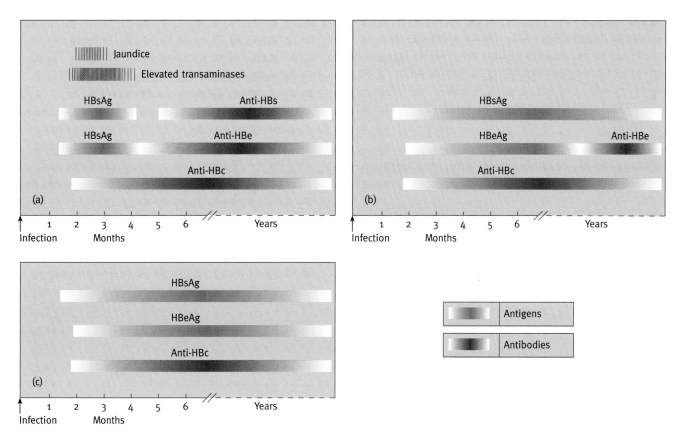

Fig. 22.5 Course of acute and chronic hepatitis B. **(a)** Acute hepatitis; **(b)** chronic antigenaemia and persistent hepatitis; **(c)** chronic aggressive hepatitis.

Chronic aggressive (or active) hepatitis is a different story, and these patients create the great bulk of the problems surrounding hepatitis B. They fail to produce either anti-HBs or anti-HBe (Fig. 22.5(c)). As a result, they continue to carry both HBsAg and infectious virions in their blood, and are thus **infectious for others**; they are sometimes referred to as 'super carriers'. There is significant damage to the liver parenchyma and raised transaminase levels indicate impaired function. These patients are liable to repeated episodes of hepatitis and are at risk of developing **cirrhosis**; some may eventually succumb to malignant disease of the liver.

HCC may result from integration of viral genome into the DNA of the hepatocytes (Chapter 6), but the pathogenesis is not fully understood. It is clear, however, that HCC arises only after a chronic infection with continuing production of complete virions that has been in progress for at least 2 years. It is often, but not always, preceded by cirrhosis of the liver. Cofactors, such as aflatoxin contaminating groundnuts, may be contributory causes, but there is now no doubt that HBV itself is the primary carcinogen.

Perinatal infections

Infants born to a mother with acute hepatitis B may themselves become acutely infected. By contrast, infants born to mothers who are HBeAg-positive carriers do not develop the acute disease, but 95 per cent of them become infected. Of these, ≈10 per cent are infected in the uterus of mothers acquiring infection during the first trimester of pregnancy. More often, however, it is transmitted either from **contact with blood and body fluids at birth** or within the next few months by close contact with the mother and siblings. The acquisition of maternal anti-HBc across the placenta seems to impair the normal immune response; nearly all such infants proceed themselves to become HBeAg-positive carriers, and many die later in life of cirrhosis or liver cancer. The outlook for boys is worse than for girls: 50 per cent of males eventually die of these complications, compared with only 15 per cent of females, who seem to mount a better immune response. The preponderance of surviving females favours perpetuation of the carrier state in populations with a high prevalence of the disease, as it is they who pass the infection to the next generation. As infection acquired early in life does not present as an acute infection with jaundice, the clinical pictures of hepatitis B in areas of high and low endemicity differ considerably.

2.2 Epidemiology

Mode of transmission

HBV is transmitted only in blood and other body fluids. Concentrations are high in blood and serum, moderate in semen, vaginal fluid and saliva, and low or undetectable in urine, faeces, sweat, tears, and breast milk. Because the titres of virus are so high in body fluids (10^6–10^8 per ml), invisibly small quantities—0.00001 ml or even less—can transmit the infection. It is therefore easy to understand that minor abrasions or cuts can serve as portals of entry. HBV is readily spread by **sexual intercourse**, particularly among male homosexuals, and in **intravenous drug abusers** by sharing of needles and syringes. It may even be transmitted by splashes of minute droplets into the eye. There are now quite a number of reports of healthcare workers becoming infected from acute or chronic carriers of HBV, and of patients acquiring the virus from their surgeons or dentists.

The worldwide impact of HBV infections—some facts and figures

The prevalence of hepatitis B in a community can be estimated by the presence of anti-HBs, or, more readily and informatively, by the proportion of the population who are HBsAg-positive carriers. Figure 22.6 shows that the carrier rates vary widely in different parts of the world.

- The **high** prevalence areas (10–20 per cent) are East and South-east Asia, the Pacific Islands, and tropical Africa.

- Russia, the Indian subcontinent, parts of Africa, eastern and south-eastern Europe, and parts of Latin America are areas of **medium** prevalence (2–20 per cent).

- The prevalence is **low** (<1 per cent) in the rest of Europe, Australia and New Zealand, Canada and the USA.

- In the UK, the HBsAg carrier rate in the general population is less than 1 per cent; higher rates in the various ethnic minorities reflect to some extent the prevalences in their countries of origin.

The following figures will some idea of the devastating effect of HBV infections throughout the world:

- It is estimated that there are 350 million HBV carriers; of these, 75 per cent were infected at birth.

- There are about 950 000 new cases every year in the WHO European region, of whom 90 000 become carriers; of these, 19 000 eventually die of cirrhosis and 5000 of liver cancer. In the USA the annual incidence of new cases is 200 000, with corresponding mortality rates for cirrhosis and HCC.

- The global death rate from HCC is estimated at 250 000 per annum.

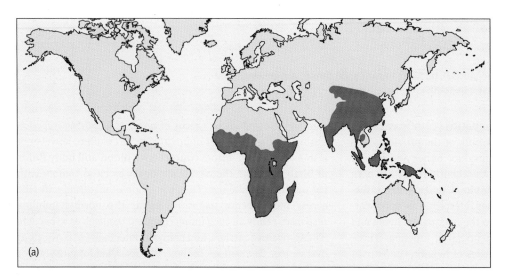

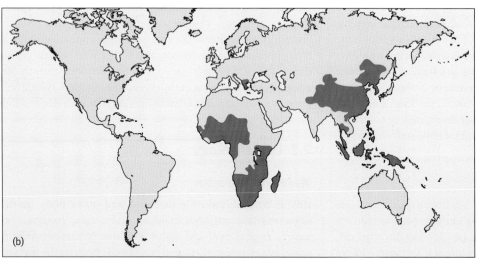

Fig. 22.6 Hepatitis B and liver cancer. Geographical distributions of: **(a)** HBsAg carriers (prevalence 5 per cent or more), and **(b)** primary hepatocellular carcinoma (annual incidence 10 cases or more per 100 000 population).

Table 22.3 Groups at higher than average risk of HBV infection

Category	Risk factors or group
General community	Sexually promiscuous people Intravenous drug abusers Partners of HBeAg-positive carriers Infants of HBeAg-positive mothers
Patients	Repeated blood transfusions Long-term treatment with blood products, e.g. haemophiliacs Chronic renal failure
Healthcare staff	Work in mental institutions Tours of duty in high endemicity areas Surgical and dental operations Some pathological laboratory work, including autopsies Work in STD clinics Prisoners and staff in contact with them

High-risk groups

This term applies to people who by reason of their country of birth, way of life, or type of work are at higher than average risk of acquiring HBV infection or of passing it on.

We have already described one such group, babies born to carrier mothers in high endemicity areas. Table 22.3 gives examples of high-risk groups in areas of low endemicity; all, in one way or another, are liable to come into contact with infective blood or body fluids. At this point, we recall that the first clue to the nature of HBV was the reaction between surface antigen in the serum of an Australian aborigine and what we now know to have been anti-HBs in the blood of a haemophiliac, both of whom would have been in high-risk groups.

2.3 Pathogenesis and pathology

HBV is even more difficult to propagate in the laboratory than HAV and many aspects of pathogenesis remain obscure, in particular, exactly what happens to the virus during the long incubation period. Very many complete virions and even more HBsAg particles are liberated into the blood stream.

In the acute phase, the pathological changes in the liver (Fig. 22.7(a)) are similar to those seen in hepatitis A (Chapter 23), except that a number of the hepatocytes are stuffed full of viral surface antigen, which gives them a 'ground-glass' appearance when stained with haematoxylin and eosin. Orcein stains the HBsAg brown (Fig. 22.7(b)). In chronic aggressive hepatitis B (Section 2.1), there may be cirrhotic changes, which, in a proportion of those thus affected, are a precursor of primary liver cancer.

2.4 Immune response

Although the appearance of anti-HBs indicates recovery, it plays little part if any in that process, which is primarily effected by

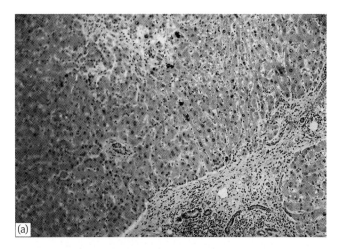

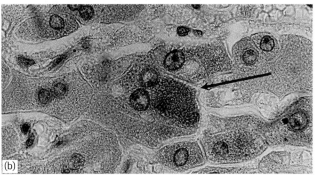

Fig. 22.7 Section of liver from a case of hepatitis B. Orcein stain. **(a)** Low power. Some of the hapatocytes are necrotic and others contain darkly stained HBsAg. Note the dense infiltration with mononuclear cells. **(b)** High power. HBsAg in a hepatocyte (arrowed).

cytotoxic (CD8+) T cells. We explained in Chapter 5 how T_c lymphocytes act on infected cells only if the viral antigen is presented in association with class I histocompatibility antigen. Hepatocytes are normally not well endowed with this antigen, but HBV infection stimulates production of IFN-α, which in turn increases the display of class I antigen on the liver cells and thus permits their lysis by the cytotoxic lymphocytes (Chapter 5).

As with many other infections, the cell-mediated immune response (CMI) may enhance as well as cure the illness, depending on the balance of forces involved.

Immunopathological damage is a major component of the response to HBV, and is notably diminished in those with defective immunity, e.g. those with Down's syndrome or AIDS.

2.5 Laboratory diagnosis

Specific tests

The first test to be performed is for surface antigen. This is normally done by **ELISA**, but if the result is needed urgently, more rapid tests are available. They might be needed when, for example, a patient from a high-risk group needs emergency surgical or dental treatment and his or her carrier status must be determined to protect the operator. They can be done by **reverse passive haemagglutination**, in which commercially available erythrocytes coated with anti-HBs are mixed with the test serum; any HBsAg present will attach to the antibody and agglutinate the cells within 20 min. A **latex slide test** based on the same principle can be read in 5 min.

A positive rapid test for HBsAg must always be confirmed by ELISA. The finding of HBsAg does not in itself mean that the patient is infective for others, although he or she should be treated with appropriate precautions until the result of a test for HBeAg is available. This takes longer, for it too must be done by ELISA. Some laboratories also test for viral **DNA or DNA polymerase** as a measure of virus replication. The full marker profile is established by testing, by variants of ELISA, for the three antibodies, **anti-HBs**, **anti-HBe**, and **anti-HBc**.

EM can be used to test quickly both for HBsAg and infective Dane particles, as they are so numerous when present that finding them in serum is easy; but this method is unsuitable for large numbers of specimens and is not in routine use.

Non-specific tests

These are useful for assessing liver function but do not distinguish between the various forms of hepatitis. In the acute phase or in exacerbations of chronic aggressive hepatitis **the levels of alanine aminotransferase and other liver enzymes are raised** and prothrombin is depressed. Serum bilirubin is also increased.

2.6 Control

Specific treatment with antivirals

The acute infection does not normally demand treatment, but the threat of an HBeAg-positive carrier state demands action. Some at least of those who become carriers in adult life are naturally deficient in IFN, and some cures have been obtained with large doses of **IFN-α**. Treatment should be prolonged for at least 6 months. Unfortunately, it is of no use in those who become infected in infancy.

Various DNA polymerase inhibitors have also been established; **lamivudine** and **famciclovir** are useful in those receiving liver transplants, but reduce viraemia only temporarily unless combined with IFN.

The first molecule to be investigated in patients infected with hepatitis B was IFN-α. Only a minority of patients responded and, worryingly, when the drug was discontinued viral replication restarted. However, these important and pioneering studies showed that antiviral chemotherapy could have a future role in the management of this disease. The primary goal is to reduce the adverse pathology of the liver and hence reduce clinical complications. What is not so clear is whether reduction in viral load will translate into clinical benefit. Large doses of IFN-α (6–10 MU three times weekly) reduce viral load, HBeAg and HBsAg. A remission is maintained for most patients who responded initially and histological progression of the disease is slowed. Patients most likely to respond more had HBV DNA levels below 200 pg/ml, whereas Asians who had acquired virus perinatally did not respond so effectively.

A new era opened when the nucleoside analogue lamivudine, known as an HIV RT inhibitor, was shown to inhibit RT of HBV and decreased HBV DNA levels by 1000–10 000-fold. But after cessation of therapy a viral rebound was found. Histological improvement was noted in half the patients. However, drug resistant mutants were soon detected and this has lead to combined therapy with IFN-α and lamivudine.

Following this initial success with drug combinations other nucleoside analogues are now being investigated including fialuridine (FIAU), adenine arabinoside (Ara A), adefovir (PMEA), and the antiherpes drugs famciclovir and ganciclovir.

Immunization

We are fortunate in having two highly effective means of preventing hepatitis B: **vaccines** prepared from HBsAg, which are both safe and effective; and human **immunoglobulin** with a high titre of anti-HBs (HBIG), which can be used in combination with vaccine to provide immediate passive protection.

Hepatitis B vaccine

The 'first generation' vaccines were prepared from the blood plasma of carriers. This method was adopted because of inability to propagate HBV in quantity in the laboratory. It included elaborate purification and safety procedures to ensure the elimination of infective HBV and other viruses. These hazards have now been eliminated by the introduction of **genetically engineered vaccines**. The gene coding for HBsAg has been cloned into yeast cells, which are cultured on a mass scale and produce large quantities of the antigen. The dosage of the vaccine employed in the UK is 20 μg of HBsAg given intramuscularly at 0, 1, and 6 months, with boosters at 5-year intervals for those at special risk. The third dose is essential to secure full protection. Some people, especially those aged over 40 years, fail to respond in terms of forming anti-HBs.

Although hepatitis B vaccines are in general highly effective, there have been reports of mutant strains against which they do not protect. In one such strain, the mutation affected only one amino acid in the HBsAg, a situation reminiscent of that with influenza (Chapter 10). It seems likely that such 'escape mutants' are rare, but clearly, a careful watch for them must be maintained. New approaches to the preparation of hepatitis B vaccines are discussed in Chapter 37.

Candidates for vaccination

In areas with high prevalences of carriers, the first priority is immunization of newborn infants, with the ultimate aim of reducing the incidence of liver cancer. In the developed countries, they are primarily

- the high-risk groups listed in Table 22.3;
- neonates born to mothers who are carriers, or who had acute hepatitis B in pregnancy (see also 'Perinatal infections', p. 229);

Table 22.4 HBV prophylaxis for reported exposure incidents (reproduced with permission from *Immunization against infectious disease*, p. 106. HMSO, 1996)

HBV status of person exposed	HBsAg positive source	Significant exposure		Non-significant exposure	
		Unknown source	HBsAg negative source	Continued risk	No further risk
⩽ 1 dose HB vaccine pre-exposure	Accelerated course of HB vaccine* HBIG × 1	Accelerated course of HB vaccine*	Initiate course of HB vaccine	Initiate course Reassure	No HBV prophylaxis
⩾ 2 doses HB vaccine pre-exposure (anti-HBs not known)	One dose of HB vaccine followed by second dose one month later	One dose of HB vaccine	Finish course of HB vaccine	Finish course of HB vaccine	No HBV prophylaxis Reassure
Known responder to HB vaccine (anti-HBs > 10 miU/ml)	Consider booster dose of HB vaccine	Consider booster dose of HB vaccine	Consider booster dose of HB vaccine	Consider booster dose of HB vaccine	No HBV prophylaxis Reassure
Known non-responder to HB vaccine (anti-HBs < 10 miU/ml 2–4 months post-immunization)	HBIG × 1 Consider booster dose of HB vaccine	HBIG × 1 Consider booster dose of HB vaccine	No HBIG Consider booster dose of HB vaccine	No HBIG Consider booster dose of HB vaccine	No prophylaxis Reassure

* An accelerated course of vaccine consists of doses spaced at 0, 1, and 2 months.
A booster dose may be given at 12 months to those at continuing risk of exposure to HBV.

- people who have undergone a significant exposure to risk of infection. In this context, 'significant exposure' means a penetrating injury with a potentially contaminated sharp object; mucocutaneous exposure to blood; or unprotected sexual exposure.

The schedules for **postexposure prophylaxis** depend on various factors, including the HBV status of the source and of the person exposed and the period elapsed since exposure. They are summarized in Table 22.4.

General measures

Person-to-person transmission

Horizontal spread of infection is blocked by preventing blood or body fluids from an infected person gaining access to the circulation of someone else. Degrees of infectivity can be assessed from the marker profile (Table 22.2 and Fig. 22.5).

Healthcare staff must take the obvious personal precautions, such as keeping cuts and abrasions covered and **wearing gloves** when injecting or operating upon actual and potential high risk patients. All hospitals should have detailed **codes of practice** for use in wards, theatres, clinics, and laboratories and it goes without saying that these must be meticulously observed. They include instructions for the use, whenever possible, of disposable equipment; sterilization by heat; chemical disinfection with hypochlorites or glutaraldehyde; and for the action to be taken in the event of spillages or injury of staff.

Special care is taken to exclude carriers from entering **renal dialysis units**, where, because of the depressed state of immunity of the patients, HBV infection readily becomes established with risks both to patients and staff. Stringent control measures

have eliminated hepatitis B from dialysis units in the UK, but it is still prevalent in some other countries.

3 Properties of delta virus

3.1 Classification

This curious little agent was first detected in 1977, in people undergoing exacerbations of chronic HBV infections. It is ≈40 nm in diameter and contains **ssRNA** only 1.7 kb pairs in size. This is much too small to code for the usual virus functions and its replication depends on that of HBV itself. Delta agent is thus an incomplete virus, reminiscent of the *Dependoviruses* described in Chapter 13. Its outer coat is in fact formed from HBsAg, the specific delta antigen itself being within the core. It is known as hepatitis D virus or HDV and has been provisionally recognized as a separate genus, *Deltavirus*.

3.2 Morphology

The small virions appear to be spherical and consist of a ssRNA core surrounded by a delta virus-coded antigen (HDAg) and an outer coat of HBsAg.

3.3 Genome

The negative-sense ssRNA genome is unique among animal viruses in being **circular**, in this respect resembling certain plant pathogens, the viroids (Chapter 2). There appear to be a number of forms of the ssRNA: the genome, a complementary copy, or antigenome; and a third, linear, form that mediates translation of the HDV antigen.

3.4 Replication

After entry into cells the genome is transcribed in the nucleus into a full length circular positive-sense RNA and a shorter linear transcript that acts as an mRNA for the delta antigen.

Packaging of the viral genome, the delta antigen and the HBsAg takes place in the cytoplasm and the complete virion is released from the cell.

4 Clinical and pathological aspects of hepatitis delta virus infections

4.1 Clinical features

This agent is **transmitted along with HBV**, either at the time of first infection with the latter (co-infection) or during a subsequent exposure (superinfection). It may have little or no effect on the associated hepatitis B infection, but sometimes causes **fulminant hepatitis** and death. The incubation period is ≈3–7 weeks, after which there is a prodromal phase with malaise, nausea, and loss of appetite. Jaundice is accompanied by biochemical evidence of liver damage, and fulminant hepatitis may develop at this point. HDV infections superimposed on chronic hepatitis B are also liable to become chronic: titres of anti-IgM and IgG remain high indefinitely.

4.2 Epidemiology

The infection is especially prevalent in Italy where it was first discovered—parts of the Middle East, Asia, Russia, and Latin America. Those mainly at risk are **intravenous drug abusers**, and epidemics among them have been documented in Scandinavia and elsewhere.

On the basis of sequence differences, HDV isolates have been divided into three genotypes, 1, 2, and 3, which vary in their geographical distribution. Thus type 1 is widely distributed in Europe, the USA, North Africa, and the Middle East, whereas types 2 and 3 are prevalent in the Far East and Latin America respectively.

4.3 Pathogenesis and pathology

As far as we know, HDV, along with HBV, replicates *in vivo* only within hepatocytes. It is difficult to assign HDV a specific role in pathogenesis when its replication is so closely linked with that of the accompanying HBV. There is nothing special about the pathological changes in the liver, which are those to be expected of hepatitis B. Concurrent or superinfections with HDV tend to be more severe than those caused by HBV alone.

4.4 Immune response

Both IgM and IgG antibodies are formed. Nothing is known of any cell-mediated response specific to HDV.

4.5 Laboratory diagnosis

Diagnosis depends mainly on tests **for IgG and IgM antibodies**. Both the delta antigen and genomic RNA can also be detected in the blood.

4.6 Control

Immunization

Immunization against hepatitis B also protects against infection with HDV.

General measures

These are similar to those for hepatitis B, the most important being the elimination of syringe and needle sharing by drug addicts.

5 Reminders

- **HBV** belongs to the family *Hepadnaviridae*, genus Orthohepadnavirus. It is a DNA virus with a circular genome and RT is used to replicate progeny DNA from an RNA intermediate.

- Transmission is by **blood** or **body fluids**, very small amounts of which may be infective for others. Hepatitis B is readily transmitted by **sexual intercourse**.

- During active infection the blood contains numerous infective virions (Dane particles) and smaller spheres and tubules of surface antigen (**HBsAg**). The presence of HBeAg indicates that the blood contains Dane particles and is infective for others. The core antigen, **HBcAg**, is not detectable in the blood.

- The antibodies **anti-HBc**, **anti-HBe**, and **anti-HBs** appear in that order and indicate recovery. People who fail to form anti-HBe or anti-HBs become chronic carriers.

- HBe-positive carriers are at risk of **cirrhosis of the liver** and **HCC**. Babies acquiring the infection at birth nearly all come into this category. The high carrier rate in some countries, e.g. Africa, is correlated with a high incidence of liver cancer.

- **Treatment** of chronic hepatitis acquired in adulthood with IFN-α is often successful.

- **Prevention** of hepatitis B depends on blocking person-to-person transmission and, particularly for large-scale control, **immunization**.

- **Delta agent** is an incomplete RNA virus dependent on HBV for replication. It may be transmitted along with hepatitis B, and exacerbates its course. It is prevalent in **intravenous drug abusers**. Diagnosis depends mainly on tests for IgM and IgG antibodies. Hepatitis B vaccine also protects against HDV.

Chapter 23

The enteric hepatitis viruses A and E

1 Properties of hepatitis A virus

1.1 Classification

HAV, formerly enterovirus 72, has now been assigned its own genus, *Hepatovirus*, on the basis of its distinctive nucleotide sequence.

1.2 Morphology

The virions have cubic symmetry and are 27 nm in diameter; they resemble those of other members of the family (Chapter 16).

1.3 Genome

The nucleic acid is ssRNA with positive polarity approximately 7.5 kb in length. It codes for four polypeptides: VP1, VP2, VP3, and VP 4. There is only one serotype.

The genome can be divided into three sections: (1) A 5' non-coding region, which is uncapped and has a viral protein Vpg covalently linked at the 5' terminus; (2) an ORF coding all the viral proteins; and (3) a short 3' non-coding region. It is similar in its general structure to the picornavirus genome.

1.4 Replication

HAV cannot be propagated in the laboratory as readily as other enteroviruses. It can be grown with difficulty in monkey kidney and human diploid cells.

Little is known about the mechanism of entry into cells and whether a specific receptor is involved. It is presumed that, in common with other picornaviruses, genome multiplication occurs entirely in the cytoplasm where the genome RNA can act as mRNA directly. The incoming viral RNA strand directs the synthesis of a large viral polyprotein, which is then cleaved into segments. Translation is a crucial step because synthesis of new picornaviral RNA cannot begin until the virus has translated an RNA-dependent RNA polymerase.

The initial step in the production of new viral RNA is to copy the incoming genome RNA to form complementary negative-strand RNA. This serves as a template for synthesis of positive-strand genome RNAs. The entire procedure in picornaviruses occurs in the cytoplasm on the smooth endoplasmic reticulum.

Picornavirus assembly is complex with formation of non-infectious 'provirions', which require a 'maturation' cleavage of one of the structural polypeptides. The new virions are usually released by an infection-mediated disintegration of the host cells. Hepatitis A, exceptionally in the family, can establish a persistent infection with much reduced cell destruction.

2 Clinical and pathological aspects of hepatitis A virus infections

2.1 Clinical features

The incubation period is 2–6 weeks. Many infections are silent, particularly in young children. Clinical illness usually starts with a few days of malaise, loss of appetite, vague abdominal discomfort, and fever. The urine then becomes dark and the faeces pale; soon afterwards jaundice becomes apparent, first in the sclera and then in the skin; if severe, it may be accompanied by itching. The patient starts to feel better within the next week or so and the **jaundice** disappears within a month. Hepatitis A is nearly always self-limiting, but relapses have been reported. The severity of illness is less in children than in adults. Complications such as fulminant hepatitis, fortunately rare, are seen mainly in older people. Mortality is only about 1/1000.

2.2 Epidemiology

The main mode of spread is that of other enteroviruses, i.e. transmission is by the **faecal–oral route** (Chapters 4 and 16). Like them, HAV survives for long periods in water and wet environments. Large quantities of virions are excreted in the **faeces** for several days before and after the onset of jaundice, but after a week the patient's stools may be regarded as non-infectious. Other routes of transmission include transfusion of blood or blood products inadvertently collected during the viraemic phase; sharing of needles by drug abusers; and **sexual contact**, particularly between male homosexuals.

The geographical distribution of hepatitis A follows the patterns described for other enteroviruses, notably poliomyelitis (see Chapter 16). Thus it is widespread in countries where sewage treatment and hygiene generally are inadequate, most persons acquiring it as a subclinical infection in early childhood. In more developed areas, outbreaks are liable to occur in mental institutions and the like where personal hygiene is poor. It occurs both in endemic form and as epidemics, some of which have been traced to infected shellfish.

2.3 Pathogenesis and pathology

The virus replicates primarily in the **hepatocytes**, from which it passes through the bile duct to the intestine, and is shed in large quantities in the faeces. There is necrosis of hepatocytes, particularly in the periportal areas, accompanied by proliferation of Kupffer and other endothelial cells. Temporary damage to liver function is indicated by **elevated liver enzymes** in the blood. However, unlike infections with HBV and HCV, there is no tendency to chronicity, cirrhosis, or malignant change.

2.4 Immune response

Specific IgM appears during the prodromal phase, is present at high titre by the time jaundice is apparent and persists for several months. **IgG neutralizing antibody** is detectable for many years after infection and protects against further attacks. Cytotoxic T cells lyse virus-infected hepatocytes, and these, together with IFN and other cytokines are important in the **cell-mediated immune response**, which in turn seems to be a major factor in pathogenesis.

2.5 Laboratory diagnosis

During the acute phase, liver dysfunction is indicated **by raised serum bilirubin and transaminases and a depressed prothrombin level**. The specific diagnosis is readily made by an **ELISA test for specific IgM**. During the early stage of jaundice the virus can be identified in the faeces by IEM.

2.6 Control

Immunization

Passive protection

Individuals travelling from temperate to subtropical and tropical countries can be given an injection of **human normal immunoglobulin (HNIG)** shortly before departure. This contains enough anti-HAV antibody to confer sufficient passive immunity to prevent or modify an attack during the next 3–6 months. It may also be used for postexposure prophylaxis, e.g. for healthcare workers and relatives at risk of infection during an outbreak. By and large, however, active protection with vaccine, or vaccine plus HNIG, is preferable to the use of immunoglobulin alone.

Hepatitis A vaccine

For practical purposes there is only one serotype, and various **formalin-inactivated vaccines** prepared from HAV grown in human diploid cells induce good antibody responses; such vaccines are licensed for use in the UK and elsewhere.

General measures

Control of infection in the community depends on maintenance of hygiene, a counsel of perfection that is often very difficult to achieve.

A **food handler** with hepatitis A must be kept away from work for 2 weeks after the onset of jaundice. Fellow workers should **not** be given immunoglobulin as prophylactic as this may merely mask an attack without completely preventing it, an obviously dangerous situation; they should be kept under surveillance and asked to report any illness during the next 12 weeks.

In **hospitals**, patients should be nursed with appropriate precautions against the spread of an enteric infection, with particular attention to **safe disposal of faeces** during the infective period.

3 Reminders

- Hepatitis A is an **enterovirus** transmitted by the faecal–oral route. The incubation period is 2–6 weeks. Jaundice lasts about a month, after which recovery is complete in the great majority of cases. There is **no carrier state** and no tendency to chronicity or malignancy.
- Laboratory diagnosis is made by finding **specific IgM antibody** in the serum or by **IEM** of faeces.
- There is an effective **inactivated vaccine. Normal human immunoglobulin** confers temporary passive immunity and is useful for travellers going to highly endemic areas and postexposure prophylaxis.

4 Properties of hepatitis E virus

HEV was identified by a unique combination of EM and nucleotide sequence analysis of a cDNA library. The clinical material originated from the bite of an infected macaque and subsequent hybridization with cDNA from a human liver identified the agent as a calicivirus. Most probably the virus is zoonotic, originating in swine. Other caliciviruses cause outbreaks of D&V (see Chapter 11, where the *Caliciviridae* are described).

4.1 Genome

A single stranded positive sense RNA, 7.2 kb in length, containing a short 5′ UTR, three open reacting frames, a short 3′ UTR and terminated by a poly(A) tract.

5 Clinical and pathological aspects of hepatitis E virus infections

5.1 Clinical features

The course of HEV infection is generally similar to that of HAV. The main differences are

- the incubation period is rather longer (about 6 weeks);
- infection is generally acquired in adolescence or adulthood, rather than in infancy. Person to person transmission rates are low;
- in women becoming infected during the later stages of **pregnancy** the mortality rate is approximately 20 per cent;
- fulminant disease is more common than in HAV infections.

5.2 Epidemiology

In 1955, following a breakdown in the water supply and sewage systems of Delhi caused by floods, there was a huge epidemic of water-borne hepatitis affecting more than 30 000 people, which affected pregnant women particularly severely. HAV was blamed at first, but years later, retrospective serological tests excluded this possibility (and showed the value of keeping specimens for long periods). In 1989 the cause was identified as a new agent, HEV. Since then outbreaks have occurred in most developing countries. The mode of spread is not so well understood as that of HAV, but certainly involves the **faecal–oral route.** Subclinical infections are common and may be as high as seven times the clinical incidence. Based on sequence analysis HEV isolates have been classified into four genotypes.

5.3 Pathogenesis and pathology

The pathology of HEV infections broadly resembles that of HAV disease.

5.4 Immune response

Apart from the fact that antibodies to HEV can be detected in the serum, little is yet known about the humoral and cell-mediated responses to HEV.

5.5 Laboratory diagnosis

The diagnosis depends on finding serum antibody to IgM.

5.6 Control

Immunization

There is as yet no vaccine to protect against HEV infection.

General measures

These depend on the maintenance of a clean water supply, and generally resemble those used to control HAV.

6 Reminders

- **HEV is a calicivirus.**
- Clinically and epidemiologically, HEV infections resemble those due to HAV, but are **severe in pregnant women** and are more likely to cause fulminant disease.
- Apart from the IgM test mentioned above, there is as yet no satisfactory diagnostic method.
- There is no vaccine or specific treatment.

Chapter 24

The blood-borne hepatitis flaviviruses

This virus is the leading cause of liver disease globally and is estimated to infect more than 170 million people. Chronic HCV leads to liver fibrosis and cirrhosis and hepatocarcinoma. The virus is a leading cause of chronic liver disease.

1 Properties of hepatitis C virus

1.1 Classification

This virus is a member of the *Flaviviridae*, genus *Hepacivirus* (see Chapter 27—Arboviruses).

1.2 Morphology

The virions are about 50 nm in diameter, and are enveloped. The core is about 30 nm in diameter.

1.3 Genome

Hepatitis C has a positive-sense ssRNA genome 9.6 kb in size (see Fig. 24.1). There are untranslated 5' and 3' ends and the 3' end is not polyadenylated. The UTRs are important for viral RNA translation and replication. 5' terminus of the genome has a complete secondary structure functioning as an internal ribosome entry site—which mediates viral protein translation in a cap independent manner.

Similarly to other flaviviruses, the gene order from the 5' to the 3' end is C, E1, E2, p7, NS2, NS3, NS4A, NS4B, NS5A, and NS5B; E1 and E2 are the virion glycoprotein spikes, C is the core and NS5 is the RNA-dependent RNA polymerase. The genome has a large ORF that encodes a polyprotein, which is processed into the four structural and six NS proteins.

The viral envelope proteins are E1 and E2. The C protein core is the major component of the nucleocapsid. This may inhibit host response and is thought to bind to viral RNA during assembly. This protein forms a self-modulating mechanism to maintain a low level of viral replication and hence persistence. NS3 is a bi

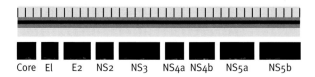

Fig. 24.1 Hepatitis C genome.

functional protease/helicase while NS4B and NS5A are part of the viral replicase complex.

1.4 Replication

The virus receptor is CD81 or the low-density lipoprotein receptor of the cell (LDLR). Viral replication is cytoplasmic. The genome acts directly as an mRNA and a single polyprotein is translated and cleaved by both viral and cellular proteases.

1.5 Variants of hepatitis C virus

There are six major genotypes, or **clades** (phylogenetic variants) with a large number of subtypes. The distributions of the major genotypes are to some extent related to the various risk groups, response to antiviral therapy and geographical areas of prevalence. For example, the response to treatment is worse in the widely distributed genotype 1b infections than with other genotypes; and genotype 5a is common only in South Africa. Clades differ from each other by about 20 per cent at the nucleotide level.

A number of similar viruses designated GBV-like agents have been identified in New World monkeys; their role in human infections is not clear.

Unfortunately, there is no cross-protection between the various genotypes, which militates against the development of a vaccine, as does the inability to propagate these agents in cell cultures.

2 Clinical and pathological aspects of hepatitis C virus infections

2.1 Clinical features

Mode of onset

The **incubation period** is about **8 weeks**. Only 10–20 per cent or so of those infected have symptoms, e.g. anorexia and nausea, which resemble those caused by other hepatitis viruses; frank jaundice is uncommon. Therefore, the term acute hepatitis C is misleading. When jaundice does occur symptoms and biochemical changes are identical to other forms of hepatitis. Alanine aminotransferase levels begin to increase shortly before symptoms and a 10-fold elevation can be detected.

Persistent infection

Hepatitis C becomes chronic in about 80 per cent of those infected, irrespective of the mode of onset. After many years, sometimes as long as four decades, **cirrhosis of the liver** may supervene in 10–20 per cent of patients, but death from this cause alone is rare. Even so, the development of cirrhosis is sinister because it is often a precursor of **HCC**, which develops in 1–5 per cent of those with chronic infection and, of course, has a very poor prognosis.

Complications

In a minority of HCV infections, liver disease is accompanied by glomerulonephritis and various forms of vasculitis, of which some at least are caused by deposition of immune complexes. HCV is also involved in the pathogenesis of type 2 cryoglobulinaemia, which often gives rise to a purpuric rash.

2.2 Epidemiology

WHO estimates that about 170 million people, or 3 per cent of the world's population, are infected with HCV. Of these, a substantial proportion are at risk of HCC (Table 24.1).

The groups at risk

The groups at risk are broadly similar to those listed for hepatitis B, but their relative proportions are different. Most cases of hepatitis C **are intravenous drug abusers**. Transmission via inadequately sterilized needles and body-piercing, tattooing, and circumcision have also been implicated. Sexual transmission and congenital infections are less important; and now that blood can be screened for HCV, infections from this source and from blood products are much less frequent than they used to be. Organ transplants have also transmitted HCV infections.

The geographical distribution

The geographical distribution, as measured by serological surveys, is lowest in northern and western Europe, the USA and Australia, and highest in Japan and the Middle East. There is a pronounced variation in the prevalence of the six various genotypes in different regions. The virus probably emerged about 2000 years ago from an animal reservoir. The genome is remarkably heterogeneous (Fig. 24.2), and there are at least six genotypes recognized with 70 different subtypes. Genotypes 1–3 are most widely distributed in the world. Genotype I is mainly detected in the USA and Europe, types II and III in the USA, and type IV in North and Central Africa. Eighty per cent of

Table 24.1 The world prevalence of hepatitis C

WHO region	Total population (millions)	Hepatitis C prevalence (rate per cent)	Infected population (millions)
Africa	602	5.30	31.9
Americas	785	1.70	13.1
Eastern Mediterranean	466	4.60	21.3
Europe	858	1.03	8.9
Southeast Asia	1500	2.15	32.3
Western Pacific	1600	3.90	62.2
Totals	**5811**	**3.1**	**169.7**

Data from WHO Weekly Epidemiological Record, 10 December 1999.

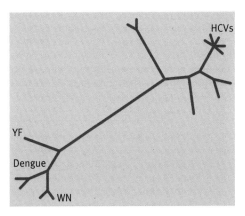

Fig. 24.2 Phylogenetic tree of hepatitis C within the flavivirus family.

infected persons develop viral persistence. It is unclear why such a high proportion fails to abrogate infection. Possible reasons are high genetic variability of an extra hepatitis replication, lack of early immune response.

2.3 Pathogenesis and pathology

In most instances there is a slowly progressive asymptomatic hepatitis, with persistent viraemia. Those with chronic active disease are liable to proceed to cirrhosis, but this process is slow, taking as long as 20 years. Periodic exacerbations are marked by rises in alanine aminotransferase values. Histologically, there is little to distinguish HCV infections from other forms of viral hepatitis, except for the presence **of lymphoid follicles within the portal tracts**. There is also intense periportal infiltration with lymphocytes, and damage to the lining of the bile ducts. The 'ground glass' appearance of liver cells infected with HBV, due to accumulation of surface antigen, is of course absent.

HCC seems to be a direct consequence of the cirrhosis, rather than integration of nucleic acid sequences into the host-cell genome, as is the case with hepatitis B.

2.4 Immune response

The cell-mediated response is more prominent than humoral immunity, but active proliferation of T-helper and cytotoxic lymphocytes seems insufficient either to clear the infection or to prevent reinfection. There is some evidence that HCV can mutate *in vivo*, thus escaping immune surveillance. Indeed, the immune response to HCV seems unusually inefficient, which accounts for its long-term persistence.

2.5 Laboratory diagnosis

Tests for antibodies

A number of **ELISA** and immunoblot tests have been developed for detecting antibodies to various viral protein epitopes, some of which are in the form of recombinant proteins. The antibody test is very valuable for diagnosis.

Tests for genome

Tests for genome by quantitative RNA **PCR** provide valuable confirmatory evidence of infection and allow sensitivity to 100 RNA genome copies/ml plasma.

2.6 Treatment

IFN-α together with ribavirin is moderately effective in 30–50 per cent of those with chronic hepatitis C, but many cases relapse during treatment; and if it is stopped; only about 15 per cent appear to be permanently cured. The results of chemotherapy with IFN are improved by using IFN in its pegylated form, i.e. attached to molecules of polyethylene glycol. Side-effects are similar to those seen with unmodified IFN, e.g. malaise, fever, fatigue, and psychiatric symptoms. Treatment for acute hepatitis C is best initiated early; a commonly used dosage is 6 mU of IFN-α three times weekly for 16–24 weeks. Pegylated IFN-αs have longer half lives and slower clearance. There is a sustained virological response in up to 60 per cent of treated patients.

Liver transplantation has proved of short or medium term benefit in some cases of cirrhosis or HPC, but reinfection of the graft probably always occurs.

2.7 Control

Immunization

As we have seen, the development of a vaccine is hindered by the number (six) of genotypes and by inability to propagate the viruses readily *in vitro*; and although some encouraging results have been obtained in the laboratory, it will certainly be some time before a good immunizing agent becomes generally available.

General measures

The detection of HCV by the above methods is of course particularly important in relation to the screening of blood donors and blood products, and has greatly diminished the chances of infection from these sources; thus control of transmission between intravenous drug abusers remains the most important target for public health measures. The virus is difficult to cultivate and the main model is the chimpanzee, which can only be used in restricted numbers. Transgenic mice have been constructed as well as mice with livers infiltrated with human hepatocytes.

3 The GBV viruses

So far, the alphabetic designations of the various hepatitis viruses has been reasonably simple. A confusing situation arose when yet another virus was isolated from the blood of a surgeon with acute hepatitis. It is perhaps unfortunate that it was termed GB, the patient's initials. Soon afterwards, similar agents were detected in New World monkeys and provided with further alphabetic designations, so that we now have a group of viruses labelled GBV-A, GBV-C, and so forth.

The roles of all these agents in causing clinical disease has yet to be elucidated. The main thing to remember is that sequence analysis of their genomes shows them to be closely related to known **flaviviruses**.

4 Reminders

- **Hepatitis C**, a blood-borne flavivirus, is transmitted in a fashion similar to HBV (Chapter 22) and is mainly prevalent in **intravenous drug abusers**. This agent, and others labelled GBV-A, GBV-B, and so forth resemble flaviviruses, of which the type species is YF virus. There are six major genotypes and many subtypes. The role of the GB viruses in disease of humans is not yet clear. All these agents are classified in the genus *Hepacivirus*.

- HCV infections tend to become chronic, with eventual **cirrhosis** and sometimes **HCC**. Chronicity may be due in part to the poor immune response, and possibly to mutations in the viral genome. A rise in incidence of HCC worldwide is thought to be associated with infection with the virus.

- The infection is diagnosed by ELISA and other tests, RNA genome copies quantified by RT–PCR.

- IFN-α, particularly in its pegylated form, and given with ribavirin, is useful in treatment but often does not effect a complete cure.

Retroviruses and AIDS

1 Introduction

The first discovery of a retrovirus was made as long ago as 1910 by Peyton Rous, working at the Rockefeller Institute for Medical Research in New York. This agent, avian sarcoma virus, induced tumours in muscle, bone, and other tissues of chickens (Chapter 6). He received the Nobel Prize for this discovery, but it was not until the 1930s that other retroviruses, causing tumours in mice and other mammals, were discovered. But these viruses were regarded as laboratory curiosities until the description of feline leukaemia virus, which appeared to spread naturally in household cats. Perhaps as a portent for the later discovery of HIV-1 in humans, it caused an immune deficiency in infected animals. Retroviruses possess a unique enzyme, RT, which uses the viral RNA as a template for making a DNA copy, which then integrates into the chromosome of the host cell and there serves either as a basis for viral replication or as an oncogene (see Chapter 6). Howard Temin and David Baltimore both received Nobel Prizes for their spectacular discovery of this enzyme, which overturned a central dogma of molecular biology—that genetic information flows in one direction only, from DNA→RNA→protein. However, of course, the discovery of HIV-1 and later HIV-2, the causative agent of AIDS, resulted in a huge surge of scientific and medical interest in this previously rather obscure family of viruses.

1.1 The controversy surrounding the discovery of AIDS virus

In 1981 a new clinical syndrome, characterized by profound immunodeficiency, was recorded in male homosexuals and was termed **AIDS.** The Centers for Disease Control in Atlanta reported an unusual prevalence of *Pneumocystis carinii* **pneumonia** in a group of young, previously healthy, male homosexuals. Before then, this parasite had been associated with disease only in patients whose immune systems had been seriously impaired as a result of drug therapy or by congenital cellular immune deficiency. At the same time came reports of previously healthy young homosexuals in New York and San Francisco who had developed a rare cancer, **Kaposi's sarcoma**. The first isolation of a retrovirus **(HIV-1)** from an AIDS case was made by Luc Montagnier and Barré-Sinoussi at the Pasteur Institute in Paris early in 1983 and quickly confirmed by Robert Gallo in the USA. Unfortunately, scientific squabbles about priority last until this day. The first case of AIDS in the UK was diagnosed in late 1981 in a homosexual from Bournemouth, after he returned home from Miami. An AIDS research trust was established in his name, Terrence Higgins. From this small outbreak has developed an epidemic, involving people of every nation of the world, men, women, and children. Now 5000 new cases occur daily in the world and 41 million people have been infected.

A fourth human retrovirus, **HIV-2**, was isolated from mildly immunosuppressed patients in West Africa and appears to be less pathogenic than HIV-1. Fewer people succumb to HIV-2 than HIV-1 and prior infection with HIV-2 may even help to prevent infection with HIV-1. However, the incidence of HIV-2 is growing. In Guinea Bissau, a former Portuguese colony, there is an 8–10 per cent prevalence. Countries with a past link with Portugal, including south-west India, Angola, Mozambique, and Brazil, and all have significant numbers of infected people. Portugal has the highest prevalence of HIV-2 in Europe, accounting for 4.5 per cent of AIDS cases.

2 Properties of HIV

2.1 Classification

The family *Retroviridae* is so named for its possession of a **RT** (Latin *retro* = backwards) (Table 25.1). Of the seven genera now recognized, only two cause disease in humans:

- *Lentivirus*, containing HIV-1 and 2 (Latin *lentus* = slow). The lentiviruses are distinguished by the presence of a vase or cone-shaped nucleoid, absence of oncogenicity, and the lengthy and insidious onset of clinical signs.
- 'BLV-HTLV retroviruses', which contain HTLV-I and -II. They are distinguished by their characteristic genomes and their ability to cause tumours rather than immunosuppression.

The spumaviruses (Latin *spuma* = foam) cause a characteristic foamy appearance in infected primate cell cultures. As far as we know, they are not pathogenic.

2.2 Morphology

The typical HIV particle is 100–150 nm in diameter with an outer envelope of lipid penetrated by 72 glycoprotein spikes, the envelope (env) protein (Fig. 25.1). The env polypeptide is composed of two subunits, the outer glycoprotein knob (gp120) and

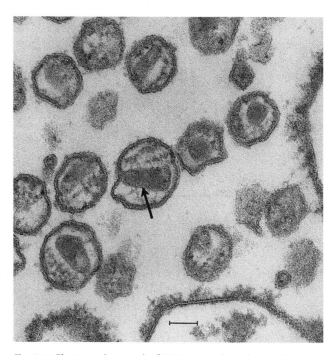

Fig. 25.1 Electron micrograph of HIV-1, vase-shaped core of the virion is arrowed. (Courtesy of Dr David Hockley.) Scale bar = 50 nm.

Table 25.1 Classification of primate retroviruses

Genus	Virus	Disease caused	Natural hosts
BLV-HTLV retroviruses (formerly *Oncovirinae*)	Human T-cell leukaemia virus (HTLV-1)	Adult T-cell leukaemia/lymphoma; tropical spastic paraparesis	Humans
	Human T-cell leukaemia virus (HTLV-2)	Hairy cell leukaemia (very rare)	Humans
Lentivirus	Human immunodeficiency virus (HIV-1)	Immune deficiency, encephalopathy Virus can infect chimpanzees but causes no clinical signs	Humans and chimpanzees
	Human immunodeficiency virus (HIV-2)	Immune deficiency. Less pathogenic than HIV-1	Humans and monkeys
	Simian immunodeficiency virus (SIV-1)	Immune deficiency. No disease in wild African green monkeys but AIDS in rhesus monkeys	Monkeys
Spumavirus	Human spumavirus	Inapparent persistent infections	Primates and other animals

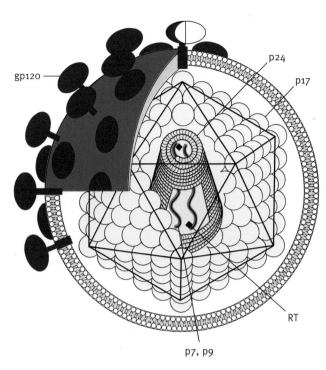

gp120

p24

p17

RT

p7, p9

Fig. 25.2 Structural features of human immunodeficiency virus. The glycoprotein (gp120) spikes protrude though the lipid membrane. An icosahedral shell (p17) underlies the membrane and itself encloses a vase-shaped structure. The diploid RNA is enclosed in the 'vase'.

a transmembrane portion (gp41), which joins the knob to the virus lipid envelope. The receptor binding site for CD4 is present on gp120 as well as very important antigens such as the V3 loop.

The inner surface of the virus lipid envelope is lined by a matrix protein (p17). There are also abundant cellular proteins, notably MHC class I and class II antigens in the lipid envelope. In the case of HIV-1 the lipid envelope encloses an icosahedral shell of protein (p17), within which is a vase- or cone-shaped protein core (p24 and p7 and p9 proteins) containing two mole-

cules of ssRNA in the form of a ribonucleoprotein. Bound to the diploid positive sense ssRNA genome are several copies of the RT, integrase, and protease enzymes (see also Fig. 25.2).

2.3 Genome

The organization of the positive sense ssRNA genome of HIV-1, approximately 10 kb in size, is well investigated (Fig. 25.3). Unlike certain oncogenic viruses in the family, it has no onc gene, but has some unique features, particularly the possession of control genes which can enhance viral replication (such as rev (regulator of virus), tat (transactivation), and vif (viral infectivity)) and a repressor gene, nef (negative factor) (Table 25.2). The genome is flanked at each end by LTRs. The 3' LTR has the polyadenylation signal while the 5' LTR has the enhancer promoter sequences for viral transcription.

The pol gene codes for at least three proteins, the largest being RT; another is an integrase with the important function of integrating the HIV proviral genome into cellular DNA; and the third is a viral protease, which has an important cleaving function, after release of the virus from the cell. All these enzymes are the targets of novel antivirals.

HIV-1 binds specifically to the CD4 receptor, which is expressed on the surface of certain T lymphocytes—the T-helper cells (Chapter 5). It also infects B lymphocytes, macrophages, dendritic cells, and brain cells. In common with most viruses the complete replication cycle takes only 24 hours. An important extra for the virus, however, is the ability to integrate into the chromosome of memory T cells and other cells.

An important second or subsidiary receptor belongs to the chemokine receptor family. T-cell tropic HIV-1 viruses use the chemokine receptor CXCR4 as a co-receptor, whereas macrophage-tropic (M tropic) primary isolates use CCR5. Individuals with defective CCR5 alleles exhibit some resistance to HIV-1 infection, which suggests CCR5 has an important role in HIV-1 replication. Both CXCR4 and CCR5 receptors help promote efficient infection of the CNS by HIV-1.

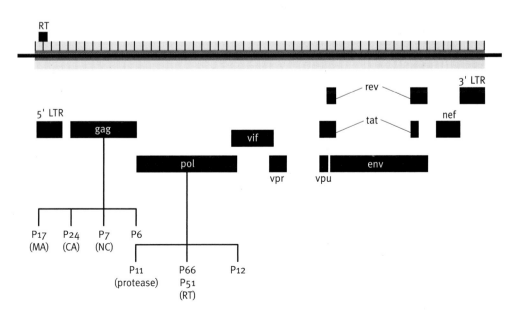

Fig. 25.3 HIV-1 genome and encoded proteins. Labelled genes are gag, pol, and env (structural proteins), vif, nef, vpu, rev, vpr, and tat (regulatory proteins).

Table 25.2 HIV genes and proteins

Gene	Virus protein	Function
Structural		
Gag	Matrix p17	Structural
	Capsid p24	Structural conical core
	Nucleocapsid p7, p6	Structural
Pol	Protease p12	Enzyme
	Reverse transcriptase p66, p51	Enzyme
	Integrase p32	Enzyme
Env	Envelope glycoprotein 120	Structural spike
Regulatory		
*tat**	p14	Transactivates transcription
Rev	p19	Transports unspliced mRNA to cytoplasm
Vif	p24	Promotes virus infectivity
Nef	p27	Promotes virus infectivity, T-cell activation, and downregulates MHC class I
Vpu	p16	Promotes virus release
Vpr	p15	Promotes virus entry into cell nucleus, arrests cell cycle in G_2
Vpx	p14	Promotes virus replication

* *tat* and the genes subsequently listed all code for small peptides with molecular weights of 14–27 kDa.

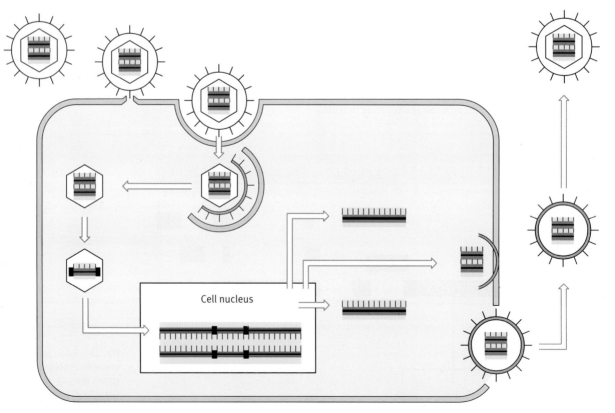

Fig. 25.4 Simplified version of replication of retrovirus (for details see text).

After attachment the virus penetrates the cell by 'fusion from without' (Chapter 3) mediated by fusogenic motif of gp41. Interaction with the secondary receptor and gp120 causes conformation changes and exposure of the fusion peptides of gp41. Synthesis of viral cDNA starts in the entered virions in the cell cytoplasm (Fig. 25.4). The viral RT enzyme directs the synthesis of a cDNA strand (minus strand) using the host positive RNA as a primer and the viral RNA as template. Then viral RNAase enzymatically removes the original viral RNA while the RT now synthesizes a second DNA strand (the plus strand). The association of newly synthesized viral dsDNA and parental viral input proteins is called the pre-integration complex. The complex M, Vpr, and integrase is conducted to the nucleus as part of the dsDNA where integration into the host chromosome occurs to form a proviral DNA. Postintegration, both viral and cellular factors, are needed to activate HIV transcription. Initial expression of viral RNAs is stimulated by Vpr and is further stimulated by the juxtaposition of cellular transcription factors such as NF-κB, AP-1, Spl, and NFAT. The primary RNA transcript is spliced to give 30 plus viral mRNAs. Early viral mRNA transcripts encode Tat, Rev and Nef. Tat is known to increase viral transcription by recruiting cellular factors. Rev is important to aid export of viral RNAs to the cytoplasmic ribosomes, where the so-called accessory proteins Vif, Vpr, and Vpu are synthesized as enzymes. We are viewing here an important milestone in the replication cycle, as in so many viruses, whereby early gene expression is converted to late gene expression. Late gene products for HIV are Gag, Pol, and Env proteins. The time is now 8 hours postinfection. Assembly of new virions can now begin with a proteolytic cascade by viral proteases. The different virus structural proteins begin to assemble with the p24 as a core and also the p7 enclosing the viral RNA. More of less simultaneously the virion buds through the plasma membrane, probably where lipid rafts already occur.

The proviral DNA may reside quietly in the chromosome for years or may be activated. Most cell transcription factors such a NF-κB bind to regulatory sequences in the proviral LTR inducing formation of tat, which binds to the tar region of the LTR and amplifies transcription of all viral genes.

As well as mRNA splicing another important method of extending the capacity of the rather small genome is that of ribosomal frame shifting exploited by the gag-pol RNA transcript. There is a

'stuttering' mechanism and the ribosome is retarded or alternatively jumps forward one nucleotide base to commence reading the triplet in a different frame. Hence two viral proteins can be translated from a single mRNA.

The viral genome assembles in the cytoplasm while env proteins migrate to the plasma membrane. Pol is cleaved by protease to produce four viral enzymes including a viral protease, which carries out an important cleavage function after budding and during maturation. Retroviruses, including HIV, are released from the infected cell by budding from the plasma membrane.

3 Clinical and pathological aspects of HIV

3.1 Clinical features of AIDS

Table 25.3 summarizes a generally accepted scheme for staging the disease. After a mild acute influenza-like illness with an incubation time of about 3–4 weeks, a viraemia spreads virus throughout the body. There is a vigorous immune response resulting in dramatic fall of virus until virus levels reach the so-called set point. A correlate of disease progression is the steady-state viral load (set point) after this primary infection. The disease *then* becomes quiescent (stage A1). Approximately 60 per cent of asymptomatic cases move into the **AIDS-related complex (ARC)** stage B of the disease within the next 4 years. This is characterized by **fever, weight loss, persistent lymphadenopathy, night sweats,** and **diarrhoea.** The most important factor here is gradual loss of CD4 cells. Virus replicates continuously although there is clinical latency. There is tremendous variation in the length of this period between patients. Patients then proceed inexorably to full-blown **AIDS (stage C)** commonly heralded by thrush, herpes zoster, and more serious, *Pneumocystis carinii* **pneumonia**. In untreated patients the time from infection to death may be as long as 10 years and is inevitable in 70 per cent of infected persons. The remainder may live as long as 17 years and form the 'long-term survivors' or 'non-progressors' group.

The signs and symptoms of AIDS may vary somewhat in the different categories of persons infected with the virus. Kaposi's sarcoma is less common, for example, in haemophilia patients, who have been infected as a result of infection of virus-contaminated factor VIII preparations. In Africa most patients die from tuberculosis, whereas superinfection with pneumocystis is more important in Europe. The clinical manifestations of AIDS are protean, but can be summarized as malignant, infective, and neurological.

Malignant disease

The most common of the malignant tumours is Kaposi's sarcoma but aggressive B-cell lymphomas, non-Hodgkin's lymphoma and genital cancers may also appear.

Infective manifestations

These are frequent and include tinea, gingivitis, oral and oesophageal candida, chronic sinusitis, and other infections of the

Table 25.3 Classification system for HIV infection

CD4+ cells per μl of blood	Clinical categories		
	A Asymptomatic acute (primary) HIV or PGL	B Symptomatic	C AIDS
1 ≥500	A1	B1	C1
2 200–499	A2	B2	C2
3 <200	A3	B3	C3

PGL, persistent generalized lymphadenopathy
Data from Centers for Disease Control and Prevention (1992). *Morbidity and Mortality Weekly Reports*, **41**: 1–19.

Table 25.4 Treatment of HIV-1 and accompanying opportunistic infections

Infective agent	Drug
HIV-1	Zidovudine with didanosine (ddI), ddc, 3TC, non-nucleoside inhibitors, protease inhibitors, fusion Inhibitors
Herpes simplex	Aciclovir or penciclovir
Varicella-zoster	Aciclovir or penciclovir
Cytomegalovirus	Foscavir® (retinitis), ganciclovir (pneumonia)
Cryptosporidium	Amphotericin
Toxoplasma gondii	Sulphadiazine and pyrimethamine
Pneumocystis carinii	Trimethoprim, sulphamethoxazole, pentamidine
Mycobacteria	Streptomycin, isoniazid, rifampicin, *p*-aminosalicylic acid (PAS)

skin and mucous membranes. Several latent viruses are activated including herpes simplex and zoster and papillomaviruses. Tuberculosis is a frequent complication, even in the USA. Common opportunistic infections are *Pneumocystis carinii*, EBV interstitial pneumonitis, cryptosporidia and microsporidia, CMV retinitis, enteritis and infection of the brain by *Toxiplasma gondii*, and *Cryptococcus neoformans*. Table 25.4 summarizes some antimicrobial therapies in AIDS patients.

Neurological sequelae

These are also common, and include dementia, severe encephalopathy, myelopathy, and motor dysfunction. There may be diminished memory, tremors, and loss of balance as well as signs of peripheral neuropathy.

Physicians caring for these patients soon become knowledgeable about the microbiological aspects of AIDS, and, until recently, the most important survival factor for a patient was not an antiviral drug but a doctor experienced in this field. The situation has now changed with combination chemotherapy (HAART).

AIDS in children

Without antiretroviral therapy 13–40 per cent of babies born to HIV positive mothers acquire infection. There is clear evidence of transplacental HIV infection; indeed, this is now recognized as the second most common mode of transmission. It is probable that transmission can also take place during delivery or from breast milk. The course of disease is accelerated and 20 per cent of infected infants develop AIDS in the first year of life and approximately one-third die in the first 5 years.

A child is considered to have ARC if interstitial pneumonitis, persistent candidiasis, or parotid swelling is present for 2 months together with two or more of the following:

- persistent general lymphadenopathy;
- recurrent bacterial infection; e.g. *Strep. pneumoniae*, *H. influenzae*, *Salmonella*, and *P. carinae* pneumonia;
- hepatic or splenic enlargement;
- chronic diarrhoea;
- growth failure.

The mortality of children with AIDS is high but the outcome in those with less severe disease or symptomless infection is less certain. The risk of paediatric AIDS is certainly higher in babies born to mothers who are symptomatic rather than simply seropositive but on a more optimistic note, administration of azidothymidine (AZT) to the mother during pregnancy reduces the transmission of virus very significantly.

3.2 Pathogenesis

HIV-1 and HIV-2

HIV-1 and HIV-2 enter the body via the bloodstream either during **sexual intercourse, needle drug abuse, transfusion with contaminated blood products,** or **via the placenta** (maternal–fetal transmission). There have been a number of instances of patients infecting healthcare staff or vice versa, during surgical or dental procedures. Virus-infected lymphocytes are present in sperm and may infect via microscopic breakages in the endothelial lining of the vagina or rectum. It is assumed that, initially, CD4+ lymphocytes, macrophages and dendritic cells are infected by the virus. But as viral antigen has been found in only about 1/10 000 lymphocytes, the reason for their ultimate dysfunction and death is a subject of some speculation. HIV-1 is strongly cytopathic in the laboratory and can cause cell-to-cell fusion resulting in the formation of giant syncytia and cell death. Viral glycoprotein present on the surface of an infected cell can interact with the CD4 receptors on many adjacent uninfected cells, thus multiplying the effect. But the virus seems to be less aggressive to cells when actually in the body because there have been no reports of syncytia, for example in AIDS patients. Moreover, many of the CD4+ lymphocytes that die have not been infected by HIV; they are innocent 'bystander' cells. Some immunologists have therefore proposed that there is an autoimmune component in the pathogenesis.

Virus replication occurs mainly in peripheral lymphoid organs, spleen, lymph nodes, and gut-associated lymphoid tissue. High rates of viral replication occur early after infection and ensure future destruction of CD4+ lymphocytes. Massive lymphocyte destruction occurs daily accompanied by equally massive cellular regeneration.

The replication of the HIV genome is enhanced in antigen-stimulated T cells and it is assumed that persons with concomitant infections that stimulate T-cell replication have a greater chance of succumbing to AIDS. Macrophages are also infected with HIV and, are themselves similarly stimulated by other antigens. They may act as a reservoir of the virus as integrated proviral DNA, as may T lymphocytes and memory cells in the lymph nodes and microglia in the brain. As infection progresses, B lymphocyte functions are affected through their regulation by CD4+ (T$_h$) cells (Chapter 5). The destruction of the CD4+ helper cell subset is particularly damaging to the overall orchestrated immune response of the host. This malfunction of the immune response leads to the appearance of opportunistic organisms which are normally held in check by immune T cells.

3.3 Immune response

Figure 25.5 summarizes the rather complicated serological response of the host to HIV-1 infection. The dynamics are important for diagnostic purposes and most diagnostic kits take advantage of the high levels of anti-env antibodies and their longevity. Antibodies to the env protein develop slowly and remain at high levels throughout the infection. Antibodies to the internal p24 protein have a different temporal pattern and rise during the early stages of the infection, only to decrease in parallel with the onset of serious signs of the disease. An antibody-mediated cytotoxic response is also generated as well as a host-restricted cytotoxic T-cell response to the structural env and gag proteins. It is considered that cytotoxic T cells directed towards the internally situated gag protein may be important in the development of antiviral immunity.

Much less is known about the dynamics of the immune response to the other human retroviruses. Antibodies to the respective env proteins can be clearly distinguished and hence are useful for differential diagnosis of the two lentiviruses and the T-cell leukaemia viruses.

3.4 Epidemiology

Origin of HIV-1 and HIV-2

Both viruses are zoonoses, infecting primates in the wild, often asymptomatically and then opportunistically crossing the species barrier. The cut/slash method whereby chimpanzee hunters were bitten during capture of these chimps for food is

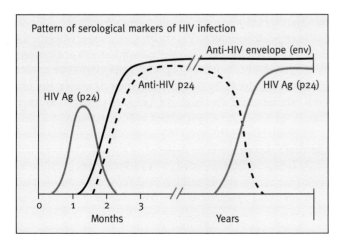

Fig. 25.5 The time course of development of HIV antigens and antibodies.

Table 25.5 Individual actions for preventing AIDS

Needle-borne transmission	Needles or syringes must not be shared
Sexual transmission	A reduction in the number of sexual partners to decrease the chance of being exposed to an infectious person. The following guidelines can be used to decrease the risk of infection
Absolutely safe	Mutually monogamous relationship
Safe	Sexual intercourse using a condom containing spermicide; non-insertive sexual play
Risky	Oral, vaginal, or anal intercourse. Virus is present in vaginal secretion and seminal fluid and in minute traces in saliva
Prenatal transmission	Those at possible risk of HIV infection should be tested for antibody. Antibody-positive women should not become pregnant. Those who do should be treated with AZT to reduce the risk of transmission to the neonate

generally accepted as the point of transfer. HIV-1 is genetically close to retroviruses from the Sootey Mangabey monkey. There may have been seven independent transmissions to humans resulting in HIV-1 serotypes A–G.

In 1990, there were 2200 diagnosed cases of AIDS in the UK and by 1998, 32 000. The actual number of persons infected is a matter for conjecture but may reach over 2 million in the USA alone, and 40 million worldwide.

In the absence of effective vaccines infection can be prevented by individual action (Table 25.5) combined with screening of potentially contaminated blood and blood products to prevent iatrogenic infections. There is evidence of modified sexual behaviour in the USA and certain African countries, which leads to reduced incidences of infection. Transmission most commonly occurs during sexual intercourse with exchange of virus contaminated semen, genital secretions, or blood. Unprotected receptive anal intercourse is the most risky activity. The risk is probably 1 percent or higher. The second most risky behaviour is via direct inoculation with blood by reusing contaminated needles. The risk here is 0.3 per cent. The third primary mode of transmission is from an infected mother to her child where the risk is 13–40 per cent. Treatment of the mother during pregnancy with antiviral drugs and the newborn at birth can significantly reduce this risk, which rises again if the mother breast-feeds.

There is considerable genetic variation between isolates of HIV-1 virus. In the case of the env protein, the degree of variation is comparable with that between subtypes of influenza A virus, namely amino acid sequences differing by up to 25 per cent. Two distinct genetic groups of virus are now recognized,

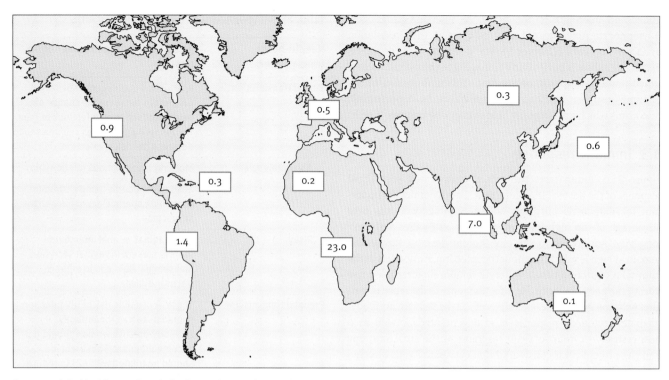

Fig. 25.6 Global incidence of HIV infection and AIDS. The numbers in boxes represent millions.

namely the M (major) and the outlier (O). Group M is further divided into eight genetic subtypes or clades (A–H). These clades have different geographical locations; for example, clade B is spread by homosexual activity in Europe and the USA, whereas clades C and E have a predilection for heterosexual spread in Africa. By far the most infections are caused by these groups.

The most explosive outbreaks of HIV-1 (Fig. 25.6) have occurred in the so-called Group III countries in Asia, including India, Thailand, Eastern Europe, Middle East, and North Africa caused predominantly by clade A spreading heterosexually. The intermediate, Group II nations include Central and East Africa where the virus has spread for the last 25 years, mainly by heterosexual intercourse and by infection of babies. Finally, in western Europe, USA, and Australia the virus has spread mainly by homosexual intercourse and the number of cases is expected to decline.

In West Africa another virus, HIV-2, has been isolated from persons at special risk for sexually transmitted disease, such as prostitutes; however, it has not been associated with such severe clinical illness as HIV-1. Moreover antibody is detected in many asymptomatic elderly persons. There is some evidence that prior infection with HIV-2 may protect against subsequent infection with the more virulent HIV-1. Many virologists would doubt whether a virus such as HIV will even remain stable. It is quite possible that virulence may become enhanced because of mutation and selection.

In the subtropical south-western part of Japan, particularly the islands around Okinawa, the prevalence of HTLV-I antibody is as high as 15 per cent; the rates increase with age and are higher in men than in women. In Jamaica, the prevalence of antibody is about 6 per cent and, in expatriate Caribbean communities, 1–4 per cent; the rates are similar in West African countries.

3.5 HIV vaccines

As well as abstinence from sexual intercourse or the use of condoms, an effective vaccine might be very useful in preventing further spread of HIV-1. However, complete protection is unlikely to be achieved against a hypervariable virus infecting a mucosal surface.

A chemically inactivated whole virus vaccine (a so-called therapeutic vaccine) has been tested in individuals already infected and induces a weak immune response. Some progress has been made with recombinant DNA techniques whereby the gene for HIV env has been transferred to yeast cells or E. coli and large quantities of pure viral spike protein (gp160 or gp120) have been produced by deep fermentation. However, the first such vaccine tested on a high-risk group of male homosexuals failed to give satisfactory protection against the virus.

A live attenuated HIV vaccine is under investigation in which the viral nef gene has been mutated or altered. This gene normally enhances viral infectivity and therefore any interference with functioning would reduce viral replication and spread. Probably most research is directed towards a prime boost approach in which the HIV env gene has been cloned into a harmless poxvirus, such as canary pox. Injection into the arm and subsequent replication of the poxvirus DNA containing the HIV env gene primes the immune system of the individual.

A boost to the immune system then follows by later injection of HIV *env* protein, itself produced by recombinant DNA technology. The two separate antigens stimulate T- and B-cell immune responses.

3.6 Antiviral chemotherapy

No cure exists for this retroviral infection and it is difficult to envisage the development of any antiviral drug, which will both repress viral replication and also excise an integrated viral genome. The antiviral compound **zidovudine** (AZT, 'Retrovir'), is still a cornerstone of treatment; however, it must be given in combination with the chemically related dideoxynucleoside analogues, **didanosine (ddI) and 3TC** and also **protease and fusion inhibitors** (Table 25.4 and Chapter 38). Such intensive regimens are referred to as highly active antiretroviral therapy (HAART) and reduce the chances of drug-resistant virus emerging.

Destruction of virus

Fortunately HIV is not a robust virus and can be easily destroyed by 35 per cent ethanol for 5 minutes or hypochloride (25 000 ppm), or by glutaraldehyde (0.5 per cent).

3.7 Laboratory diagnosis of HIV infection

It cannot be overemphasized that laboratory investigation is needed for a definitive diagnosis of HIV infection. The diagnosis cannot be made on clinical grounds alone. Most laboratories screen blood for antibodies to viral env protein using a rapid **ELISA** method and confirm 'positives' using a more elaborate and more expensive **Western blot** analysis. In view of the great personal and social implications of a positive test for anti-HIV antibody, **it is important to carry out a confirmatory test** by a completely different technique. Modern third generation tests are 99–100 per cent specific but false negatives do occur. There may be a period of several months when the virus is present but the infected person has not yet produced detectable antibodies. If, therefore, a person is a member of the high-risk groups and is concerned about a recent sexual or other risk event, serological testing will have to be performed again after 6 or even 12 months before a negative result is acceptable.

Viral genome load assays are now routinely performed to quantify the number of viral genome RNA copies in plasma by PCR. The results correlate well with clinical prognosis; for example, a high number of RNA copies indicates a potentially rapid onset of AIDS.

Gloves and a disposable plastic apron or gown must be worn when taking blood or other specimens from ARC or AIDS patients. Eye protection is recommended. Obviously, **safety procedures for taking, packing and transporting clinical specimens must be strictly observed**.

It must be noted that in the USA home testing is being explored whereby a skin prick is made and blood dried on to a paper filter which is then mailed to a laboratory under code. Approximately 1 percent are positive for HIV-1 antibodies.

Personal accidents involving potentially HIV infected material must be reported and skin pricks treated immediately by encouraging bleeding and washing with soap and water. Some hospital pharmacies retain stocks of zidovudine, ddI, 3TC, and protease inhibitors for immediate administration to staff who have been potentially infected via skin pricks. The chance of becoming infected after a 'needlestick' with infected blood is 0.3 per cent.

4 The discovery of the other human retroviruses HTLV-I and HTLV-II

4.1 HTLV-I

In 1978, Robert Gallo, in the USA, isolated a retrovirus from the lymphocytes of a leukaemia patient that had been mainained in culture in the laboratory by a new technique involving stimulation of the cells with IL-2. Japanese workers had earlier noticed clustering of cases of adult T-cell leukaemia/ lymphoma in the southern islands of Japan. To epidemiologists this clustering hinted at an infectious aetiology. The first human retrovirus to be discovered was named HTLV-I. It proved to be endemic not only in southern Japan, where there are over one million carriers but also in parts of Central and South America, the Caribbean, and Africa. It has been suggested that HTLV-I originated in Africa, where it infected Old World primates; after transmission to humans, it may have reached the Americas along with the slave trade, and then the southern islands of Japan with early Portuguese explorers who had previously been in Africa. Clusters in families show that vertical transmission or close contact is needed for spread. The important mode of transmission is sexual intercourse. Prevalence in blood donors may reach 5 per cent in epidemic areas.

4.2 HTLV-II

A second virus, HTLV-II, was isolated in Seattle, USA, from the cells of a patient with a rare 'hairy cell' leukaemia, but little is known about it at present. It is prevalent in intravenous drug users in the USA but is not known to cause disease in them.

4.3 Transmission

HTLV-I is transmitted by **intravenous drug abuse, sexual intercourse**, and **blood transfusion** and enters the body inside infected CD4+ lymphocytes in semen or blood as well as vertically from mother to infant via breast milk and possibly via the placenta,

The prime suspect for initiating disease must be the HTLV-I-infected lymphocyte, transformed in adult T-cell leukaemia/ lymphoma and presumably chronically activated in **tropical spastic paraparesis** (TSP). The product of the virus regulatory gene *tax* transactivates transcription from the viral LTR and also from cellular oncogenes. Neuronal damage and demyelination are probably consequences of the inflammation, so that HTLV-I may not be truly neurotropic. As only a few cases of both diseases in the same patient have been reported, despite the many hundreds of each in Japan and the Caribbean, infected lymphocytes seem to be committed to produce one disease or the other, or, much more often, neither.

Little is known about the pathogenesis of HTLV-II.

4.4 Clinical features of HTLV-I and HTLV-II infections

HTLV-I

Most persons infected with HTLV-I remain asymptomatic for life but in about 5 per cent overt disease may appear after an incubation period of 10–40 years: there are two distinct clinical manifestations.

Adult T-cell leukaemia/lymphoma

HTLV-I frequently presents in middle-aged adults as acute **aggressive lymphoma** of the skin and most viscera including particularly the liver, spleen, and lymph nodes. A further important diagnostic feature is hypercalcaemia, with or without bone lesions. The leukaemic phase of the disease is not always evident. Variants of what is usually an acute and aggressive disease occur and include a chronic T-cell lymphocytosis.

A form of 'smouldering' adult T-cell leukaemia/lymphoma is also seen, in which the patients present with persistent lymphocytosis, with or without lymphoma.

HTLV-I-associated myelopathy

The other clinical form is seen in Martinique, West Indies, and here most patients have the chronic neurological disease, **TSP,** sometimes called **HAM.** Progressive demyelination of the long motor neurone tracts in the spinal cord results in spastic paraparesis of both lower limbs. Women are affected more often than men.

HTLV-II

This is known to cause a 'hairy T-cell' leukaemia, but very few cases have been described.

5 Reminders

- Retroviruses are enveloped and contain **diploid RNA** of approximately 10 kb in size; they possess a **RT** able to catalyse transcription of viral RNA into DNA (proviral DNA).

- HIV-1 causes slow persistent infection. A substantial proportion of those infected develop **AIDS**.

- The three stages of HIV-1 disease are: (1) the asymptomatic phase; (2) ARC with persistent lymphadenopathy, night sweats, and diarrhoea; and (3) full-blown AIDS with a plethora of opportunistic infections.

- There is a group of HIV-positive individuals who after 25 years have not developed AIDS, the so-called long-term survivors.

- Laboratory studies are required to confirm infection with HIV-1 or HIV-2. **ELISA** detects specific antibodies to these retroviruses. Determination of **viral RNA load** as measured by number of viral RNA copies is an important prognostic test.

- The life of AIDS patients may be prolonged by treatment with **combinations of the antiretroviral drugs zidovudine, ddI, 3TC,** and **protease and fusion inhibitors** and prompt treatment of bacterial, parasitic, and viral opportunist infections. There are no vaccines at present.

- The individual can take important actions to prevent infection both by using **safe sex procedures** and by **not sharing needles and syringes**. Fortunately, the virus has low infectivity.

- Worldwide, 80 per cent of HIV infections are transmitted by heterosexual intercourse. Perinatal and blood transfusions account respectively for 10 per cent and 5 per cent of infections.

- Three groups of nations have been identified in which the epidemiology of HIV has varied: in Group I (Europe, the USA, and Australia) the cases are mainly homosexuals and numbers are decreasing. Group II nations are Central and East Africa, where virus is spread heterosexually and by infection of babies. The most explosive outbreaks are occurring now in India, Thailand, and North Africa, where the spread is predominantly among heterosexuals.

- HTLV-I causes cancer (**adult T-cell leukaemia lymphoma**) and also a chronic neurological disease, TSP, or HTLV-I-associated myelopathy (HAM). HTLV-II causes a rare hairy cell leukaemia.

Lyssavirus and rabies

1 Introduction

This awesome disease of animals, comparatively rarely transmitted to humans, has been recognized since the dawn of history and references appear in the Babylonian Eshnunna Code before 2300 BC. Celsius first described hydrophobia in AD 100 and recommended cautery of animal bites with a hot iron; this remained the treatment of rabid animal bites until 1884, when Louis Pasteur introduced his famous rabies vaccine. With very rare exceptions, the disease is fatal in humans and many people still die each year, especially in the developing countries.

2 Properties of the virus

2.1 Classification

Rabies virus belongs to the *Rhabdoviridae* (Greek: *rhabdos* = a rod), a family of characteristically **bullet-shaped RNA** viruses, that contains over 150 animal, fish, insect, and plant viruses. Rabies and other viruses of the genus *Lyssavirus* (Greek: *lyssa* = madness) infect vertebrates; seven species are known (Table 26.1). Vesicular stomatitis virus belongs to the genus *Vesiculovirus* and affects horses and cattle; it may cause a mild febrile illness in humans exposed to it. Other genera in the family affect only insects or plants.

Table 26.1 Some members of the family *Rhabdoviridae*

Genus	Members
Lyssavirus	Rabies
	Lagos bat virus
	Australian bat lyssavirus
	Mokola
	Duvenhage
	European bat virus 1; virus 2
	Australian bat virus
Vesiculovirus	Vesicular stomatitis virus and other viruses infecting vertebrates and invertebrates

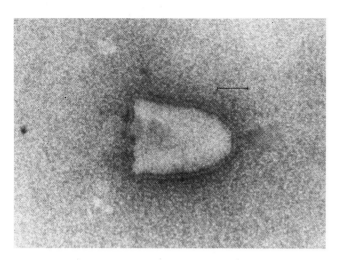

Fig. 26.1 Electron micrograph of rabies virus. Note the characteristic bullet shape and the fringe of glycoprotein spikes on the surface. (Courtesy of Dr David Hockley.) Scale bar = 50 nm.

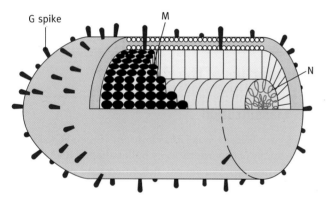

Fig. 26.2 Structural features of rabies virus. Glycoprotein (G) spikes protrude through the lipid of the bullet-shaped virion. The M protein subunits are represented as short cylinders. The nucleoprotein (N) is closely associated with the RNA.

2.2 Morphology

*The rabies virion consists of a **helical** nucleocapsid contained in a bullet-shaped lipoprotein envelope (Fig. 26.1) about 180 nm in length. Protruding from the lipid envelope are approximately 200 glycoprotein (G) spikes of the virus, responsible for viral attachment to cellular receptors and subsequent fusion activity. G also has HA activity and has important antigenic sites which are neutralized by specific antibody.*

The M or matrix protein is the major structural protein of the virus; lying internally beneath the lipid membrane; it may contact the end of the G spike, helping to stabilize the structure of the virion (Fig. 26.2). The nucleoprotein (N) encapsidates and protects the RNA from degradation by RNAase enzymes. Closely attached to the RNA and N protein in the virus particle is the L or large protein which functions as the virus RNA transcriptase and also has 5′ cap methylase, 3′ poly(A) polymerase, and protein kinase activities.

2.3 Genome structure

Rhabdoviruses contain an ssRNA genome of negative polarity and 11–12 kb in size. Viruses in this class contain a virion-associated RNA transcriptase (the L protein), which is responsible for the production of viral mRNAs in infected cells (Chapter 3). Five monocistronic virion mRNAs are synthesized and the gene order from the 3′ end is promotor, N, P, M, G, and L. Polyadenylation may occur by RNA polymerase slippage or 'stuttering' at each inter-gene stretch of seven U residues and the enzyme then moves on to the next gene. There is higher molar abundance of gene products at the 3′ end of the genome. In contrast, full-length complementary copies of genomic RNA are presumably synthesized by complete read through of intergene regions by a modified RNA replicase enzyme (L+P) coded by the virus.

2.4 Replication

Rabies virus attaches via the G spike to a cellular ganglioside receptor molecule the nicotinic acetylcholine receptor and then enters a susceptible cell by viropexis, in much the same way as influenza virus. A coated pit is formed which then fuses with a lysosome. Uncoating and release of the virus ssRNA occurs in the cytoplasm and replication of the viral RNA genome in the nucleus. Positive-strand mRNA migrates from the nucleus to the cytoplasmic ribosomes for translation of viral proteins. The newly synthesized minus strand viral RNA genome migrates to the cytoplasm. Minus strands of ssRNA associate with the M protein and trigger budding at areas of the plasma membrane where G protein is already inserted. The virus is released by budding from the plasma membrane of the infected cell. The cell may not die but continues to act as a source of budding viruses.

3 Clinical and pathological aspects

3.1 Clinical features

Humans

Rabies is usually acquired from the bite of an infected animal, but simple licking of abraded skin may also transmit the virus; the infection has also been acquired from aerosols in bats' caves.

Human-to-human transmission of rabies via infected transplant donors is an unusual mode of acquisition and depends on the unfortunately timed transfer of tissue from a donor who is incubating the disease. There have been several such episodes involving transplants of corneal tissue and of lung, liver, and kidney.

The **incubation period** in humans varies from 10 days to a year or more, but is on average 1–3 months, the time depending on the quantity of virus deposited and—because the virus has to reach the brain via the peripheral nerves—on the distance of the bite from the head. As quantity of virus is so important multiple bites may transmit the disease more readily than single bites.

The onset is usually insidious, with a 1–10-day prodromal period of malaise, fever and headache, and hypersalivation.

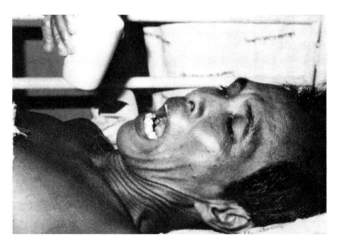

Fig. 26.3 Patient with rabies (from Kaplan, C. *et al* (1977). *Rabies: the Facts*. Oxford University Press, Oxford).

There may also be psychological disturbances including anxiety and aggression; indeed, one case in the UK was at first misdiagnosed as acute schizophrenia. Pain and tingling around the area of the bite, sometimes accompanied by small jerky movements, are particularly suggestive of incipient rabies. The subsequent course may take one of two forms.

Furious rabies

The patient passes into the 'stage of excitement', with anxious and apprehensive expression, fast pulse, and rapid breathing (Fig. 26.3). The physical signs are protean, their nature depending on the areas of brain affected. Cranial nerve and other paralyses are frequent, and there may be greatly increased activity of the autonomic nervous system and hyperpyrexia. The classical sign, present in most cases, is **hydrophobia**; this is particularly distressing, as the patient needs to drink, but any attempt to do so, or even the sight of water, elicits violent spasms of the respiratory and other muscles, accompanied by a feeling of extreme terror. Periods of lucidity alternate with impaired consciousness; after a week or so, the patient dies in coma with generalized paralysis and cardiovascular collapse. About one-fifth of infected patients present with this form of the disease.

Paralytic ('dumb') rabies

The course is less dramatic. An illness lasting as long as a month is characterized by ascending paralysis; hydrophobia is not a prominent feature. In these cases, the spinal cord and medulla are affected more than the brain. They are particularly associated with bites from vampire bats rather than dogs. As with furious rabies, death is inevitable.

Animals

Both forms of the disease occur in dogs and cats, 'dumb rabies' predominating. The incubation period in dogs can be as long as 8 months. The first sign is usually a change in behaviours. It should be remembered that the classical image of a rabid dog running amok and biting all and sundry is not always true; there may be intervals in which both dogs and cats become abnor-

mally friendly and make repeated attempts to lick those near them. A small proportion of dogs may recover from rabies. Most rabid cats enter a furious phase, scratching and biting without provocation.

3.2 Pathogenesis

Following an animal bite, rabies virus reaches the CNS in humans by way of **peripheral nerves** and is a classical example of centripetal spread of a virus followed by centrifugal spread from the CNS. The virus first replicates in epithelial or striated muscle cells at the site of the bite or in the mucosal cells of the respiratory tract and gains access to the peripheral nervous system via the **neuromuscular spindles**. In another major site of neuronal invasion the virus binds specifically to the cholinesterase-positive binding sites at neuromuscular junctions. The rate of centripetal progress of the virus along the axons of the peripheral nerve has been estimated experimentally in mice as 3 mm per day. Once the virus has replicated in the spinal cord and throughout the CNS it may spread centrifugally along the neuronal axons of the peripheral nerves to other tissues, including the salivary glands and hair-bearing tissues. In persons infected by aerosols, e.g. in bat-infested caves or in laboratory accidents, the virus probably reaches the CNS via nerves supplying the conjunctiva or the upper respiratory tract, including the olfactory nerves. The unfortunate victim almost invariably dies of encephalitis. Strangely, there is comparatively little pathological evidence of neuronal necrosis, but the virus may interfere with neuronal transmission. Therefore the precise pathology still remains a mystery. Myocarditis is often present and the characteristic cytoplasmic inclusions (Negri bodies) are detectable in the hearts of some patients.

3.3 Epizootology

Rabies vectors are mainly carnivores (Fig. 26.4), but the virus may transmit to 'cul de sac' animals such as ourselves. The virus

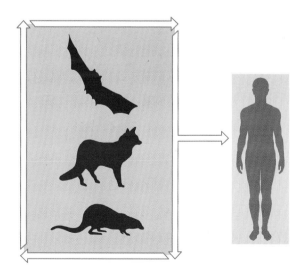

Fig. 26.4 Cycling of rabies to humans.

has two epidemiological forms: urban rabies mainly with domestic dogs as reservoirs and transmitters; and sylvatic rabies with various wild life species fulfilling these roles. Rabies virus is capable of infecting all warm-blooded animals. The reservoirs of infection vary according to the geographical area; dogs and cats are the most important sources of human infection, which is nowadays most frequent in developing countries. The main sylvatic reservoirs are wolves in eastern Europe, the red fox in western Europe, mongooses and vampire bats in the Caribbean, skunks and racoons in the USA and Canada, and vampire bats in Latin America.

Except for New Zealand, Norway, Australia, and the UK, rabies is present in every continent (Fig. 26.5). The UK has, however, remained rabies-free because of its strict quarantine regulations, which are, of course, relatively easy to enforce in an island. Elaborate precautions have been taken to prevent wild fauna getting to the UK from continental Europe via the Channel Tunnel.

However, with the introduction of highly effective rabies vaccines, combined with confirmation of vaccination in the form of an implanted microchip, and serological evidence of vaccination, the need for maintaining quarantine in the UK has now vanished.

About 700 rabies deaths are officially reported each year worldwide, but these probably represent only a fraction of the total number, which is estimated at 100 000, mainly in the developing world. In contrast only one to two cases per year are reported in the USA. Over 40 per cent of human cases are in children aged 5–14 years; most cases are male, presumably because of greater contact with animals.

The epizootology of the rabies-related viruses is not clear; but Duvenhage virus, carried by bats, has been recovered from cases of rabies in South Africa, Finland, and the USSR (now CIS).

3.4 Laboratory diagnosis of rabies

Fortunately, virus isolation is rarely, if ever, needed for diagnostic purposes. However, if necessary, samples of brain tissue, saliva, CSF, or urine may be injected intracerebrally into newborn mice. This can only be performed in a high security Category IV laboratory. Only a handful of such laboratories are in operation around the world. The central feature of laboratory diagnosis is **demonstration of rabies antigen by immuno-fluorescence** in cells obtained from **corneal impressions** or **hair-bearing skin**. This method may also be used on brain smears obtained post mortem from humans or animals. A less sensitive, but useful post mortem technique is the search of brain smears for the eosinophilic **cytoplasmic inclusions** known as **Negri bodies** named after the Italian physician who first discovered them. The tissue is taken from the Ammon's horn region of the hippocampus and stained with Mann's stain. These diagnostic procedures for rabies or for virus isolation may be undertaken only in specialized, high-security laboratories.

3.5 Prophylaxis in humans using vaccines

The original Pasteur rabies vaccine

Until recently, immunization regimens had changed little from those originally proposed by Pasteur in the late nineteenth century. The strain of rabies virus which Pasteur employed for his now famous immunization experiment was isolated from the brain of a rabid cow. Rabies viruses isolated from the wild are called 'street viruses'. After passage in the laboratory their virulence is reduced and stabilized. The Pasteur virus was

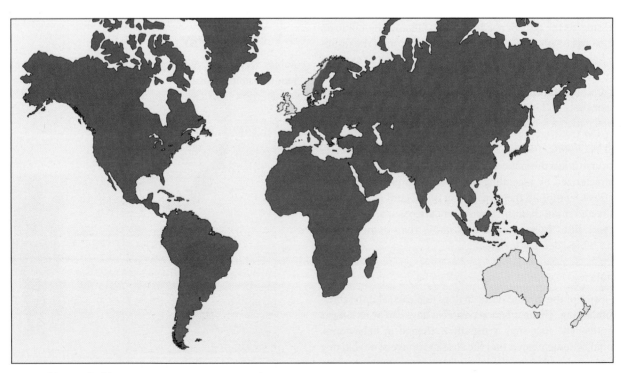

Fig. 26.5 **World map of rabies.**

passaged many times intracerebrally in rabbits, by which time the incubation period had become shorter and **fixed** at 6–7 days; hence the designation 'fixed' virus. The spinal cords of infected rabbits were dried in air at room temperature, the virulence of the virus contained in them decreasing rapidly with progressive desiccation. In July 1885, a 9-year-old boy, Joseph Meister, was admitted to hospital with multiple and severe bite wounds from a presumed rabid dog. For the next 10 days Pasteur administered a course of 13 injections of rabies-infected cord suspensions, the earliest preparation having been desiccated for 15 days, the subsequent ones for period decreasing to 1 day. Joseph Meister survived. Pasteur noted, 'The death of this child seemed inevitable and I decided not without lively and cruel doubts, as one can believe, to try in Joseph Meister the method which has been successful in dogs.' A year later Pasteur reported the result of treatment of 350 cases; only one person in this group had developed rabies, a child bitten nearly 4 weeks before treatment commenced. Contemporary figures show that 50 per cent of those bitten should have developed rabies. 'The prophylaxis of rabies is established. It is time to create a centre for vaccination against rabies.' Within a decade there were Pasteur Institutes around the world and, by 1898, 20 000 persons had been treated, with a mortality of only 0.5 per cent. Of course, no one knew about viruses at the time and, as Pasteur was unable to cultivate bacteria from the rabbit spinal cord, he concluded that 'one is tempted to believe that a microbe of infinite smallness having the form neither of bacillus nor a micrococcus is the cause'.

Rabies vaccines derived from infected animal nervous tissues (Semple vaccine) continue to be widely used today (Table 26.2), but it was recognized that neurological reactions in one in every thousand or so recipients limited their acceptability. In the 1950s a rabies vaccine grown in duck embryos also became available and replaced nervous tissue vaccine in the USA and some European countries; it was, however, relatively ineffective and is no longer used.

Table 26.2 Historical development of human rabies vaccines

Date introduced	Vaccine and comments
1884	**Pasteur vaccine.** Historical interest only
1911	**Semple vaccine.** Phenol-inactivated virus vaccine prepared in brains of rabbits, sheep, or goats. Widely used in developing countries. Cheap. Liable to cause neuroparalytic reactions
1957	**Duck embryo vaccine.** Virus inactivated with β-propiolactone. Free from neural tissue, but caused allergic reactions and was a relatively ineffective antigen. Discontinued
1964	**Human diploid cell strain virus (HDCS).** Virus inactivated with β-propiolactone. Few side-reactions. The most widely used vaccine in developed countries. Expensive

Modern rabies vaccines

A major advance in rabies vaccines was cultivation of the virus in **human diploid cells (HDC)** such as WI-38. This method provided a potent vaccine which is considerably less reactogenic than those preceding it. **Human diploid cell strain (HDCS) vaccine** (Table 26.2) has become the vaccine of choice for prophylactic and therapeutic use. The vaccine is given prophylactically to veterinary surgeons, animal handlers, or others at risk from rabies in three doses 1 month apart with a booster at 2 years. Some Asian countries have developed rabies vaccines from virus-infected hamster kidney cells, which are less costly to produce than those made in WI-38 cells.

If a person is unfortunate enough to be bitten by a suspected rabid animal, the wound should be thoroughly washed with soap and water, alcohol, iodine, or a **quaternary ammonium compound** (to which rabies virus is particularly susceptible). Good wound care remains the cornerstone of rabies prevention and is thought to reduce the risk of rabies by 90 per cent. Appropriate **antitetanus treatment** should be given to those not immunized against this infection within the past 3 years. The management then follows the scheme in Table 26.3. A full

Table 26.3 Treatment of people in contact with animals with suspected or actual rabies

Nature of contact	Status of animal*	Treatment of patient†
Indirect contact *only*	Appears healthy *or* has signs suggesting rabies	Not needed
Licks to skin	Appears healthy *or* has signs suggesting rabies	
	(a) under observation for at least 10 days after the contact	Start vaccine immediately. Stop only if animal is normal 10 days after the contact
	(b) escaped	Full course of vaccine immediately
	(c) killed	Start vaccine immediately. Stop only if laboratory tests on animal for rabies are negative
Bites	Schedules as for 'Licks to skin' *plus* human rabies immunoglobulin (HRIG), 20 international units/kg body weight, of which half is injected around the bite(s) and half is given intramuscularly	

* Note that the risk of contracting rabies from a wild animal is significantly greater than from domestic dogs and cats.

† Regardless of any pre-exposure prophylaxis, persons exposed to a significant risk of contracting rabies should be given at least two doses of HDCS rabies vaccine.

course of HDCS vaccine consists of six doses given intramuscularly on days 0, 3, 7, 14, 30, and 90 days after exposure. This modern vaccine is free of unpleasant side-effects.

Rabies is one of the few diseases in which vaccine is effective when administered during the incubation period. Over 1.5 million people are still immunized yearly throughout the world, often with the Semple-type vaccines (Table 26.2), which are given as 21 daily injections subcutaneously. Side-effects, particularly encephalomyelopathies, are not uncommon with such vaccines. They are due to an allergic response to myelin which is present as an impurity in the vaccine, but these vaccines are so much cheaper than the cell culture preparations that the risk of side-effects is judged to be the lesser evil.

3.6 Principles of rabies control in animals

Domestic animals

The removal of stray animals and vaccination of all domestic dogs and cats are essential features of control programme in rabies-endemic areas. As a result of these procedures, rabies in dogs has decreased dramatically in the USA. Immunization of cats is now being encouraged.

Any domestic animal that is bitten and scratched by a bat or by a wild carnivorous mammal is regarded in the USA as having been exposed to a rabid animal and unvaccinated dogs and cats are destroyed immediately or quarantined for 6 months. Vaccinated animals are revaccinated and confined for 90 days.

Wildlife

The control of rabies in wild life is a difficult and, some might say, an impossible task. In the USA, continuous trapping or poisoning as a means of rabies control is not recommended, but limited control is maintained in high-contact areas such as picnic or camping grounds in National Parks. Similarly, bats are eliminated from houses.

In Europe, attempts are being made to control rabies in foxes by a unique immunizing technique. Chicken heads are impregnated with **live attenuated rabies vaccine and tetracycline** and dropped by helicopter into remote mountainous areas. The foxes eat the heads and become infected and hence vaccinated with the attenuated rabies strain; concomitantly, the tetracycline is deposited in their bones. A simple fluorescence test on the bone tissue of captured foxes can detect tetracycline and indicate whether they have been immunized. By this method, rabies has been drastically reduced in parts of Switzerland, and many other European countries are now trying the system, but unvaccinated foxes often move into areas where it was previously considered that all foxes had been vaccinated.

4 Reminders

- The genus *Lyssavirus* belongs to the family *Rhabdoviridae* and contains rabies and other viruses that infect vertebrates. Another genus within the family, *Vesiculovirus*, causes a febrile illness with vesicular lesions in horses and cattle. The viruses are **bullet-shaped** and its glycoprotein spikes project from the lipid envelope. The genome is **ssRNA of negative polarity** and 11–12 kb in size.

- A series of five monocistronic mRNAs are transcribed by the virion associated RNA transcriptase. RNA transcriptase 'stuttering' at intergene poly U residues results in addition of poly(A) tails to the preceding mRNA and initiation of transcription at the next gene. Full-length copies of genomic RNA are synthesized by read-through of intergene regions by the newly synthesized viral RNA replicase.

- The natural reservoir of rabies is the wild animal population and the animal involved varies in different continents. In Europe **domestic dogs** are an important source of infection for humans, whereas the main reservoir in the wild is **foxes**. Some countries, including Australia and New Zealand, impose a strict **quarantine**, but the advent of effective **vaccines** and techniques for confirming that immunization has been performed are making this method of control unnecessary in the UK.

- Following a bite, virus replicates in muscle and moves along **peripheral nerves** to the CNS. Centrifugal spread along peripheral nerves to other tissues follows. The **incubation period** varies from 10 days to a year or more with an average of **1–3 months**, the time depending upon the distance of the bite from the CNS.

- The onset of clinical disease is insidious with malaise, fever, and headache. The 'stage of excitement' is characterized by local paralysis, swallowing difficulties, and **hydrophobia**. The patient dies within 1 week of cardiovascular collapse and coma. The illness may also take a predominantly paralytic form ('dumb rabies').

- Rabies may be prevented by immunization after infection. The safest vaccine is the **HDCS** virus inactivated with β-propiolactone. At least six doses of vaccine are given by deep intramuscular injection, in combination with **human rabies immunoglobulin (HRIG)**. The vaccine is also used prophylactically to protect persons, such as veterinary surgeons, at special risk.

Arthropod-borne viruses

1 Introduction

The viruses to be considered in this chapter are diverse, but we shall deal with them together because their epidemiology is similar and there is much overlap in the syndromes that they cause. They were indeed once classified together as 'arboviruses', i.e. arthropod-borne viruses, but it is now clear that several families fall into this category, of which four are important in relation to infections of humans: they are the *Bunyaviridae*, *Togaviridae*, and *Flaviviridae*, which have many points of resemblance; and the *Reoviridae* (Table 27.1). 'Arbovirus' is, however, still a useful umbrella term and we shall use it when convenient. It should be borne in mind that, although the number of arboviruses runs into the hundreds, only a minority cause disease in humans. Indeed, in view of their wide geographical distribution it is fortunate for mankind that for every serious arbovirus illness there are something like 1000 inapparent or minor infections.

The natural reservoirs of these viruses are in animals, birds, and even reptiles, among which they are transmitted by the bites of blood-sucking arthropods, usually mosquitoes, sand

Table 27.1 Arboviruses pathogenic for humans

Family	Genus	Approximate number of viruses	Important illnesses
Togaviridae	*Alphavirus*	30	Equine encephalitides, O'nyong-nyong fever
Flaviviridae	*Flavivirus*	70	Yellow fever, dengue, Japanese and other encephalitides, including West Nile
Bunyaviridae	*Bunyavirus*	170	California encephalitis, Oropouche fever
	Phlebovirus	50	Sandfly fever, Rift Valley fever
	Nairovirus	35	Crimea-Congo haemorrhagic fever
Reoviridae	*Coltivirus*	15	Colorado tick fever

flies or ticks; humans are infected only if they get in the way of their natural cycle by entering areas where they are prevalent and then bitten by an infected arthropod. Infection is often inapparent or trivial; but some of these viruses can cause very severe illnesses with high mortality rates.

Some are considered resurgent viruses because of their ability to cause new problems and an example is West Nile, which is currently spreading very widely in the USA, being carried by birds and then moving to humans via mosquitoes.

2 Properties of the viruses

2.1 Togaviruses and flaviviruses

Classification and morphology

The family Togaviridae

Derives its name from the closely fitting envelope surrounding the virions; it contains two genera, of which only *Alphavirus* concerns us here. The other is *Rubivirus*, which is not arthropod-borne and causes rubella (Chapter 12).

The family Flaviviridae *(formerly classified with the* Togaviridae)

Contains the following three genera, of which only the first contains arboviruses.

- *Flavivirus*, of which there are many serotypes. The prototype virus causes YF (Latin: *flavus* = yellow).

- *Pestivirus*, which affects only cattle.

- *Hepacivirus* and related viruses, which are dealt with in Chapter 24.

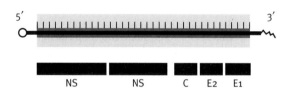

Fig. 27.1 Togavirus genome and encoded proteins. Labelled proteins are E1 and E2 (enveloped spikes), C (capsid), and NS (non-structural proteins).

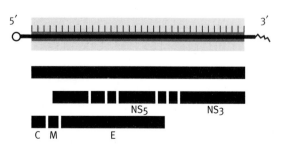

Fig. 27.2 Flavivirus genome and encoded proteins. Labelled proteins are E (envelope), M (membrane proteins), C (capsid protein), and NS (non-structural proteins). Other proteins are not labelled.

These viruses are enveloped and have cubic symmetry; they range from 40 to 70 nm in diameter.

Genomes

*Toga- and flaviviruses have single **positive-sense RNA genomes** 11–12 kb in size; they are 5′ capped and have a 3′ poly(A) tail (Figs 27.1 and 27.2). The RNA codes for a single ORF flanked by 5′ and 3′ non-translated regions (NTRs). Precursor proteins are cleaved by viral and cell proteases.*

Replication

The viruses attach to cellular receptors and enter by receptor-mediated endocytosis. The genome is released into the cytoplasm of the cell by fusion mediated by a low pH in the phagolysosomes. Replication takes place exclusively in the cytoplasm.

Most of the flavivirus genome from the 5′ end is translated directly into a polyprotein, which is then cleaved into four viral NS proteins, namely RNA polymerase, a methylation and capping enzyme, a protease and a helicase. The full length minus strand is synthesized using these viral enzymes. Subsequently a full length positive genomic strand is transcribed; in addition, a subgenomic mRNA is synthesized, mainly from the 3′ end of the genome. This codes for a polyprotein, which is cleaved to produce the viral structural proteins, the nucleocapsid (C) glycoprotein spikes (E1 and E2) and a transmembrane protein. There are seven NS proteins.

Virus self-assembly begins in the cytoplasm and is completed after 15 hours or so at the plasma membrane by the incorporation of a lipid containing viral glycoprotein spikes.

The virions are spherical and enveloped, 40–90 nm in diameter. The nucleocapsid has cubic symmetry and contains a single molecule of positive-sense RNA.

2.2 Bunyaviruses

Classification and morphology

The family takes its name from the prototype Bunyamwera virus, which, like many arboviruses, is named after the place where it was first isolated. There are five genera, of which three are arboviruses pathogenic for humans (Table 27.1). The largest group is the *Bunyavirus* genus, of which about 50 species cause disease in humans.

The other two genera are *Hantavirus* (Chapter 19) and *Tospovirus*, which infects only tomatoes and thus may now be forgotten.

The viruses are 90–100 nm in diameter, are spherical, and have a lipid envelope through which protrude stubby glycoprotein spikes.

Genome

The bunyavirus genome is negative-sense ssRNA in three circular segments of 7, 4, and 2 kb (Fig. 27.3).

Replication

The viruses attach to a cellular receptor and enter by endocytosis. Replication is entirely cytoplasmic. Similarly to influenza virus,

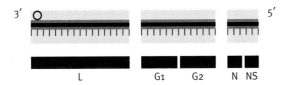

Fig. 27.3 Bunyavirus genome and encoded proteins. Labelled proteins are G1 and G2 (envelope spikes), N (nucleocapsid), L (polymerase transcription protein), and NS (non-structural protein). O , RNA transcriptase.

12–15 nucleotides are cleaved from the 5' end of cellular RNA molecules. These 'snatched caps' are then used as primers for transcription of each of the negative-sense RNA gene segments on to subgenomic mRNAs. The large mRNA codes for the L protein, the medium sized mRNA for the two glycoproteins and an NS protein and the small mRNA for the nucleocapsid, another NS protein. Different start codons are used and are encoded in different ORFs, the NSs being located within the N ORF.

Genomes and antigenomes are encapsidated by the N protein to form biologically active RNPs. The L and N proteins are responsible for transcription and replication of the artificial mini genomes.

Thereafter secondary transcription of negative-stranded genome RNAs is accomplished. The virus glycoproteins accumulate in the Golgi apparatus, associate with nucleocapsids, and are eventually released by budding at the Golgi apparatus

2.3 Orbiviruses and coltiviruses

Classification and morphology

These agents belong to the family *Reoviridae*, which contains nine genera, of which only one, *Coltivirus*, is an arbovirus. Other reoviruses cause gastroenteritis and are described in Chapter 11.

These viruses are doughnut-shaped and are approximately 80 nm in diameter. They do not possess an envelope.

Table 27.2 Arboviruses associated with fever/rashes/arthritis

Family	Virus	Geographical distribution	Vector
Togaviridae	O'nyong-nyong	E. and W. Africa	Mosquito
	Chikungunya	E. Africa, India,	Mosquito
	Ross River	S.E. Asia Australia, Oceania	Mosquito
Flaviviridae	Dengue (four types)	Entire tropical zone	Mosquito
Bunyaviridae	Sandfly fever	S. Italy, Sicily	Sandfly
Reoviridae	Orbiviruses Colorado tick fever	N.W. America, E. Europe	Tick
	Kemerovo viruses	CIS (USSR)	Tick

Genome

The genome is negative-sense dsRNA in 12 segments.

Replication

The replication of coltiviruses has not been studied in detail, but is probably similar to that of other reoviruses. The virus attaches to cellular receptors and enters the cell by endocytosis. Replication is cytoplasmic with residual virus cores acting as factory sites. The virion-associated transcriptase transcribes 5' capped mRNAs which are extruded and translated. Later, mRNA positive-stranded molecules form a template for transcription of genomic negative-strand RNAs. Virus self-assembly begins in the cytoplasm and the newly formed virions are released by disruption of the host cells.

3 Clinical and pathological aspects of arbovirus infections

3.1 Clinical syndromes

Table 27.1 lists the arboviruses pathogenic for humans and the main illnesses that they cause. Because of their large number, running well into the hundreds, it is pointless trying to describe the various clinical syndromes individually. However, the more severe illnesses can conveniently be divided into three main groups, each of which may be caused by a number of unrelated viruses (Tables 27.2–27.4).

Group 1: febrile illnesses with rashes and arthritis
(Table 27.2)

Anyone doing medical work in Africa will be struck by the many villagers who complain of fever and aches and pains in the joints. It is likely that a number of these minor illnesses are caused by arboviruses. They can, however, be more severe and characterized by **arthritis, myositis**, and itchy **maculopapular rashes.** Their names sometimes graphically describe the agonizing symptoms: O'nyong-nyong, for example, means 'breakbone' fever, and Chikungunya, 'doubled-up'. But despite the acute discomfort, recovery is complete.

Epidemics of these infections can be massive: in 1959 about 2 million people were affected by an outbreak of O'nyong-nyong fever in Central and East Africa.

Group 2: meningitis, encephalitis, and encephalomyelitis
(Table 27.3)

By contrast with these benign infections, involvement of the CNS may cause severe sequelae or even death. The viruses concerned invade the CNS directly during the initial viraemia, lysing neurones and causing the usual pathological changes seen in viral encephalitis, i.e. lymphocytic infiltration, activation of microglia, and perivascular 'cuffing'; there may be petechial haemorrhages in the pons, medulla, and cord. Clinically, a febrile illness is followed shortly by neck rigidity, convul-

Table 27.3 Arboviruses associated with meningitis/encephalitis/encephalomyelitis

Family	Virus	Geographical distribution	Vector
Togaviridae	Eastern, Western, and Venezuelan equine encephalomyelitis	USA, South America	Mosquito
Flaviviridae	Japanese B and Murray Valley encephalitis	Far East, Australia	Mosquito
	St Louis encephalitis	Canada to Argentina, Northern Britain	Tick
	West Nile	USA, Africa, Central Asia	Mosquito
Bunyaviridae	California and La Crosse	USA	Mosquito
Reoviridae	Orbiviruses		
	Colorado tick fever	USA	Tick
	Kemerovo viruses	Eastern Europe, CIS (USSR)	Tick

sions, disturbances of consciousness and various pareses; the **sequelae** include **motor, sensory,** and **psychological defects.**

Epizootics and epidemics of arboviral encephalitis may be widespread. For example, more than 200 000 horses died in an epizootic occurring in Peru and Texas during 1969–71; the

Table 27.4 Arboviruses associated with haemorrhagic fevers

Family	Virus	Geographical distribution	Vector
Flaviviridae	Yellow fever	Tropical Africa and S. America	Mosquito
	Dengue (four types)	Entire tropical zone	Mosquito
	Chikungunya	India, S.E. Asia*	Mosquito
	Omsk	Siberia	Tick
Bunyaviridae	Crimean-Congo	Crimea, Central and S. Africa, Iraq, Pakistan	Tick
	Rift Valley	Africa, Egypt	Mosquito
	Hantavirus	Korea, E. Europe, CIS (USSR), Scandinavia	None

* Does not cause haemorrhagic fever in Africa; cf. Table 27.2.

associated epidemic affected several thousand people. More recently, an epidemic of Venezuelan equine encephalomyelitis in Latin America caused an estimated 75 000 human infections.

Coltivirus infections of humans are transmitted from small rodents by ticks. They cause febrile illnesses, often with meningitis or meningo-encephalitis, and are seen in the north-western USA and Canada (Colorado tick fever) and in the CIS and eastern Europe (Table 27.3).

Group 3: haemorrhagic fevers (Table 27.4)

This term is applied to a group of illnesses with similar clinical features, caused not only by some of the arboviruses described in this chapter but also by members of the *Arenaviridae* and *Filoviridae* (see Chapter 19).

In general, these illnesses carry mortalities of the order of 20 per cent; the initial febrile episode is followed by bleeding into the skin and mucous membranes, **haemorrhagic rashes** and **haemorrhages from body orifices,** notably those of the gastrointestinal tract. There is thrombocytopenia and sometimes disseminated intravascular coagulation. Some infections have special features and are described in more detail.

Yellow fever (Table 27.4)

As its name implies, this infection is characterized by **jaundice,** the result **of mid-zone necrosis of the liver;** the flavivirus responsible also damages the kidney and heart and bleeding from the gastrointestinal mucosa may cause '**black vomit**' and melaena. In terms of people killed, YF is historically the most important of the arbovirus infections. It seems to have originated in Africa, from whence the mosquito vector, *Aedes aegypti,* was spread to the New World during the seventeenth century in sailing ships; the unsuspected importation of a deadly disease along with the slaves that many of these boats carried might be regarded as poetic justice. The virus is endemic in Central Africa and South America, where it exists mainly as a zoonosis in monkeys and only occasionally transmits to humans.

There are two forms of YF, which differ only in their epidemiology. The so-called **urban** variety is unusual in that the only hosts are humans. Urban YF has caused huge epidemics when introduced into populations with no herd immunity. During the nineteenth century its ravages in newly arrived foreign workers completely halted construction of the Panama canal for some time; more recently, there were major outbreaks in Ethiopia and West Africa during the 1960s, with thousands of deaths.

By contrast with urban YF, which as its name implies mainly affects inhabited places, the **sylvan** (or sylvatic) form occurs in forested areas; here the epidemiology more closely follows the classical arbovirus pattern as there is an animal reservoir, namely monkeys, among which the virus is spread by a variety of mosquitoes; men—and here the term is used to imply gender rather than species—are infected when they venture into forests, usually to hunt; women are much less often the victims.

YF is still prevalent in Africa and Latin America (Fig. 27.4(a)); why it does not occur in the Indian subcontinent, where there

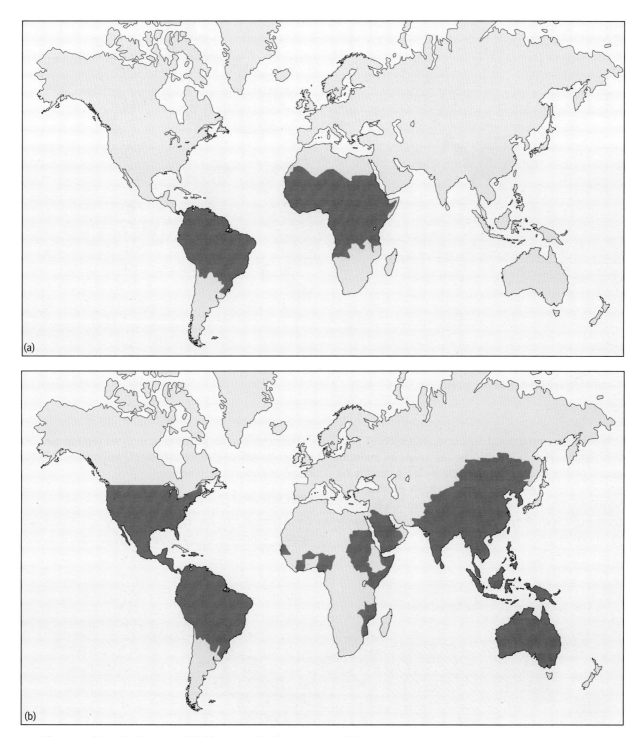

Fig. 27.4 **(a)** Geographical distribution of YF. **(b)** Geographical distribution of dengue.

is no shortage of susceptible mosquitoes, is something of a mystery.

Dengue (Table 27.2)

Like YF, this 'classic' arbovirus infection is also caused by a flavivirus and transmitted by *Aëdes aegypti* mosquitoes (Fig. 27.4(b)). In adults, the clinical features are usually similar to those of the fever/rash syndrome described above, with severe joint and muscle pains; lymphadenopathy and altered perception of taste are common. Children may suffer from **DHSS.** This is a dangerous complication with a mortality of 4–12 per cent and it is worrying that it appears to be on the increase, notably in Southeast Asia. It affects 50 million people annually. In Malaysia, for example, over 6000 cases per annum are not unusual in a busy year. A brief febrile illness is followed by collapse with shock, low blood pressure, and haemorrhagic

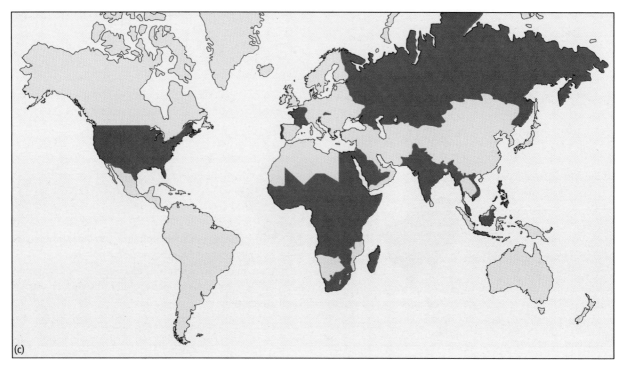

Fig. 27.4 **(c)** Geographical distribution of West Nile.

signs. There are four serotypes of dengue virus (numbered 1–4), and it is thought that DHSS may be the result of **immune enhancement** due to a second infection with a heterologous serotype: the virus forms complexes with pre-existing non-neutralizing antibody to the first virus and then, via Fc receptors, gains access to monocytes, in which it multiplies very easily and becomes widely disseminated.

Treatment is quite effective; it involves replacement of fluid loss, correction of electrolyte balance, and transfusion of whole blood if haemorrhage is severe.

West Nile virus (Table 27.3)

This flavivirus, like others, has a wide geographical distribution, causing outbreaks in Africa, Asia, and Europe (Fig. 27.4(c)).

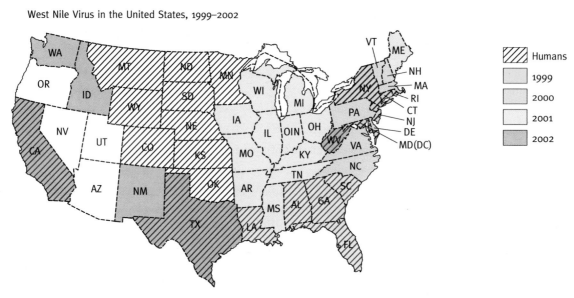

Fig 27.5 Spread of West Nile virus in the USA.

It deserves special mention because in 1999 it became the first of these agents to cause major outbreaks in the Western hemisphere, affecting a number of states in eastern USA. Birds and culicine mosquitoes are the main alternate hosts.

The virus is endemic in Africa and the Middle East and probably was imported into the USA via a sick bird. It is transmitted from birds to humans by *Culex pipiens*, which is a hybrid mosquito feeding off birds and mammals. Two human cases were found in New York in 1999 but the virus spread rapidly carried by birds and by 2002 there were over 4000 cases with 284 deaths in 44 states in the USA (Fig. 27.5).

This is now a very widespread virus causing problems as far afield as the USA, Central Asia, Africa, India, and Australia.

The disease is characterized by fever after an incubation period of 1–6 days. Often the patient has a fever, headache, backache, and generalized myalgia for a week. Nearly half of the patients have a rosealar rash involving the chest, back, and arms while many person also suffer with pharyngitis, nausea, and diarrhoea. There are many subclinical infections, perhaps as many as 250 per clinical case. The case fatality rate is about 1–3 per cent and the elderly are particularly at risk.

The virus

The spherical virion is 50 nm in diameter with a host-derived lipid membrane surrounding a nucleocapsid core.

The genome

Approximately 10 000 nucleotides as a piece of ssRNA of positive sense polarity. It has a short 5′ non coding region followed by a single ORF coding for three structural and seven NS proteins.

Replication

Occurs in the cytoplasm in association with the rough endoplasmic reticulum. Virus assembly takes place in the endoplasmic reticulum lumen and virus is released from the cell through the cell secretory pathway.

Louping ill (Table 27.3)

This virus is of some interest because it is the only arbovirus infection seen in the UK. It is a tick-borne flavivirus causing serious infection of the CNS of sheep in northern England and Scotland. The occasional infection of a human characteristically presents as a biphasic febrile illness with meningitis; complete recovery is the rule.

3.2 Epidemiology

This section should really be entitled 'epizootology' because these infections occur primarily in animals and are thus examples of zoonoses. Replication of the viruses in these hosts causes **viraemia**, thus permitting their spread to other hosts by the bites of blood-sucking arthropods, which are referred to as **vectors** of infection.

The large variety of vectors, viruses and mammalian, avian, and reptilian hosts makes for complex and variable epidemiological situations. Here, we can give only a generalized picture of the factors that affect transmission.

The ability of the vector to spread infection is determined by its feeding preferences, range of mobility, and whether the virus concerned can be transmitted to the next generation, thus enabling it to 'overwinter' between one breeding season and the next. Unfortunately, arboviruses do not kill their insect vectors, thus ensuring their own survival.

The **reservoir** is usually a wild bird or small mammal, which acts as an **amplifier of infection** (Fig. 27.6). Sometimes, as for example in equine encephalomyelitis, mosquitoes transmit infection from wild to domestic animals, in this instance horses, causing a local epizootic that presages an epidemic in a nearby human population. Another example is seen in Japan, where epidemics of Japanese B encephalitis have been predicted by testing locally kept pigs for recent seroconversion.

Humans may also acquire arboviruses by entering an area harbouring infected arthropods, either for work or recreation. Their susceptibility will depend on their state of immunity: by contrast with new arrivals, locals who have had subclinical infections in the past are protected.

Given this mode of transmission, it is apparent that direct person-to-person infection cannot take place unless there is actual transfer of blood, e.g. by a 'needle-stick' injury to a medical attendant during the viraemic stage of an illness. In Crimean-Congo haemorrhagic fever abdominal pain may be severe, and there have been several deaths among theatre staff who mistakenly operated on such patients.

The many arboviruses shown in Table 27.1 do not all cause significant illness in humans. Some affect both humans and animals, others animals only, and others again are known only because they have been isolated from arthropods. The proportion of viruses pathogenic for man in each family roughly corresponds with their relative importance in terms of numbers of cases world-wide, the flaviviruses being the leaders, followed by the alphaviruses.

3.3 Pathogenesis and immunity

After the virus is introduced into a subcutaneous capillary in the saliva of an infected arthropod there is an incubation period of a few days during which it replicates in the lymphatic system and endothelium; the first signs of illness are usually malaise and fever caused by the subsequent viraemia. Characteristically, signs of infection of the target organs follow 4–10 days later, resulting in a **biphasic illness**. Immunity to reinfection is mediated by the antibody response, which may also confer some protection against related viruses, but its role in recovery is not clear.

3.4 Laboratory diagnosis

Manipulation of the viruses described in this chapter is dangerous and a number of laboratory workers have become their victims. Tests involving virus isolation or demonstration of

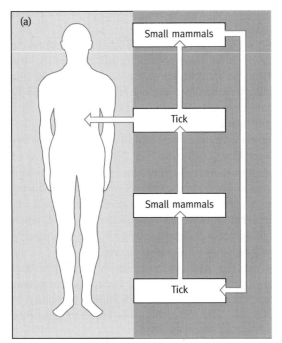 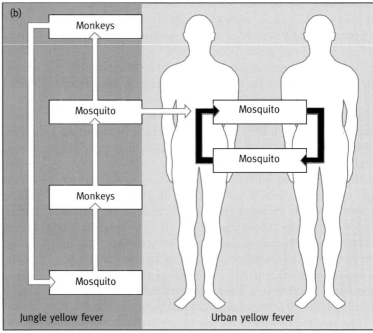

Fig. 27.6 Transmission cycles of arthropod-borne virus infections. **(a)** An example of a tick-borne encephalitis; **(b)** jungle and urban types of YF.

specific antigens are therefore done only in special laboratories. Viruses can be isolated by intracerebral inoculation of newborn mice, a method now being superseded by culture in mammalian or insect cells, or by inoculation of mosquitoes. A method for isolating dengue virus recently developed in Malaysia is of particular interest. We have seen how, in dengue, DHSS may be precipitated by antibody-assisted replication of the virus in macrophages. The technique involves inoculating a mouse macrophage cell line with the patient's blood plus specific antibody to flavivirus. Dengue virus could be demonstrated 2–4 days later by immunofluorescence staining; the method is claimed to have an efficiency of 80 per cent, much higher than mosquito inoculation. Serological tests, especially demonstration of specific IgM antibody, are also widely used.

3.5 Control

The only ways at present open to us for controlling arbovirus infections are (1) eradication of vectors, and (2) immunization.

In view of the great diversity of vectors and viruses, both approaches present formidable problems; efforts must therefore be both directed to the most serious infections and guided by what is practicable. The most outstanding success has been the combination of vector control and immunization in the fight against urban YF. Chemical warfare against adult mosquitoes has been hindered by the emergence of resistant strains, but much can still be done by spraying or eliminating both large and small pools of static water, thus preventing development of the larvae. Not unexpectedly, large urban developments, deforestation, irrigation, and resettlement programmes, which disturb

the sylvan cycle of the virus all contribute toward outbreaks of arbovirus infections in humans.

The development in 1937 of a highly effective **attenuated YF vaccine** by Theiler and Smith was a landmark in the history of immunization. This vaccine, prepared from the 17D strain in chick embryos, has had a major impact on the incidence of urban YF. The immunity induced is very durable, perhaps life-long. The vaccine is not heat-stable and an extensive 'cold chain' (i.e. refrigeration during transport and storage) is needed; this is often a problem in tropical countries and a compromise now often reached is to introduce mass vaccination only when an outbreak is spotted in an urban area.

Both preparation and administration of YF vaccine are strictly controlled and limited to government-approved centres. Apart from use in the face of an epidemic as described above, people who should be immunized include (1) those living or travelling in endemic areas, including tourists, and (2) laboratory staff working with the virus.

Vaccinees must have an International Certificate of vaccination signed and stamped at an approved vaccination centre. It is valid for 10 years. Persons arriving from an endemic area in a country free from YF will need such a certificate.

Both live and inactivated vaccines effective against several encephalitis viruses are available in countries where they are prevalent, notably Japan and the USA: but it is clearly impossible to eliminate all the vectors or to provide vaccines against the hundreds of different viruses implicated in these infections; so despite these important but limited successes it looks as though arboviruses will continue to plague mankind for the foreseeable future.

4 Reminders

- Members of four families contain **arboviruses** pathogenic for humans: the *Togaviridae*, *Flaviviridae*, *Bunyaviridae*, and *Reoviridae*. Of these, the *Togaviridae* and *Flaviviridae* are the most and the *Reoviridae* the least important in terms of their potential for causing disease in humans.

- The **toga- and flaviviruses** have **positive-sense ssRNA** genomes, which are 5′ capped and 3′ polyadenylated. Those of **bunyaviruses** are segmented **negative-sense ssRNA**; and the genomes of **coltiviruses** are segmented **dsRNA**.

- These infections are **zoonoses**, with reservoirs mostly in **small mammals** and **birds**. They are transmitted by the bites of blood-sucking arthropods, i.e. **mosquitoes**, **sandflies**, and **ticks**.

- Arboviruses are found in all tropical and temperate zones but are more prevalent in hotter than in cooler countries.

- The illnesses they cause are often **biphasic**, an initial **viraemia** being followed some days later by infection of the target organs.

- Many infections are **inapparent**, but some are more severe, resulting predominantly in
  - fever/rashes/arthritis/myositis; *or*
  - meningitis/encephalitis/encephalomyelitis; *or*
  - haemorrhagic fevers.

- Two dangerous flavivirus infections to be noted particularly are:
  - **YF**, a haemorrhagic fever affecting the liver and other viscera, and its two epidemiological forms, urban and sylvan;
  - **dengue** and its **haemorrhagic shock syndrome**, which probably results from immunopathological damage due to consecutive infections with different serotypes.

- West Nile virus is spreading widely in the USA and is an example of how these ancient viruses can emerge in a new community.

- Because these viruses are dangerous they can be handled only in high-security laboratories. **Laboratory diagnosis** is therefore usually based on **serological tests**.

- **Control** depends, when practicable, on **vector control** and on **immunization**. Highly effective **vaccines** are available for some infections, notably **YF**, and some of the encephalitides.

Chapter 28

Exotic and dangerous infections: filoviruses, arenaviruses, and hantaviruses

1 Introduction

Most of the viruses described in this chapter (Table 28.1) have been isolated and characterized in the last two decades, although there is no reason to think that they have not existed and evolved over many thousands of years. They cause haemorrhagic fevers in tropical countries and their common link is existence in an animal reservoir in which they exist quietly until disturbed by human intrusion. They are known as **exotic viruses**; some are named after the town or area where an outbreak was first investigated. An example is the filovirus 'Marburg', named after the town in Germany where seven persons died of what was, at that time, a new and unrecorded disease. In this outbreak the common link between the infected persons was the handling of monkeys or monkey tissues. The monkeys had been imported from Africa to provide kidney tissue for preparing poliomyelitis vaccine. Nearly 10 years later an outbreak of an even more lethal haemorrhagic disease caused by a filovirus was described in Zaïre and the Sudan—'Ebola disease', named in this case after a river in Zaïre. Members of another virus family described in this chapter, the *Arenaviridae*, also cause outbreaks with disturbing frequency. The filo- and arenaviruses are so dangerous that only high-security category

Table 28.1 Exotic and dangerous viruses

Family	Genus	Important viruses
Filoviridae	*Filovirus*	Marburg Ebola
Arenaviridae	*Arenavirus*	Lassa Junin Machupo Lymphocytic choriomeningitis (LCM)
Bunyaviridae	*Hantavirus*	Hantaan

IV laboratories handle them. Hence, 20 years after their discovery, they have still not been as thoroughly studied as some viruses that were isolated much later. However, the chain of clinical transmission in nature can be quite easily broken and in relation to the number of viruses there have been very few deaths over the last 30 years.

2 Filoviruses

2.1 Properties of the viruses

Classification

The family *Filoviridae is* composed of extremely pleomorphic viruses: its name derives from the Latin *filum*, a thread, which refers to their morphology (see below). The family belongs to the order *Mononegavirales*. Marburg and Ebola viruses can be distinguished from each other by the size of their genomes and their different protein composition; they also differ serologically.

Morphology

These viruses have an extraordinary filamentous morphology and are sometimes longer than common bacteria, up to 1400 nm, often with branched, circular, and bizarre-shaped forms (Fig. 28.1). They have lipid envelopes, beneath which a nucleocapsid structure containing RNA can be visualized by

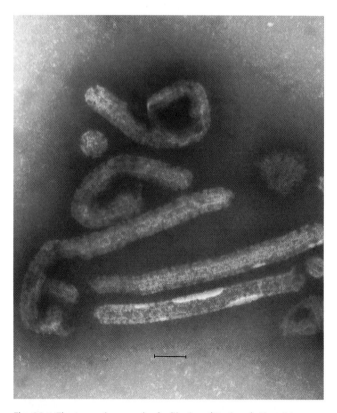

Fig. 28.1 Electron micrograph of a filovirus (Marburg). The virions are highly pleomorphic. (Courtesy of Dr Anne M. Field.) Scale bar = 100 nm.

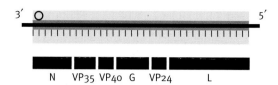

Fig. 28.2 Filovirus genome and encoded proteins. Labelled proteins are N (nucleoprotein), G (glycoprotein spike), and L (polymerase). Other proteins are not illustrated or labelled. O, RNA transcriptase.

EM. The nucleocapsids have **helical symmetry**. The virion surface is covered by GP spikes 10 nm in length.

Genome

The genome is negative-sense ssRNA, 19 kb in size (Fig. 28.2). It is the largest genome of all the viruses in this group. It has seven ORFs coding for the seven or eight known structural proteins. There are stop and start signals at the boundaries of each gene similar to those of the paramyxoviruses rabies and measles. There is a start site at the 3' genome end and genes are terminated with a transcription stop site. Termination of transcription occurs at a series of 5–6 Us where 'stuttering' (repeated copying) by the viral RNA polymerase results in the addition of long poly(A) tails to the transcripts.

Replication

The viruses infect and enter cells by endocytosis: transcription and genomic RNA replication takes place in the cytoplasm. Transcription starts at the 3' end of the genome, synthesizing a leader RNA and several poly(A) forms. Translation leads to accumulation of NP and VP35, which trigger a switch to production of full length antigenomes, which in turn act as templates for genome synthesis. During cellular infection the viral glycoprotein (G) spikes insert into the plasma membrane and nucleocapsids (NP) accumulate in the cytoplasm. The two come together at the inner cell surface just before budding and virus release. Other viral proteins are the small secreted sG, VP40, VP24 matrix protein, L protein and VP35 (an RNA dependent RNA polymerase), NP and VP30 (nuclear proteins), and finally a VP24 of unknown function. The cycle is complete in 12 hours.

2.2 Clinical and pathological aspects

Clinical features

The illnesses caused by the Marburg and Ebola viruses are very similar, with abrupt onset after an incubation period of 3–16 days. Severe frontal headache, high fever, and back pains characterize the early phase. The patient is rapidly prostrated with D&V lasting about a week; conjunctivitis and pharyngitis are usually present. A transient non-itching **maculopapular rash** may appear after 5–7 days. At this time **severe bleeding** starts in the lungs, nose, gums, gastrointestinal tract, and conjunctiva in a large proportion of patients, preceded and accompanied by **thrombocytopenia**. Deaths in cases with severe shock and blood loss usually occur between days 7 and 16. The mortality may be high, ranging from 25 to 90 per cent.

Pathology

Both Marburg and Ebola are so-called pantropic viruses: they infect and cause lesions in many organs, but especially the liver and spleen, which become enlarged and dark in colour. In both these organs severe degeneration and necrosis occur. The actual mechanism of pathogenesis remains obscure but clearly damage to endothelial cells resulting in **increased vascular permeability** followed by haemorrhage and shock is a central feature. Infected cells release large quantities of TNF-α, MCP (monocyte chemotactic protein)-1, and MIP (major intrinsic protein)-α, whereas IFN-α and -β are blocked. Cytokines stimulate endothelial cells to produce cell surface adhesion and pro-coagulant molecules. Disseminated intravascular coagulation and platelet dysfunction also occur.

Epidemiology

Apart from the first recorded episode, known outbreaks of clinically apparent Marburg disease have been limited to a few individuals in Africa, most likely from bats (Fig. 28.3). The disease is usually brought to attention by infection of hospital staff. It appears to be entering the Congo. By contrast, there have been large outbreaks of Ebola infection in the Sudan and Zaïre, where, on the basis of serological surveys, the virus seems to be endemic (the viruses are slightly different and are called Ebola S and Ebola Z; Fig. 28.4). The outbreak in a primate facility in Reston, USA has led to identification of a third virus, Ebola-Reston. In this outbreak in a monkey colony in the USA many macaques died, but in the four employees who were diagnosed as infected there were no clinical signs. This is an encouraging observation and may indicate that certain strains are non-path-

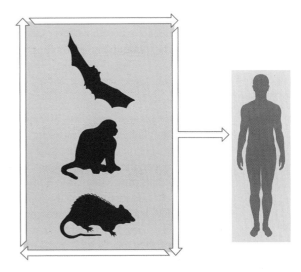

Fig. 28.3 Transmission of filovirus Ebola from an, as yet, unidentified reservoir, but most likely a fruit bat.

ogenic. The virus is spreading among chimpanzees and gorillas in the wild in Central Africa. It is not clear whether the great apes form the normal host or whether rats or bats are the reservoir in nature.

The disease in the Reston outbreak was a zoonosis and although monkeys were also involved in the Marburg outbreak, the precise animal reservoir is still unknown. Virus is spread mainly by close contact with infected blood, although it can also be detected in body fluids: in one case in the Marburg outbreak there was laboratory evidence of spread from semen during sexual intercourse. The virus may persist in infected individuals for at least 2 months, which presents an additional transmission

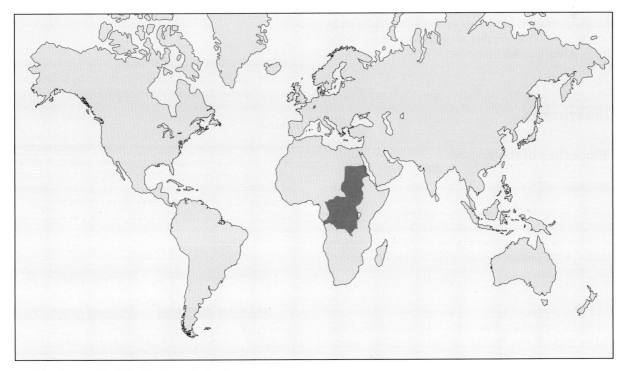

Fig. 28.4 Geographical distribution of Ebola virus.

hazard. Apart from direct contact with animals, very close contact with an infected patient is a prerequisite for infection, and normal isolation and barrier-nursing methods prevent transmission.

Laboratory diagnosis

Only certain laboratories designated category IV have the experience and high-level containment facilities to propagate these viruses in quantity. There are only a handful of these facilities in the world, including two in the USA, one in Canada and Europe and three in the UK. **Virus may be isolated** from blood and autopsy tissue in Vero cells and identified by its characteristic morphology under the **EM** or by **immunofluorescence** of impression smears of infected tissues. Specific **antigen** can also be detected by **ELISA**, and **RT–PCR** can be used to detect viral RNA. A significant rise in **antibody**, as measured by ELISA, is also diagnostic.

Young guinea pigs can be infected by intraperitoneal injection and these diagnostic procedures can then be applied to their tissues.

Prevention and treatment

No vaccines or specific chemotherapeutic agents are available at present, although ribavirin is often administered and adenosine analogues are active *in vitro*. Since the Reston outbreak further controls have been imposed on export and import of primates and stricter regulations introduced to protect workers in monkey units. However, outbreaks of Ebola continue to occur in Africa with regularity. Transmission is by direct contact, droplet infection or contact with body fluids. Fortunately the Ro value is very low, about 2 or 3. **Healthcare staff are particularly at risk**, as most or all infections involve close contact with sick patients. In hospitals with adequate facilities the attack rate in hospital staff is low but where they are not, transmission rates to staff of 80 per cent have been recorded.

3 Arenaviruses

3.1 Properties of the viruses

Classification

The family *Arenaviridae* contains a number of viruses (Table 28.2) with a distinctive 'sandy' appearance (Latin *arena* = sand) when virus sections are examined by EM. The viruses have ssRNA in the form of two segments with predominantly negative-sense polarity.

Morphology

The virions are somewhat pleomorphic and range in diameter from 50 to 300 nm (Fig. 28.5). Glycoprotein spikes project through the virus envelope and on their inner ends presumably contact the internally situated nucleoprotein. The nucleo-

Table 28.2 Arenaviruses that infect humans

Virus	Geographical distribution	Disease
Junin	Argentina	Argentinian haemorrhagic fever
Machupo	Bolivia	Bolivian haemorrhagic fever
Lassa	West Africa	Lassa fever
Lymphocytic choriomeningitis	Worldwide	Lymphocytic choriomeningitis

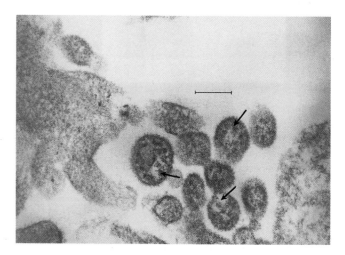

Fig. 28.5 Electron micrograph of an arenavirus (Lassa). This is a thin section of virus in an infected liver. The granules (arrowed) are host-cell ribosomes that have become incorporated in the virions. (Courtesy of Drs David Ellis and Colin Howard.) Scale bar = 100 nm.

protein has a rather unusual structure of two helical closed circles. The 'sandy' appearance is caused by the inclusion in the virion of cellular ribosomal material during virus budding.

Genome

Arenaviruses are unusual negative-stranded RNA viruses with two ambisense ssRNA segments, (L)ong and S(hort); both have a small positive-strand RNA (at the 5' end) and a large negative-strand RNA (at the 3' end) (Fig. 28.6). Similarly to influenza, the mRNA derives its 5' cap by 'cap snatching' short cellular heterogeneous RNAs. The L (7.2 kb) and S (3.4 kb) segments of

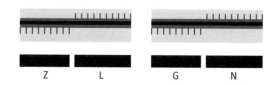

Fig. 28.6 Arenavirus genome and encoded proteins. Labelled proteins are N (nucleoprotein), G (glycoprotein spike), L (polymerase), and Z (zinc-binding protein).

RNA form circles by hydrogen bonding of the ends of the molecules.

Replication

A subgenomic mRNA coding for the N (nucleocapsid) protein is transcribed by the virus-associated transcriptase from the 3' minus-sense half of the S segment. At the same time a subgenomic L (transcriptase) mRNA is transcribed from the 3' minus-sense L segment and translation of both these mRNAs proceeds prior to replication of the viral genome. Only at this stage can the mRNA for the G spike protein and another protein called Z be transcribed from the other end of the S and L segments.

Replication is confined to the cytoplasm and budding takes place at the plasma membrane of the infected cells. Replication of the genome needs the synthesis of full-length complementary copies of both ambisense genome segments. Presumably it is at this stage that cellular ribosomes are incorporated, by chance, into the budding virion. Genetic reassortment can easily occur if a cell is infected with two arenaviruses.

3.2 Clinical and pathological aspects

Clinical features

Lassa, Argentinian, and Bolivian haemorrhagic fevers

In endemic areas, subclinical infections are frequent (Fig. 28.7). Clinically apparent disease may be severe; the fatality rates in hospitalized patients with Lassa fever range from 15 to 25 per cent. The incubation period is commonly 1–2 weeks and the first signs are non-specific, including fever, headache, and sore throat. A **rash** on the face and neck and a worsening of the patient's general condition usually signals the next stage. In the second week of the illness there may be **gastrointestinal and urogenital tract bleeding** and a **shock syndrome**. Even if the patient survives, the convalescence is prolonged; **neurological sequelae** are a prominent feature, especially in Lassa fever. Argentinian and Bolivian haemorrhagic fevers are similar clinically.

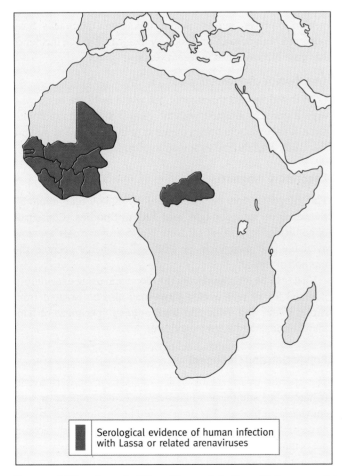

Serological evidence of human infection with Lassa or related arenaviruses

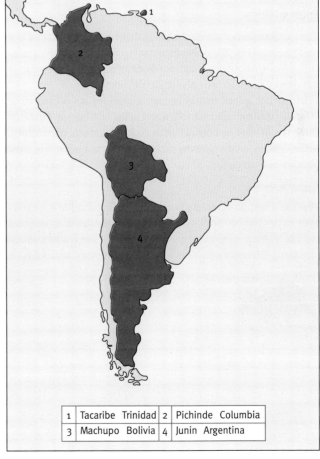

1	Tacaribe	Trinidad	2	Pichinde	Columbia
3	Machupo	Bolivia	4	Junin	Argentina

Fig. 28.7 **(a)** Prevalence in Africa of human infection with Lassa or related arenaviruses, as shown by serological tests. **(b)** Prevalence in South America of arenaviruses. Only the Machupo and Junin viruses are known to infect humans.

Lymphocytic choriomeningitis

By contrast with these haemorrhagic fevers, LCM is a comparatively mild infection, beginning with headache, fever, and malaise. The illness usually resolves after this stage, but a small proportion of patients develop **meningitis** or **choriomeningitis**, which again usually resolves without sequelae; deaths are rare.

Pathology

Extrapolation of data from experimental infections of primates suggests that viral replication in humans occurs in the hilar lymph nodes and lungs following an aerosol infection. The subsequent **viraemia** causes wide dissemination to other organs including **liver, spleen, heart,** and **meninges. Bronchopneumonia**, either primary viral or secondary bacterial, is a common finding. Large amounts of viral antigen are detected in autopsy samples of spleen, bone marrow, and viscera.

Exactly how these arenaviruses cause haemorrhagic fevers is an open question. Extensive macrophage infection causes release of TNF and other cytokines, and platelet-activating factor. Immune complexes, complement activation, or disseminated intravascular coagulation are not thought to play any role in the pathogenesis.

Epidemiology

The distribution of arenaviruses is determined by that of the host rodents (Fig. 28.8). Persistent infection of the rodent reservoir, often without overt signs of disease, maintains the virus in nature and humans are only incidental hosts.

In rodents, infection may be transmitted vertically *in utero* or via milk; transmission via saliva and urine also occurs. Humans catch the disease by **contact with rodent excreta**, particularly urine, which contaminates surfaces and may enter via skin abrasions or aerosols.

Lassa fever

This has a certain notoriety because of its first dramatic appearance in the USA in 1969, when, following the death of hospital staff in Nigeria, clinical samples were sent to the world-famous arbovirus laboratory in Yale where they infected and killed a technician and laid low the well known virologist who was head of the unit.

The infection is endemic in rural West Africa (Fig. 28.7(a)), particularly Nigeria and Sierra Leone, where subclinical infections are frequent, but where there have also been a number of outbreaks with high mortality rates. There are more than 100 000 new infections yearly in this area with thousands of deaths. It is the only viral haemorrhagic fever to have reached the UK, where 10 imported cases have been diagnosed in the last 20 years Although this number is small, the serious nature of the disease dictates continued vigilance when dealing with febrile illnesses in patients arriving from endemic areas within the previous 3 or 4 weeks. Rarely, it may spread from person to person.

Argentinian haemorrhagic fever

This is caused by the **Junin** arenavirus (Fig. 28.7(b)). Those predominantly infected are male field workers who come into contact with the excreta of chronically infected wild rodents. Thousands of cases may occur when the maize is harvested in late spring and early summer; the case fatality rate is 10–20 per cent.

Bolivian haemorrhagic fever

This (Fig. 28.7(b)) is due to another arenavirus, **Machupo**, which again is transmitted from rodent excreta, although person-to-person spread is not unknown. Outbreaks have occurred both in town and country dwellers, but the incidence has greatly diminished in recent years.

Lymphocytic choriomeningitis

LCM is widespread throughout the world in house mice, who are chronically infected without clinical signs. Contact with mice or their excreta brings the virus to humans as a 'dead end' infection, with no further spread to others.

Laboratory diagnosis

The diagnosis can be established by ELISA and immunofluorescence tests for **IgM and IgG antibodies**. Consensus oligonucleotide primers for New World arenaviruses are now available and **diagnosis by PCR** will probably become the method of choice.

Virus can be recovered from the blood and urine of acutely ill patients for several weeks. Virus may also be isolated from throat swabs and urine and from autopsy specimens of lymphoid tissue, bone marrow, and liver.

Prevention and treatment

The specific treatment of choice of Lassa fever is **ribavirin** (Chapter 38) administered intravenously, either alone or with convalescent plasma. The drug should be administered as soon as possible after onset of the disease. Bacterial superinfections are common and need to be monitored carefully.

For all the haemorrhagic fevers, supportive care is often life saving, and comprises careful maintenance of fluid and electrolyte balance, protein replacement therapy, and appropriate support for cardiac complications. Isolation and barrier nursing

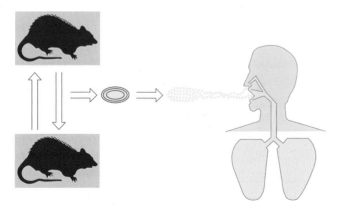

Fig. 28.8 Animal reservoir of Arena virus and transmission to humans via inhalation of dried urine.

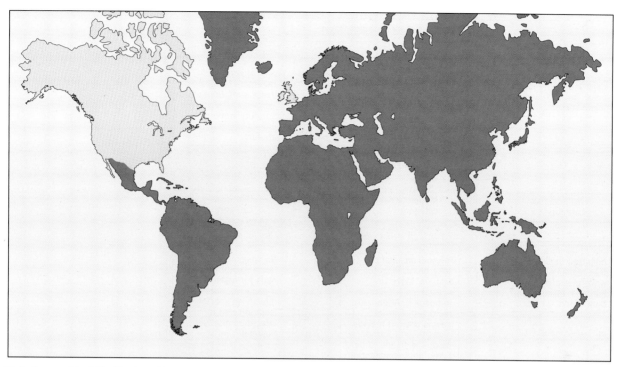

Fig. 28.9 Geographical distribution of hantavirus.

experience is vital to prevent spread to other patients and to nursing and doctoring staff. Control of rodents is an important method of controlling arenavirus infections, but may be impracticable in rural areas.

4 Hantaviruses

The great majority of bunyaviruses are arthropod-borne and cause fever and infections of the CNS, mostly in tropical or subtropical areas. They are members of the Bunyavirus family. In 1978, however, a bunyavirus isolated from field mice found near the Hantaan river in Korea was later identified as the cause of haemorrhagic fever with renal syndrome, a disease of hitherto unknown aetiology prevalent in Scandinavia, Russia, and Asia (Fig. 28.9), and also referred to as Korean haemorrhagic fever, nephropathia epidemica, and many other names. This agent—

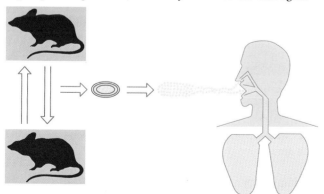

Fig. 28.10 Animal reservoir of hantavirus and transmission to humans via inhalation of dried urine.

Hantaan virus and subsequent isolates—differed sufficiently from other bunyaviruses to be classified as a new genus, *Hantavirus*. More recently, hantaviruses were found to cause another severe illness, hantavirus pulmonary syndrome (HPS). Unlike other bunyaviruses, hantaviruses are spread not by arthropod vectors but by contact with rodent excreta (Fig. 28.10). The rodent carriers remain symptomless. Serological evidence suggests that many infections are subclinical.

4.1 Properties of the viruses

Classification

The genus **Hantavirus** belongs to the family *Bunyaviridae*. There are at many species, mostly affecting rodents.

Morphology, genome, and replication

In so far as they have been studied in detail, these properties are generally similar to those of other members of the *Bunyaviridae*, namely enveloped spherical negative-stranded RNA viruses with three genome segments.

4.2 Clinical and pathological aspects

Clinical features

These viruses caused two severe diseases in humans.

Haemorrhagic fever with renal syndrome (HFRS)

HFRS ranges in severity from mild to a severe life-threatening infection with a mortality of ≈5 per cent. The incubation period

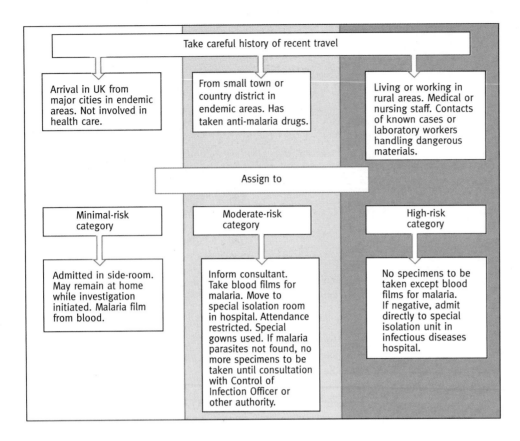

Fig. 28.11 Summary of procedures for dealing with suspected haemorrhage fevers.

varies widely, but is usually about 3 weeks. The onset is marked by **malaise, fever**, and **abdominal pain** and is typically followed by a **hypotensive phase** 5 days later. There may be thrombocytopenia, with petechiae on the face and trunk, and severe bleeding in the gastrointestinal tract and CNS. **Renal function becomes impaired** by the ninth day, with oliguria, proteinuria, and elevated blood urea and creatinine. About half the deaths occur at this time and are due to renal failure, pulmonary oedema, or shock. With good management, the mortality rate is about 5 per cent but may be higher. Recovery of renal function is signalled by copious diuresis about 2 weeks after onset. Convalescence is often prolonged.

Nephropathia epidemica is caused by the Puumala strain of hantavirus; it is prevalent in Scandinavia and western Europe and resembles HFRS but is less severe, with a mortality of <1 per cent.

Hantavirus pulmonary syndrome

In 1993, there was an outbreak of severe acute respiratory illness in the south-western states of the USA, with a mortality rate of 50 per cent. Serological and epidemiological evidence implicated other hantaviruses, which differ genetically from those causing HFRS and appear to be found predominantly in the Americas. There is, however, considerable overlapping in the geographical distribution of the viruses, which varies with the prevalence of different species of wild rodents.

This syndrome is much more severe than HFRS, with mortality rates of ≈80 per cent. The onset is sudden, starting with cough and muscle pains, followed by dyspnoea, tachycardia,

pulmonary oedema, pleural effusion, and hypotension. Blood clotting is impaired but severe haemorrhage is not an important feature. Death is due to respiratory failure.

Pathology

Haemorrhagic fever with renal syndrome

Acute tubulo-interstitial nephritis is the main feature, with infiltration by lymphocytes, macrophages, and polymorphonuclear cells. The glomeruli do not show obvious changes under light microscopy.

Hantavirus pulmonary syndrome

This is characterized by **interstitial pneumonitis**, with oedema and infiltration by mononuclear cells. Hantavirus antigen can be demonstrated in the capillary endothelium of the lung and many other organs, including the spleen and kidneys.

In hantavirus infections there is increased expression of a wide range of T-cell inflammatory cytokines, including TNF-α, and IFN-γ and -β. It is thought that some of the pathological changes may be mediated by immune mechanisms and direct interaction of viral and host cell proteins. Epithelial cells, monocytes, and macrophages are the main target cells and spread the virus within the body. Lung endothelium and kidney tubular cells are involved in HPS and HFRS respectively.

Epidemiology

Like filovirus infections, the prevalence of both hantavirus syndromes depends on the distribution of the rodent hosts (where they are persistently maintained), which include a number of species of wild rats and mice. Individual hantaviruses are associated with particular species of rodent. No symptoms are apparent in the rodents. **HFRS** first appeared in 1950, when it affected thousands of United Nations troops in Korea. In 1993 a new Hantavirus appeared in south-west USA, where it has caused well over a hundred cases of **HPS**. This agent was originally named after the township where it was first identified, but local protests prompted its renaming as 'Sin Nombre' ('No Name') virus. So far, this highly lethal infection has been confined to the USA, but the renal syndrome has been reported in the Far East, Asia, CIS, Scandinavia, the Balkans, and western Europe, notably Germany and Holland; several strains of hantavirus are involved.

Although contact with rodent excreta is the prime method of transmission, a report of a small outbreak in Argentina during 1997 suggests that HPS may occasionally spread from person to person.

Laboratory diagnosis

Serological methods include ELISA for detecting specific **IgM** or rising titres of IgG and **immunofluorescence tests** on infected Vero cells. PCR tests are now being developed.

Treatment

The therapy of hantavirus infections is largely supportive, with particular attention to maintaining the fluid and electrolyte balances. Intravenous **ribavirin** may be of benefit in cases of HFRS. There is as yet no vaccine.

5 Risk categories

Where haemorrhagic fevers are endemic or causing an epidemic, the possibility of such infections will be well to the fore and the diagnosis of moderate or severe illnesses will probably be fairly obvious. This may not be true of travellers from such areas who fall ill after arriving in a non-endemic country. **The importance of taking a careful history from anyone developing a febrile illness within a month of arrival from an endemic area cannot be overstressed.** In many cases the illness is due to malaria, which should always be tested for, but even so, the possibility of a double infection should not be overlooked. Figure 28.11 summarizes the procedures for dealing with such situations. It is most important that the patient be assigned to the appropriate risk category to avoid over- or under-reacting to the possibility of a haemorrhagic fever.

6 Reminders

- The filoviruses Marburg and Ebola (family *Filoviridae*) are **enveloped** viruses with a bizarre **filamentous morphology**. They have ssRNA genomes of positive polarity.

- The arenaviruses Lassa, Junin, and Machupo (family Arenaviridae) have a 'sandy' appearance due to incorporation of cellular ribosomes in the virion. Their genomes are segmented, and are ambisense with positive-stranded RNA at the 5′ end and negative-stranded RNA at the 3′ end.

- The **filoviruses** cause zoonotic infections in **monkeys**, and may infect other animals as yet not identified. The **arenaviruses** cause persistent infections in **rodents** and are transmitted to humans by **contact with rodent excreta** either as an aerosol via skin lesions or by ingestion of contaminated food or water. They are prevalent in Latin America and parts of Africa. LCM virus occurs worldwide.

- In humans, infections are often inapparent, but the **filoviruses** and the **Lassa, Junin,** and **Machupo** arenaviruses may cause **severe haemorrhagic fevers** with high fatality rates; **LCM** virus may cause **'aseptic' meningitis** or rarely, meningoencephalitis.

- Lassa and filovirus infections are **pantropic**, causing lesions in many organs, notably the liver and spleen. Prostration, diarrhoea, rashes, vomiting, and **bleeding** from the **respiratory, gastrointestinal,** and **urogenital tracts** are features of the haemorrhagic forms of these illnesses.

- Hantaviruses belong to the *Bunyaviridae*, but, like arenaviruses, are acquired by contact with infected rodent excreta. They cause **HFRS** characterized by haemorrhages and renal failure; and **HPS,** with severe pulmonary and cardiac involvement. The respective mortalities are ≈5 and 80 per cent.

- Prompt treatment with **convalescent plasma** and **intravenous ribavirin** may be of some value in Lassa and also Ebola fever but supportive care with careful maintenance of fluid and electrolytes are key elements for survival.

- The diagnosis of these illnesses is based on the **history and circumstances of travel in endemic areas,** the exclusion of malaria and other tropical fevers, and on isolation of virus and serological tests in a specialist high-security category IV laboratory. PCR is being used experimentally for rapid diagnosis.

Chapter 29

Prions and the spongiform encephalopathies

1 Prion diseases

In 1920 and 1921 respectively, Creutzfeldt and Jakob described the first cases of the fatal dementia that now bears their names. Forty years later a somewhat similar illness known as kuru was described in Papua New Guinea; both diseases were subsequently linked with scrapie, an infection of sheep, and with transmissible spongiform encephalopathies (TSE) affecting humans and some other animals. These unlikely partners had in common **long incubation periods**, measured in months or years; a **progressive and fatal disease affecting the CNS**; and **spongiform degeneration of the neurones.** These spongiform encephalopathies are generally believed to have as their cause an agent quite new to microbiology—the **prion**.

The rather cumbersome terms and possibly unfamiliar abbreviations used to describe prions and their diseases are listed in Table 29.1.

1.1 Infections of humans (Table 29.2)

Creutzfeldt–Jakob disease

CJD has an incubation period of several years, sometimes as many as 20 or 30. It is characterized by dementia and recur-

Table 29.1 Terminology of prion diseases

Abbreviation	Meaning
BSE	Bovine spongiform encephalopathy
CJD	Creutzfeldt–Jakob disease
CJD^{nv} (or nvCJD)	Creutzfeldt–Jakob disease, new variant
FFI	Fatal familial insomnia
GSSD	Gerstmann–Sträussler–Scheinker disease
PrP	Proteinaceous infectious particle
PrP^c	Normal cellular PrP
PrP^{Sc}	Scrapie-type PrP
PrP^{RES}, PrP^{CJD}	Synonymous with PrP^{Sc}
TSE	Transmissible spongiform encephalopathy

Table 29.2 Prion diseases of humans

Disease	Transmission
Creutzfeldt–Jakob disease	
Sporadic	Mostly unknown. 10–15 per cent are inherited
Iatrogenic	Growth hormone, dura mater transplants, inadequately sterilized instruments
New variant	Acquired from BSE
Gerstmann–Sträussler–Scheinker disease	Inherited as autosomal dominant condition
Fatal familial insomnia	Inherited as autosomal dominant condition
Kuru	Ritual cannibalism, probably via contamination of skin abrasions

rent seizures; death usually occurs within a few months of onset. Histologically, the brain shows spongiform vacuolation (Fig. 29.1), pronounced astrocytosis, and neuronal loss; in a proportion of cases, amyloid plaques are also present. CJD is a rare disease, only about 20 cases a year being reported in the UK, mostly in middle-aged or elderly people. The incidence—of the order of 1 case per million people per annum—is similar in other countries. Since the start of the bovine spongiform encephalopathy (BSE) epizootic there have been a number of cases of CJD^{nv} (see Section 6), many in young people.

In most cases of CJD the mode of transmission is unknown. There have, however, been a number of iatrogenic infections, mostly from human pituitary growth hormone and from transplants of dura mater; inadequately sterilized neurosurgical instruments have accounted for a few such catastrophes (see Section 5). One case arose in the recipient of a corneal transplant from a patient with CJD. Measures are now taken to guard

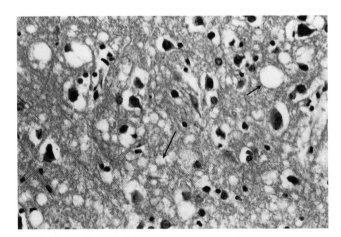

Fig. 29.1 Section of brain from a case of CJD. The 'holes' (arrowed) are characteristic of all the spongiform encephalopathies. (Courtesy of the late Dr Carl Scholtz, The London Hospital Medical College.)

against these known hazards, but it is possible—although perhaps unlikely—that there are others of which we are as yet unaware. There is no evidence of transmission to neonates during childbirth. CJD^{nv} has been transmitted by blood transfusion.

Inherited spongiform encephalopathies

Israeli Jews originating from Libya have a substantially higher than average rate of CJD; elsewhere, ≈15 per cent of CJD cases are familial. The rare **Gerstmann–Sträussler–Scheinker disease (GSSD)** somewhat resembles CJD; but has a longer clinical duration (2–10 years) than CJD; ataxia is a prominent feature. **Fatal familial insomnia**, an even more rare syndrome, is marked by severe disturbances of sleep and of the autonomic system, and by atrophy and gliosis of the medial thalamus. Cognitive impairment is slight in the early stages. These disorders are inherited as autosomal dominant conditions.

Kuru

This is—or was—another progressive and fatal dementia, usually with pronounced cerebellar involvement leading to difficulty in walking. This curious disease was limited to the Fore tribe of Papua New Guinea; it was spread by ritualistic cannibalism, during which the brains of dead relatives were eaten by the women and children only, among whom there was a very high incidence. It is thought that the infection was transmitted by contact of tissue with cuts and abrasions, and possibly ingestion. When cannibalism was stopped in the 1950s kuru started to disappear, and is now extinct. It seems that this disease is of comparatively recent origin; there is speculation that it may have been introduced into the tribe as a result of butchering someone with CJD, or who was incubating it.

Kuru has been transmitted to a number of species of primates, and CJD both to primates and other animals.

Alzheimer's disease

Alzheimer's disease, characterized by dementia and the presence of amyloid plaques in the brain, may also be a prion disease, but this is as yet unproven.

Table 29.3 Prion diseases of animals

Disease	Transmission
Scrapie (sheep and goats)	
Adult animals	Contact; grazing on infected pastures
Newborn animals	Possibly perinatal
BSE (cattle)	Foodstuffs (meat and bonemeal concentrates)
Other transmissible SE (captive or domestic animals: mink, deer, elk, and other ungulates, cats)	Probably foodstuffs

1.2 Infections of animals (Table 29.3)

Scrapie

This enzootic infection of sheep and goats is the best studied of all the spongiform encephalopathies, and from it we have gained most of our knowledge of prions. The name derives from the need of infected animals to rub themselves against objects, e.g. fences, to try and relieve the characteristic intense itching. Infection is transmitted directly or indirectly from animal to animal, and is often acquired at birth. The incubation period is 1–5 years; the onset of itching and ataxia heralds a downward, invariably fatal course lasting a few months. Scrapie has been prevalent in the UK, particularly in the north of England and Scotland, for over 200 years; some countries, e.g. Australia, are however completely free of this infection.

Other prion diseases of captive and domestic animals

Transmissible mink encephalopathy

Transmissible mink encephalopathy, chronic wasting disease of deer and elk and TSE in other ungulates have also been reported. A feline form of TSE infects domestic cats, and some large cats, e.g. cheetahs and tigers. It is significant that all these reports relate to captive or domestic animals, as they are most likely to be exposed to contaminated feed.

Bovine spongiform encephalopathy

BSE is the most serious TSE in terms both of its potential for being transmitted from cattle to humans, and of economic impact. For this reason we have devoted a separate section (6) to it, but before doing so, it is time to deal with the salient facts about prions.

2 What are prions?

Rather oddly for a virology textbook, the word 'virus' has not appeared in this chapter. The reason is that during the 1960s, it was found that the scrapie agent could not be inactivated by ultraviolet light or ionizing radiation, ruling out the presence of a nucleic acid, and by implication, any resemblance to known micro-organisms. Various ideas were advanced as to the nature of such an agent, but the one that has gained the most widespread acceptance is the prion hypothesis of Stanley Prusiner in the USA. Although still somewhat controversial, it is the one that best answers the following questions.

- How can an infective agent devoid of RNA or DNA replicate?
- How can it be inherited?
- How can it be transmitted horizontally?

The answers lay in the identification of a small (33–35 kDa) glycoprotein, **PrP^C** (c = cellular) found in normal cells, but without any apparent function. A variant, termed **PrP^{Sc}**, is present only in scrapie-infected brain (Table 29.1). Its molecular weight (27–30 kDa) is somewhat lower than that of PrP^C, its

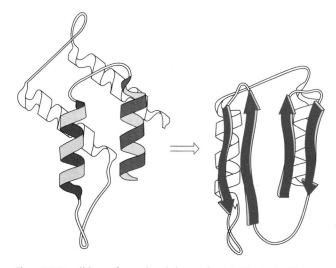

Fig. 29.2 Possible conformational change from PrP^C to PrP^{Sc}. The two α-helices, shown as spirals in the left-hand figure, are converted into a β-sheet structure in the right-hand figure during the formation of PrP^{Sc}.

molecular conformation is different (Fig. 29.2) and it is resistant to protease (hence the alternative designation PrP^{RES}). In humans, the appearance of PrP^{Sc} is mediated by a point mutation in the *PrP* gene, located on chromosome 20 (chromosome 2 in mice). The codons affected by such mutations vary with the syndrome and with the host species. In humans, there is a polymorphism between methionine and valine at codon 129 of the *PrP* gene. Homozygosity of either allele is a feature of most cases of CJD; there are many similar examples. These findings help to explain the hereditary transmission of prions and predisposition to prion diseases.

Another important piece of evidence for the causal role of prions in TSE was the finding that mice in which the *PrP* gene is ablated are resistant to prion disease.

The mechanism by which PrP^C is converted to PrP^{Sc} in other words, how PrP^{Sc} 'replicates', is of fundamental importance, but is not as yet not well understood. It probably involves a change in the conformation of the PrP^C glycoprotein: prions have the same amino acid sequence as the normal protein, but the conformation is different: about 40 per cent is in the protease-sensitive α-helical state, whereas the prion form is composed of 50 per cent β-sheet and 20 per cent protease-resistant α-helical form (Fig. 29.2).

Given that humans and animals, once 'seeded' with PrP^{Sc}, can produce it in quantity, the question of horizontal transmission is readily understandable. Prions are likely to be most abundant in nervous tissue, but lymphoid organs and possibly blood in the early stages of infection are also suspect. The most common route of infection is probably via foodstuffs, but contamination of cuts and abrasions cannot be ruled out.

Strain variation in prions

The discovery that mice and hamsters can be artificially infected with scrapie was an important step forward. The incubation period is only about 6 months, thus making practicable infectivity titrations and other studies, including research on pathogenesis. Such experiments also revealed the existence of genetically different strains of scrapie, characterized in terms of variability in incubation periods and of the patterns of histopathological lesions produced. The existence of separate strains implies a genetic mechanism for maintaining them, and in which mutations can take place. The picture is further complicated by genetic variation in the incubation times shown by different strains of mice and hamsters; in mice, these are determined by a gene, *Sinc*, which is closely linked to, or possibly identical with, the *PrP* gene.

3 Pathogenesis and pathology

Studies of the pathogenesis of scrapie in animals are important because of the light they may shed on spongiform encephalopathies (TSE) in humans. After appearing in the blood, the agent first multiplies in the spleen and other organs of the reticuloendothelial system, from which it spreads to the CNS by migrating up peripheral nerves to the spinal cord and brain. The cerebellum is particularly affected.

In addition to the spongiform lesions (Fig. 29.1) there is **astrocytosis** but little or no inflammatory reaction. The most characteristic feature is the presence of **amyloid plaques** in neural tissue, which appear to be formed from PrP^{Sc} and are particularly characteristic of GSS. EM of protease-treated brain extracts (Fig. 29.3) shows clusters of prion rods (or 'scrapie-associated fibrils').

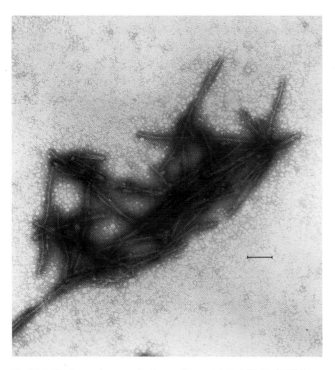

Fig. 29.3 Electron micrograph of scrapie-associated fibrils (SAF) from brain of scrapie-infected mouse. (Courtesy of Dr J. Hope, AFRC and MRC Neuropathogenesis Unit.) Scale bar = 100 nm.

3.1 Antibody response

As might be expected, there is no detectable immune response to such a small molecule. It is however possible to raise both polyclonal and monoclonal neutralizing antibody in the laboratory.

4 Laboratory diagnosis

A major hindrance to research on prion diseases is the lack of a rapid and reasonably simple test for PrP^{Sc}. So far, only surrogate tests have been described, that is, the assay of some characteristic other than the causal agent (an example is the altered CSF/blood ratio of proteins seen in viral encephalitis).

One such test is an immunoassay of a protein known as 14-3-3 (or P130/131) in the CSF or tonsillar tissue; it is found in nearly all cases of CJD. The test is not, however, specific for this disease, since it may be positive in other neurological conditions, notably viral encephalitis. The serum concentration of another protein, S100, is also claimed to be elevated in CJD, but again, the specificity is not as high as one would wish. Neither test is at present practicable for routine use.

5 Safety measures

5.1 Disinfection procedures

As there are no laboratory tests for contamination with prions and no treatment for these infections, we must for the time being concentrate on means for preventing their spread, whether by natural means or as the result of accidents.

Prions are highly resistant to the usual disinfection procedures and special care must be taken when undertaking operations or autopsies on patients likely to have CJD. In the UK, the Advisory Committee on Dangerous Pathogens (1994) has issued guidelines for safety, including recommendations for extended autoclaving of instruments used in neurosurgical procedures. Immersion in 1 N sodium hydroxide has also been recommended, but with the possible exception of this and strong hypochlorite, none of the conventional chemical disinfectants can be relied upon. It should be noted that the CJD agent can survive for years in brains preserved in formalin.

In the UK, regulations for the handling of animal carcasses are in force to protect farm and abattoir workers.

5.2 Blood transfusion

The gaps in our knowledge of the pathogenesis of CJD and methods for detecting it in body fluids and tissues mean there is an element of uncertainty in drawing up policies for preventing its spread. There has already been at least one confirmed instance of infection deriving from blood donated by a person with variant CJD (vCJD) and this possibility is of great concern to the blood transfusion service. At present, precautions include:

- withdrawal of any blood components or tissues derived from any person who later develops vCJD;
- import of plasma for fractionation from countries other than the UK;
- leucocyte depletion of all blood components.

6 The great bovine spongiform encephalopathy outbreak

The arrangement of this chapter necessarily differs from those dealing with more conventional agents. We have left this important topic until last, because it cannot be understood without some knowledge of prions and their pathogenicity.

In 1985–6 a hitherto unknown disease of cattle made its appearance in the UK; the animals affected suffered from hind-limb ataxia to such an extent that they had to be put down. Their severe state of apprehension was probably the feature that prompted its designation by the media as 'mad cow disease'. It was most prevalent in dairy herds, particularly in south-east England; bull calves were spared because they are slaughtered at about 2 years of age, before the end of the long incubation period. So far, more than 165 000 cattle have been affected.

The cause was traced to the introduction of meat and bone meal (MBM) as a dietary supplement. This material must have contained scrapie-infected offal. It seems that the hydrocarbon extraction process used originally inactivated any prions that it contained; but the abandonment of this method in favour of a cheaper system allowed infective material into the animal feed. The result was disastrous; all herds in which even a single case of BSE occurred were slaughtered, with a loss to the economy of millions of pounds. This policy, coupled with a total ban on MBM and on the sale for human consumption of meat from cattle over 30 months old eventually brought the epizootic under control. At its peak in August 1992 it attained an incidence in

England and Wales of about 36 000 (Fig. 29.4). The losses due to slaughter were compounded by a ban on British beef instituted by other countries. It is surprising that few cases of BSE have been reported in mainland Europe, despite the importation of large quantities of MBM before 1990.

6.1 Crossing the species barrier

Although scrapie has existed in the UK for more than 200 years, no human disease associated with live sheep has yet been reported. Furthermore, there is much laboratory evidence of a barrier to infection between species, conditioned in part by differences in the amino acid sequences of PrP. This barrier may be absolute, or manifested as a prolonged incubation period in the recipient species. It has been postulated that the spread of sheep scrapie to cattle was facilitated by the similarity of their respective PrP molecules.

6.2 If from sheep to cattle, why not from cattle to humans?

This has been a major worry since the start of the BSE outbreak. In theory, such infections could be acquired by various routes.

6.3 Exposure to scrapie of farmers, abattoir workers, and butchers

There is no evidence of infection being acquired in this way.

6.4 Potential contamination of cattle-derived products

These include pharmaceutical and surgical items, e.g. some sutures, albumen and other bovine blood products. The identification of such materials as posing a risk is purely speculative, due to lack of a rapid and reliable test for contamination.

6.5 Ingestion of contaminated food

Some guidance on this important possibility is provided by mouse titrations of the infectivity of various tissues from scrapie-infected mice. They show that, as might be expected, brain and spinal cord contain most infectivity, followed by ileum, lymph nodes, spleen, and tonsil. Other organs are only occasionally infected, or not at all. There is no evidence that milk is infected.

In the light of what we do know about the distribution of scrapie prions in the various tissues, there has since 1989 been a ban on the use of 'specified bovine offal' for human consumption, extended in 1990 to animals and birds. The term 'specified bovine offal' covers mainly nervous and lymphoid tissue, but its definition and the regulations for processing carcasses have both changed from time to time as new information becomes available.

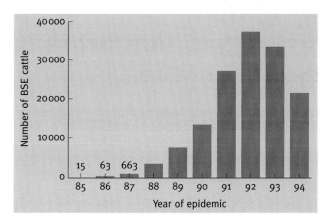

Fig. 29.4 Annual incidence of BSE in Great Britain. All cases were confirmed clinically and neuropathologically. (From Prusiner, S.B. (1998). In *Topley and Wilson's Microbiology and Microbial Infections*, (9th edn), Arnold, London Vol. 1, fig 39.9.)

6.6 A new variant of CJD: cause for alarm?

With these concerns in mind, national surveillance for new cases of CJD in the UK was implemented in 1990, since when about 150 cases have been reported that varied in the following respects from the classical pattern:

- a lower than usual age of onset (19–41 years, median 29 years);
- a longer than usual time to death;
- progressive neuropsychiatric disorder;
- amyloid plaques more typical of those seen in kuru than in classical CJD;
- absence of the electroencephalogram changes characteristic of sporadic CJD.

This syndrome is termed vCJD, or CJD^{nv} and was first reported in 1995. It is of course possible that this form of CJD has existed for some time, and has now come to light as a result of increased awareness of the possibility of CJD. Nevertheless, its occurrence does raise the possibility of acquisition by consuming BSE-infected meat or offal, with the consequent spectre of an epidemic involving young people; but because of the prolonged incubation period, we shall not know where we stand for some time to come. Several organization in various countries keep a constant watch for significant fluctuations in the incidence of the various forms of CJD, with particular attention to the variant type. In the UK, the responsible organization is the National Creutzfeld–Jakob Surveillance Unit based in Edinburgh.

So far, earlier fears of an epidemic among young people have not materialized. There was a 'blip' in the number of deaths (28) around the year 2000, but this number decreased to 18 by 2003. By the end of December 2004 there had been 147 deaths due to definite or probable vCJD in the UK. Nevertheless, many coun-

tries have banned blood donations from their citizens who lived in the UK in the 1990s who may be incubating the disease.

Figure 29.5 compares the incidence in the UK of vCJD with the sporadic form of the disease over the period 1996 to 2004 (note that these figures relate to reported deaths, not to cases).

7 Reminders

- The TSEs have in common **very long incubation periods**, a progressive, **uniformly fatal course**, characteristic **spongiform changes** in the brain, and lack of inflammatory and immune responses. They occur in humans, (kuru, CJD, GSSD) and a variety of animal species, notably sheep and goats (scrapie) and ruminants (BSE). Except in sheep and cattle, TSEs are rare.

- These syndromes are caused by an agent highly resistant to radiation, and hence not possessing nucleic acid. It is now widely accepted that it is **PrP**, a small protein normally present in the brain. In this form it is designated PrP^{C}. A mutated form, PrP^{Sc}, causes the TSEs. How PrP^{C} is converted to PrP^{Sc} is not known. **Genetic factors** are important in determining susceptibility to the TSEs.

- Scrapie can be transmitted experimentally to mice, in which most of the studies of infectivity and pathogenesis have so far been done. PrP^{Sc} appears to enter the body via skin abrasions or by ingestion, and travels to the brain via the blood, reticuloendothelial system, and peripheral nerves.

- The histopathological changes in the brain include **spongiform vacuolation, astrocytosis**, and sometimes **amyloid plaques**.

- There is no readily available diagnostic test, and no treatment.

- During 1987–8, a major epizootic of **BSE** began in the UK. This was due to contamination of feed with scrapie-infected material. The economic loss from slaughter of infected and suspect animals, together with a ban on export of British cattle, was enormous. Measures to eliminate infected feed and to control the processing of carcasses are bringing the epizootic to an end.

- Since December 2004 there have been 147 definite or probable cases of CJD in teenagers or young adults, which differ somewhat from the classical form and are termed **CJD^{nv}**. It is possible, but not proved, that CJD^{nv} is the result of eating the meat of cattle infected with BSE.

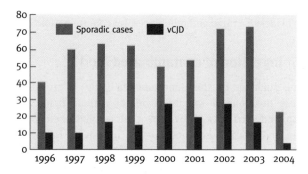

Fig. 29.5 Deaths from sporadic versus vCJD in the UK.

Part 3

Special
syndromes

Viral diseases of the central nervous system

If you are reading these chapters in sequence, you will by now have realized that many of the viruses so far dealt with can cause disease of the CNS. In fact, members of nearly all the 15 or so families of animal viruses can do so in one way or another. This propensity varies, however, from family to family: in some, for example the *Herpesviridae*, all members are potentially neurotropic; by contrast, few of the *Papovaviridae* cause CNS disease and then only rarely. Manifestations of CNS involvement caused by individual viruses are described in the appropriate chapters; here, we shall deal with the topic in a more general way so as to give you an overall picture of the kinds of lesions encountered and of the principles of laboratory diagnosis.

At first sight, the number of viruses involved and the variety of syndromes are confusing. We can simplify things by classifying these illnesses into three groups (Table 30.1). Group 1 is straightforward, comprising acute infections that directly involve the CNS; Group 2 illnesses are also acute, but are less directly related to the associated virus infections; and the chronic fatal diseases in Group 3, fortunately all rare, are caused by grossly abnormal responses to conventional viruses or by prions (Chapter 29). The pathogenesis of infections in the latter group is not yet fully understood. The alphaherpesviruses may give rise to latent infections of the CNS (see Chapter 4).

A general point to remember is that the ways in which the CNS can respond to virus infections are limited: the neurones themselves may undergo **lysis**, **demyelination**, or **spongiform degeneration** and the inflammatory response is mainly expressed by the appearance of **lymphocytes** and **activation** of microglia, the macrophages of the CNS. These inflammatory cells tend to collect in the perivascular spaces of the small blood vessels, an appearance graphically described as 'cuffing' (Fig. 30.1). Another important response of great diagnostic value is the manufacture of **specific IgM antibody** within the

Table 30.1 Virus diseases of the CNS: general classification

Virus usually demonstrable in CNS	Yes	No
Acute	Group 1	Group 2
Chronic	Group 3	

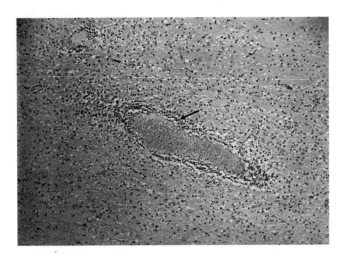

Fig. 30.1 Section of brain from a case of herpes simplex encephalitis. Note the 'cuffing' of the blood vessel with mononuclear cells (arrowed) and the intense proliferation of microglia.

CNS; as such antibody cannot cross the 'blood–brain barrier', its presence in the CSF is good evidence of an active infection by the corresponding virus **within** the CNS compartment.

A final introductory remark: please note the word 'predominant' in the headings of Tables 30.2–30.4. Like most clinicopathological syndromes, these are often not clear-cut and allowance must be made for variations on the main themes. For example, in those illnesses classified as 'meningitis' there may also be some involvement of the brain substance.

1 Acute infections (Group 1) (Table 30.2)

These syndromes all arise from direct invasion of the CNS by the virus concerned, which can usually be isolated from the CSF or brain. The routes of access to the CNS vary with the virus. Some, e.g. the arboviruses, are **blood-borne**. These viruses have to penetrate the so-called **'blood–brain barrier', which** normally stops potentially harmful micro-organisms and macromolecules from entering the brain. They appear to do so by smuggling themselves through the barrier inside macrophages or lymphocytes. This is the haematogenous route. Others—the minority—adopt the **neural route**, gaining access via the peripheral nerves. The classic example is rabies, in which the virus replicates at the site of inoculation and then travels up the axons to the brain.

Table 30.2 Virus diseases of the central nervous system. Group 1: acute infections

Predominant syndrome	Viruses	Predominant neurological lesions
Meningitis	**Enteroviruses**, especially ECHO, Coxsackie A and B, enteroviruses 70 and 71, poliovirus	Inflammation of the meninges, with or without some degree of encephalitis
	Mumps, lymphocytic choriomeningitis, louping-ill, Epstein–Barr virus, HSV-2, VZV	
Poliomyelitis	Polioviruses; occasionally other enteroviruses	Meningitis, lysis of lower motor neurons
Meningoencephalitis	HSV-1, arboviruses	Necrosis of neurons in grey matter of brain
Encephalitis	Rabies	Varying degrees of neuronal necrosis; perivascular and focal inflammation
AIDS dementia complex (ADC)	HIV-1	Meningitis; cortical atrophy; focal necrosis; vacuolation, reactive astrocytosis, and microgliosis in subcortical areas; demyelinating peripheral neuropathy
Tropical spastic paraparesis	HTLV-1	Upper motor neurone lesions

Table 30.3 Virus diseases of the central nervous system. Group 2: acute postexposure syndromes

Syndrome	Viruses	Predominant neurological lesions
Postinfection and postimmunization encephalomyelitis	Measles, rubella, mumps, varicella-zoster, rabies (killed neural tissue vaccines), vaccinia	Demyelination; pronounced microglial proliferation and lymphoctyic 'cuffing'
Guillain–Barré syndrome	Many viruses, including influenza (vaccine), enteroviruses, Epstein–Barr virus, cytomegalovirus	Polyradiculoneuritis with demyelination, inflammation, and degeneration of nerve roots and ganglia
Reye's syndrome	Influenza B, varicella, adenoviruses	Non-inflammatory encephalopathy; cerebral oedema

Table 30.4 Virus diseases of the central nervous system. Group 3: chronic infections (all rare)

Syndrome	Viruses	Predominant neurological lesions
Subacute sclerosing panencephalitis (SSPE)	Measles, rubella	Neuronal degneration, demyelination, microglial proliferation
Progressive multifocal leucoencephalopathy (PML)	Papovaviruses (JC, very rarely SV40)	Multiple foci of demyelination in brain; hyperplasia of oligodendroglia and astrocytes
Creutzfeldt–Jakob disease (CJD), scrapie, kuru, and other spongiform encephalopathies	Prions	Spongiform degeneration and atrophy of brain and anterior horn cells; astrocytosis

Although the distinction between these two modes of entry is clear enough, we cannot assume that all viruses confine themselves to one or the other. For example, herpes and polioviruses may use either route of infection.

1.1 Viral meningitis

During some virus infections of childhood, notably with **mumps** and some **enteroviruses**, there may be a degree of meningitis indicated by headache, neck rigidity, fever, and sometimes vomiting. In adults, meningitis is also an occasional feature of genital tract infection with HSV type 2. These episodes, although somewhat alarming, usually resolve quickly and have no sequelae. They are often referred to as 'lymphocytic' or 'aseptic' meningitis because of the predominance of lymphocytes in the CSF, although some polymorphs may be present in the early stages. On lumbar puncture, the opening pressure is normal or slightly raised and the fluid is clear, as opposed to the turbid CSF of pyogenic meningitis. There are several hundred cells per ml, the concentration of protein is normal or slightly raised (<100 mg/100 ml) and the sugar > 40 mg/100 ml. The associated virus can usually be isolated from the CSF. It is worth remembering that LCM, an arenavirus, produces a similar clinicopathological picture; it is acquired from animals, usually mice or hamsters, and should come to mind in case of an outbreak of meningitis in laboratory workers handling small rodents. Louping ill is caused by a flavivirus indigenous to the UK and occasionally manifests as meningitis in those in contact with sheep, particularly in northern England and Scotland.

In any case of lymphocytic meningitis the possibility of **tuberculosis** must be thought of, especially if the sugar concentration in the CSF is depressed; failure to diagnose such an infection could be catastrophic. **Leptospirosis** is another non-viral and treatable cause of lymphocytic meningitis.

1.2 Poliomyelitis

The syndromes caused by this virus are described in Chapter 16.

1.3 Meningoencephalitis

Herpes simplex virus infections

By contrast with simple meningitis, usually associated with HSV-2, the much more dangerous meningoencephalitis is nearly always caused by HSV-1 (see Chapter 18). Early diagnosis is important, because treatment at the earliest possible moment with **ACV** considerably reduces both mortality and the incidence of sequelae. Indeed, this drug is often started as soon as a reasonable suspicion of HSV encephalitis arises, without waiting for any test results, but its availability and lack of toxicity must not be allowed to dull alertness to the possibility of a quite different diagnosis. Treatment with ACV must be adequately backed up by intensive care, including energetic measures to reduce intracranial pressure.

The pathological lesions are those of an **acute necrotizing encephalitis**, characteristically most pronounced in the **temporal lobes** and accompanied by intense meningeal inflammation. There is usually severe cerebral oedema, which may mimic the clinical presentation of a space-occupying lesion. This is the classical picture, but less severe cases probably occur that are never correctly diagnosed.

The laboratory diagnosis is made by using one or more of the methods detailed in Table 30.5 to detect:

- specific antibody, antigen, or viral DNA in the CSF;
- virus or viral antigens in a brain biopsy.

Brain biopsy is rapid and definitive and has the additional advantage that it may establish an alternative diagnosis; but its

Table 30.5 Methods for detecting markers of viral infection within the central nervous system

Marker	Specimen	Test
Specific antibody generated within the CNS	Serum/CSF	Antibody – protein ratios
Characteristic inclusion bodies	Brain biopsy	Light microscopy
Replicating virus	Brain biopsy, CSF	Virus isolation PCR
Viral antigen	Brain biopsy	Immunofluorescence
Viral nucleic acid	Brain biopsy	Nucleic acid hybridization, PCR
Histological changes	Brain biopsy	Light microscopy (not specific)
Cytology, protein, sugar (not specific)	CSF	Microscopy, biochemical tests

use is somewhat controversial and is of course not possible in the absence of adequate surgical and laboratory facilities.

Arboviruses

These tropical infections are described in Chapter 27. Meningoencephalitis is a major feature in many of these infections (Table 30.3) but its severity varies considerably and the incidence of sequelae differs according to the virus involved. The clinical features in the acute stage are similar, comprising fever, headache, and meningismus; in severe cases there may be convulsions proceeding to coma and death. Laboratory identification depends on tests for serum antibody, but the diagnosis is usually made on clinical and epidemiological criteria. There is no specific treatment for any of these infections, although vaccines are available for preventing some of them, e.g. Japanese B encephalitis.

1.4 Encephalitis

The only example of a 'pure' encephalitis without meningeal involvement is rabies, which is described in detail in Chapter 26. By contrast with the other infections in this group, which spread to the CNS via the bloodstream, rabies gains access to the cord and brain by migrating up the peripheral nerves serving the site of injury.

1.5 AIDS dementia complex

The neurotropism of HIV was at first overshadowed by the associated intercurrent infections with micro-organisms that may also infect the CNS, such as herpesviruses, mycobacteria, and toxoplasma. It is now realized, however, that this virus is the direct cause of brain damage resulting in a variety of symptoms and signs including particularly psychiatric problems, motor and sensory disturbances (see Chapter 25). These have to be disentangled from the effects of opportunistic infections, so that differential diagnosis depends on the results of careful clinical examination supported by a battery of laboratory tests including computerized tomography of the brain. In AIDS dementia complex, the CSF protein is usually elevated and lymphoctyes may be present; virus can be isolated from the fluid. The histological appearances are summarized in Table 30.2. Viral antigen is detectable in the white matter of the brain and basal ganglia and is associated particularly with multinucleate cells and macrophages.

2 Acute postexposure syndromes (Group 2)
(Table 30.3)

We now come to a group of three syndromes that have three points in common:

- they are each associated with exposure to one of a number of viruses;
- the associated viruses cannot be isolated from the CNS;
- the pathogenesis is obscure.

We have coined the term 'postexposure syndromes' for this group, because they follow exposure to both live and inactivated viruses or viral antigens; the usual expression, 'postinfection' is thus inadequate for the group as a whole.

2.1 Postinfection and postimmunization encephalomyelitis

In 1905, reports started to appear of mysterious paralytic illnesses following immunization with both rabies and smallpox vaccines. The incubation periods were similar and remarkably constant: 14–15 days after the first dose of smallpox vaccine and 10–13 days after smallpox vaccination. Later, it was noticed that there were occasional similar episodes about 2 weeks after onset of the common virus infections of childhood.

It took some time to distinguish these syndromes from other untoward reactions to the vaccines and from the meningitis sometimes associated with the childhood infections described above, both of which tended to occur earlier after immunization or the onset of illness. Eventually however, a clearer picture emerged. The illness following rabies immunization presents either as an ascending Landry-type paralysis with a mortality of about 30%, a more frequent dorsolumbar myelitis with a mortality of about 5%, or a comparatively benign neuritis affecting the cranial nerves. The syndrome associated with smallpox vaccination and the childhood fevers was rather that of meningoencephalitis but in all these conditions the histological appearances are those of **demyelination, microglial proliferation**, and **cuffing** of the blood vessels. It must, however, be pointed out that, although the diagnosis of postimmunization encephalomyelitis is fairly straightforward, the clinical distinction between meningitis complicating the childhood infections and true postinfection encephalomylitis is often blurred.

How frequent are these episodes? This question raises the interesting problem of geographical association. The incidence of postvaccinial encephalitis was notoriously higher in Holland than elsewhere, about 1/4000 vaccinations compared with, for example, 1/50 000 in England and Wales. This difference was not attributable to the strain of vaccinia in use and seemed to depend on some environmental factor that remains totally obscure.

Because it is cheap, rabies vaccine prepared from neural tissue is still widely used in Third World countries. The reported incidences of neuroparalytic episodes are of the same order as those for smallpox vaccine, varying from 1/1000 to 1/10 000 courses of vaccine.

Postinfection encephalomyelitis is most common after **measles**, occurring in perhaps 1/1000 cases; it is less frequent after chickenpox, rubella, and mumps.

Clinical aspects

The onset is often abrupt and is heralded by convulsions or coma. Personality and behavioural changes are frequent and may be followed by any of a wide range of focal neurological signs, mostly motor. The severity varies considerably; the prognosis is poor when coma supervenes and neurological defects following recovery are often severe.

The pathogenesis of these conditions remains a mystery. The neuroparalytic accidents following rabies vaccination occurred with both live attenuated and killed vaccines prepared from the brains of infected animals, but are not associated with modern vaccines made in cell culture, which might suggest that injection of neural tissue is the predisposing factor; and indeed, a similar disease can be induced by injecting rabbits with rabbit brain extract. However, this does not explain the postvaccinial and postinfectious syndromes. As failure to detect the relevant viruses in the CNS seems to rule out any direct effect of viral multiplication, the activation of some unknown latent virus has been suggested, or, more plausibly, that these episodes are the result of an abnormal immune response to the viral antigen.

Apart from identifying the causal infection, laboratory tests are not particularly helpful. The CSF shows the now familiar picture of raised protein, normal sugar, and lymphocytosis. As we have seen, virus cannot be isolated from the CNS in these cases.

2.2 Guillain–Barré syndrome

This is another demyelinating disease that has features in common with the syndromes described in Section 3.1. It differs in affecting the **nerve roots** rather than the substance of the brain and cord and follows exposure to a number of viruses (Table 30.3), which again, need not be live. This was dramatically illustrated by cases of Guillain–Barré syndrome in the USA that followed mass vaccination in 1976 against a newly appeared H1N1 strain of influenza virus (Chapter 10). The incidence of this syndrome was 1 per 100 000 of those vaccinated, four to eight times higher than in the general population. The reason why this inactivated vaccine—and not others prepared subsequently—should have had such dire effects remains a mystery.

In Guillain–Barré syndrome there is no pleocytosis in the CSF, but the protein concentration is well above normal.

2.3 Reye's syndrome

This differs from the postexposure syndrome so far described, as it presents as a **non-inflammatory encephalopathy** with **cerebral oedema** and **fatty degeneration of the liver**. It affects children, in whom the mortality rate is 25–50 per cent. Survivors may have neurological damage. Again, the pathogenesis is unknown, but there has been much discussion, so far unresolved, about the possible role of virus infections, notably influenza B, varicella, and adenoviruses as precipitating factors. It has been suggested that salicylates may also be implicated, especially if given during the course of an influenza B infection. The current advice, which seems sensible, is not to give aspirin to children with febrile illnesses.

3 Chronic infections (Group 3) (Table 30.4)

As with the illnesses in Group 1, the causal agents can be demonstrated in the CNS, but there the resemblance ends

because these syndromes are all very rare and uniformly fatal. Their pathogenesis presents as many puzzles as those just discussed in Group 2.

3.1 Subacute sclerosing panencephalitis

Because of the comparatively young age group affected, its duration, and relentless downhill course, this must surely rank as one of the most distressing virus infections of the CNS. About 7 years after contracting measles (or more rarely, congenital rubella) a child starts to develop neurological signs. At first, there may be nothing more than a slight impairment of movement in one limb or another, or behaviour disorder. Within weeks or months, however, the true nature of the condition becomes apparent, with mental deterioration, myoclonic seizures, spastic paralyses, and blindness. Death occurs within 1–3 years from onset.

The incidence varies with country and with ethnic group. As a very rough guide, there is about 1 case per million of acute measles, but this figure is rather higher in Scandinavia and lower in the UK and USA. Children who acquire measles below the age of 2 years are at greatest risk, and males are more often affected than females.

The pathology is curious. There is generalized encephalitis with the usual cuffing of blood vessels with mononuclear cells. Glial proliferation is pronounced and both glia and neurones contain **inclusion bodies**. These consist of randomly arranged measles virus nucleocapsids, which do not infect cell cultures in the normal way, but can be made to express replicating virus by co-cultivating biopsied brain cells with other cells susceptible to measles infection. **There is a defect in the production of the measles virus M protein** (Chapter 9), which accounts for the difficulty in replication.

The diagnosis is readily confirmed by the finding in the serum of a **high titre of antimeasles antibody, including IgM,** and in the CSF **of measles IgG antibody lacking the normal anti-M component.**

3.2 Progressive multifocal leucoencephalopathy

Patients with lymphoproliferative disorders and other immunosuppressive conditions occasionally develop a progressive and fatal illness with gross intellectual impairment and paralyses. This syndrome is caused by a polyomavirus and is described in Chapter 15.

3.3 Subacute spongiform encephalopathies

These are rare, progressive, uniformly fatal infections that appear to be caused not by true viruses but by prions (proteinaceous infective particles). They are dealt with in Chapter 29.

4 Laboratory diagnosis

It goes without saying that where facilities for electroencephalograms, brain scans, and PCR tests are available they will be brought to bear on the diagnosis of virus diseases of the CNS. The virus laboratory can also make a useful contribution, provided that there is good liaison with the clinicians.

In the first instance, you will need to take:

- throat swabs;
- faecal samples (don't forget the enteroviruses!);
- **paired** CSF and serum samples;
- fluid from any vesicular rash present.

Table 30.5 summarizes the tests used to diagnose virus infections of the CNS

5 Reminders

- Many viruses cause diseases of the CNS, which can be classified in three groups: **acute infections, acute postexposure syndromes**, and **chronic diseases**.

- Virus can usually be demonstrated in the CNS in the acute infections, but not in the **postexposure syndromes**, in which **demyelination** is usually a prominent feature and may result from **an abnormal immune response** to live or inactivated virus.

- The chronic infections are all rare, progressive, and fatal. They include **subacute sclerosing panencephalitis**, a late result of measles infection; **PML**, a polyomavirus infection seen in immunodeficient patients; **Creutzfeld–Jacob disease,** a spongiform encephalopathy seen mostly in elderly patients; and **kuru**, a similar type of infection formerly endemic in a New Guinea tribe and spread by contact with infected human brains.

- The **laboratory diagnosis** of virus diseases of the CNS sometimes demands special techniques, including those for **detecting viruses or their antigens**, and for determining whether **intrathecal synthesis of antibody** is taking place.

Intrauterine and perinatal infections

Of all the distressing situations encountered in medical practice, the loss of a wanted pregnancy or the birth of a malformed infant are among the most poignant; the latter may indeed carry the prospect of many years of misery and hardship for both child and parents. Some of these tragedies are caused by infection with viruses, bacteria, and even protozoa; it must, however, be stressed that **microbial infection is responsible for only a small proportion of the overall total of miscarriages and damaged infants**; in the UK, the incidence of birth defects is about 20 per 1000 live births, or 2 per cent. This background level must be kept in mind before drawing overhasty conclusions about a causal relationship between an infection in pregnancy and an unfavourable outcome. Some virus infections other than those described in this chapter have been suggested as causes of fetal damage, but we feel that the evidence is not strong enough to warrant their inclusion.

The diagnosis of congenital infections has in the last few years been greatly facilitated by ultrasonic examination, the ability to take samples of blood, amniotic fluid, and chorionic villi from the fetus, and the application of the newer laboratory tests such as PCR.

In this chapter the term **intrapartum** refers to events taking place during birth, and **perinatal,** to the period from a week before to a week after delivery.

1 Pathogenesis

The pathogenesis of fetal infections is beset by uncertainties because, more often than not there is no suitable animal model, and there is an obvious difficulty in investigating them in humans. Much of what is written is thus based on inference. In this chapter we shall concentrate as far as possible on what is reasonably certain.

There are two main routes by which intrauterine and intrapartum infections are transmitted. **Transplacental infection** results from a maternal viraemia, and may take place at any time during pregnancy, the outcome depending on the virus concerned. There is little or no evidence that **ascending infection** from the cervix or vagina can penetrate the fetal membranes during pregnancy; but contact infection from these sources can certainly take place during delivery, and is facilitated by a long interval between rupture of the membranes and birth. Table 31.1 shows the ways in which the viruses most frequently implicated in these infections gain access to the embryo or fetus.

Table 31.1 Modes of intrauterine and perinatal viral infections

Virus	Transplacental	During birth	Shortly after birth
Rubella	+ +	−	−
Cytomegalovirus	+	+ +	+ + (BM)
Herpes simplex	+	+ +	+
Varicella-zoster	+ +	+	+
Parvovirus	+ +	−	−
Enteroviruses	+ (Late)	+ +	+ +
Human immunodeficiency virus	+	+ +	+ (BM)
Hepatitis B	+	+ +	+ +
Human papillomaviruses	−	+ +	−

+ +, Most frequent route; +, less frequent route; (BM), can be transmitted via breast milk.

Some of the wide range of effects exerted by viruses on the fetus are shown in Table 31.2. They may be teratogenic, resulting from a CPE during organogenesis in the first trimester of pregnancy, or from virus-mediated damage to organs that have completed their development. In practice, the distinction is often difficult; rubella and CMV are certainly teratogenic but others may or may not act in this way. Viruses, including rubella, can cause apoptosis or genetically controlled cell death.

2 Fetal immunity

The first class of immunoglobulin to be synthesized by the fetus is **IgM**, which becomes detectable at about 13 weeks of gestation and attains ≈10 per cent of the adult concentration by the time of birth. Being a comparatively large molecule, it does not cross the placenta from the maternal circulation; this is also true of IgA, which is not made in significant amounts. The fetus starts to make **IgG** at 17 weeks, but, because its cellular immune system is immature, it cannot make specific antibody in response to an infection. Its only protection—and a very important one—is maternal IgG that reaches it across the placenta. This immunoglobulin of course contains a full complement of the mother's antibodies, and we shall see later in the chapter how it comes into play.

At birth, the infant's own cell-mediated and antibody responses are relatively ineffective and IFN production is poor; however, the maternal antibodies in its circulation are—if the baby is breast fed—supplemented by **IgA antibodies in the colostrum**. These are not absorbed into the bloodstream, but protect the gut against pathogens that gain access by the oral

Table 31.2 Possible adverse outcomes of intrauterine and perinatal viral infections

Virus	Death of embryo/fetus	Clinically apparent disease at or soon after birth	Long-term persistence of infection, with or without clinical signs
Rubella	+	+	+
Cytomegalovirus	?	+	+
Herpes simplex	+	+	+
Varicella-zoster	+	+	+
Parvovirus	+	−	−
Coxsackie B and echoviruses	+	+	−
Human immunodeficiency virus	?	+	+
Hepatitis B	−	−	+
Human papillomaviruses	−	−	+

? = uncertain.

route, a particularly valuable property in areas where hygiene is poor.

3 Specific infections

3.1 Rubella

We mentioned in Chapter 7 the discovery by Gregg in Australia, 65 years ago, of the congenital rubella syndrome. This was the first recognition that fetuses can be damaged by viruses.

Congenital rubella is the result of a **primary** infection of the mother (Chapter 12) during the first 16 weeks of pregnancy. In the absence of maternal antibody, the virus readily crosses the placenta and the time at which this happens is an important factor in determining the outcome. By and large, the earlier in gestation infection takes place, the worse the result; during the first month, the infection rate approaches 100 per cent.

Full-blown congenital rubella—the 'expanded rubella syndrome'—has features in common with those of congenital infections by HSVs, CMV, and toxoplasmosis, a parasitic disease

(Table 31.3). Many systems are affected and the prognosis is very poor. Figure 31.1 gives an idea of the relative frequency of some of the major lesions; the chart is compiled from figures obtained during a major epidemic of rubella in New York during 1964, well before the introduction of rubella vaccine. It shows, for example, that of 106 infants born after their mothers contracted rubella during the second month of pregnancy, only five (4.7 per cent) were clinically normal; 58 per cent had defects of the cardiovascular system or CNS; 29 per cent had eye defects (Fig. 31.2); and 72 per cent were later shown to have sensorineural deafness. Clearly, the inner ear is susceptible to damage over a longer period than the cardiovascular system or CNS. It is interesting that the curve for clinically normal infants is a mirror image of that for deafness, perhaps implying that aural damage is the lesion best correlated with infection *in utero*.

Latent defects

Some infants who appear normal at birth are later discovered to have hearing defects, with or without some degree of mental retardation. Prenatal infection often results in prolonged

Table 31.3 Most frequent physical signs of severe congenital rubella, cytoplasmic inclusion disease, herpes simplex, and toxoplasmosis*

Defects	Expanded rubella syndrome	Cytomegalic inclusion disease	Generalized herpes simplex	Toxoplasmosis
Low birth weight	+	+		+
Hepatosplenomegaly, jaundice	+	+	+	+
Thrombocytopenia, petechiae, purpura	+	+		
Skin vesicles			+	
Microcephaly	+	+		
Intracranial calcifications		+		+
Hydrocephalus				+
Meningitis, encephalitis			+	
Pneumonitis				+
Cataracts	+			
Choroidoretinitis	+	+		+
Patent ductus arteriosis, lesions of pulmonary artery and aorta	+			
Bone defects	+			
Sensorineural deafness, speech defects, mental retardation[†]	+	+		
Insulin-dependent diabetes mellitus[†]	+			

* All these infections, when severe, involve many body systems. A blank does not necessarily mean that the relevant defect is *never* present. The table aims to show only the most important associations.

[†] Late signs, becoming apparent months or years after birth.

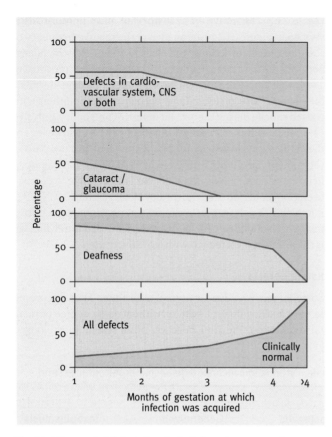

Fig. 31.1 Congenital defects in rubella-infected neonates. Data simplified from Cooper, Z. *et al.* (1969). *American Journal of Diseases of Childhood*, **118**, 18. The incidences of cardiovascular and CNS defects at the various stages of gestation were almost identical, and have been combined.

excretion of virus from the throat, a source of infection for susceptible contacts. Progressive subacute sclerosing encephalitis is a late and fortunately very rare complication.

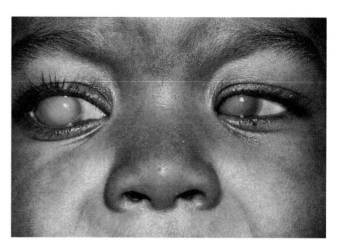

Fig. 31.2 Congenital rubella syndrome: bilateral cataracts in a 5-month-old baby (right). (Courtesy of the late Dr W. Marshall.)

Preconceptual rubella

An Anglo-German study showed no evidence of intrauterine infection in women who had rubella rashes before, or up to 11 days after, their last menstrual period.

Rubella immunization during pregnancy

There have been many instances of inadvertent vaccination against rubella during early pregnancy, followed by termination for fear of possible fetal damage by the live vaccine virus (Fig. 31.3). Although vaccine virus has been isolated from aborted products of conception, there is no evidence, from such pregnancies allowed to go to term, of rubella-associated defects, and termination should not be recommended on this ground. The figure also shows the diminishing rate of abortions undertaken because of rubella in pregnancy, or fear of its consequences.

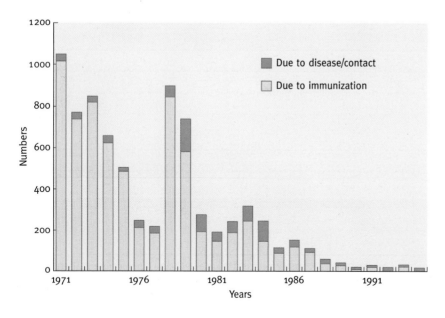

Fig. 31.3 Rubella terminations due to disease/contact or immunization, England and Wales (1971–94). (Reproduced with permission for Department of Health (1996). *Immunisation Against Infectious Disease*, p. 194. HMSO, London.)

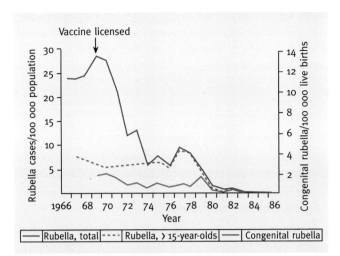

Fig. 31.4 **Effect of immunization on incidence of congenial rubella.** (Adapted from data in (1988) *Morbidity and Mortality Weekly Report*, **36**, 664.)

Incidence of congenital rubella

Figure 31.4 shows that, following the introduction of immunization in 1970, the incidence of congenital rubella in the UK is now very small; nevertheless, continued vigilance is needed to prevent these disastrous infections.

Diagnosis of the mother

Because the clinical diagnosis of rubella is not always easy, laboratory tests are essential as a guide to the important decisions that must be made following a history of contact with rubella, or of a rubella-like illness, within the first trimester of pregnancy. **Tests for specific anti-rubella IgM and IgG antibodies** are made (Chapters 18 and 36), and action is taken according to the scheme shown in Fig. 31.5. **These tests must**

be done irrespective of a history of past immunization, which is not always reliable.

The plan looks a little complicated, but is in fact quite logical; it is based on:

- the time course of the appearance of IgM and IgG antibodies; and
- the possible results of tests, arranged according to whether they are first done during, or outside the extreme ranges of the incubation period of rubella (10–21 days). There is one trap to beware. In addition to a known contact, say 14 days previously, there may have been another unsuspected contact some days later; if this seems a possibility, weekly tests for IgM antibody should be continued until the end of the longest possible incubation period has passed.

Diagnosis of the neonate

Congenital rubella is normally diagnosed by demonstrating **specific IgM antibody** in the cord or peripheral blood.

Virus isolation is used only for confirming a diagnosis of prenatal rubella by testing the tissues of an aborted fetus and monitoring the shedding of virus from a congenitally infected baby. Specimens are inoculated into Vero or RK 13 cells. Provided the culture conditions are properly controlled, a CPE is seen several days later; its specificity should be confirmed by immunofluorescence staining or by further passage in cell cultures. It is also possible to demonstrate viral RNA with a PCR test.

3.2 Cytomegalovirus

The epidemiology and pathogenesis of fetal rubella are relatively straightforward. The behaviour of CMV is much more complex. Infection of the fetus may take place *in utero* or in the perinatal period.

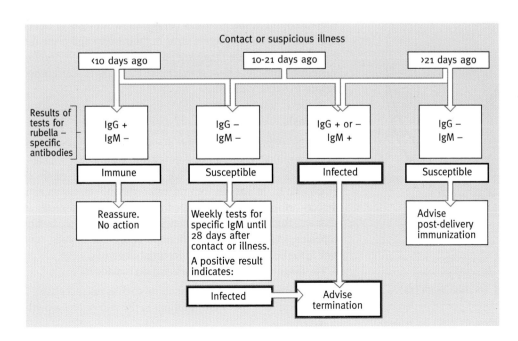

Fig. 31.5 Action following exposure to rubella in early pregnancy.

Risk of maternal infection

CMV infection is widespread, its prevalence being highest where living standards are low (Chapter 19). On average, one might expect 60–70 per cent of women of childbearing age to have serological evidence of infection. Again on average, 1–2 per cent of seronegative pregnant women have primary infections during their pregnancy. An ill-defined proportion of people undergo periodic reactivations; and something like 10 per cent of pregnant women excrete CMV in their urine at some time during pregnancy.

Risk of fetal infection

Primary maternal infection

Transmission is thought to take place as a result of maternal viraemia, followed by transplacental spread. As might be expected, the effects on the fetus are usually more serious if transmission takes place during a primary infection, and the earlier in gestation that transmission occurs, the worse the outcome for the fetus; those infected late in pregnancy tend to be born with inapparent infections. The risk of damage to the fetus as a result of primary infection in pregnancy is about 40 per cent.

Recurrent maternal infection

Unlike rubella, transmission of CMV to the fetus takes place even in strongly seropositive women, perhaps because the virus travels within leucocytes and is to some extent sheltered from the effects of antibody. It is well known that an infected woman can give birth to damaged infants in successive pregnancies. The risk to the fetus following a recurrent infection is, however, less than 2 per cent.

Figure 31.6 shows that of fetuses infected *in utero*:

- about 1 per cent die at or soon after birth with severe congenital defects;
- 4 per cent have severe cytomegalic disease;
- 15 per cent appear normal but hearing defects and perhaps some degree of mental retardation become apparent later;
- the remaining 80 per cent are clinically normal but are liable to be persistently infected.

It has been estimated that of 700 000 live infants born annually in the UK, about 2000 are congenitally infected with CMV; of these, approximately 200 are significantly damaged, making this infection a much greater hazard than congenital rubella now is.

Cytomegalic inclusion disease

This term is applied to the syndrome seen in infants born with the severe defects characteristic of CMV infection acquired early in pregnancy. It is a devastating generalized infection, liable to affect every system; Table 31.3 shows the most frequent abnormalities, but cardiovascular, gastrointestinal, and muscular defects also occur. The prognosis is poor, and some infants die shortly after birth.

Latent defects

In a small proportion of infected infants who appear normal at birth, hearing defects become apparent in early childhood; they may be associated with a degree of mental retardation.

Inapparent infection

The great majority of infected neonates (Fig. 31.6), notably those infected in the perinatal period, show no signs of infection, but continue to excrete virus in their saliva and urine for months or even years. They are potent sources of infection for susceptible people in close contact with them, particularly other infants in nursery schools.

Diagnosis

Clinically, cytomegalic inclusion disease must be distinguished from congenital rubella and toxoplasmosis, with both of which—particularly toxoplasmosis—it has many features in common (Table 31.3). In rubella, central cataracts and cardiovascular defects are particularly noteworthy, whereas toxoplasmosis is characterized by the high frequency of choroidoretinitis, hydrocephalus, and intracranial calcification. Congenital syphilis, now rare in the UK, also enters the differential diagnosis.

The diagnosis of intrauterine infection is made by

- **ultrasonography** for abnormalities such as microcephaly, calcifications, and necrotic lesions in the viscera and growth retardation;

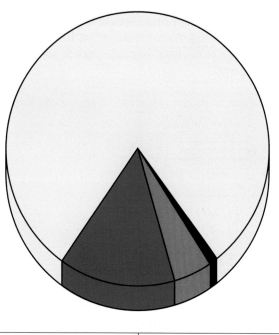

| Clinically normal, but liable to excrete CMV (80%) | Severe abnormalities (4%) |
| Hearing defects/mental retardation (15%) | Perinatal death (1%) |

Fig. 31.6 Clinical outcomes of cytomegalovirus infection *in utero*.

- detection of **specific IgM antibody** in the amniotic fluid;
- **detection of virus** in amniotic fluid and blood.

Prevention

As the vast majority of CMV infections in adults are silent, there is no practicable way of knowing if or when a susceptible woman becomes infected while pregnant; and even if there were, the position is complicated by the liability of recurrent infections to be transmitted to the fetus, and by uncertainty as to the outcome if this does happen. Under these circumstances, advice as to termination of pregnancy is fraught with difficulty.

Is it possible to immunize against CMV? A vaccine prepared from the Towne strain of CMV gave encouraging results in protecting renal allograft recipients, but in another study the antibody responses in women in contact with young children in group care were much lower than those resulting from natural infection. Furthermore, there are uncertainties about the advisability of large-scale immunization with a herpesvirus vaccine, so far an unknown quantity in humans.

Treatment of infected mothers with antivirals, e.g. ganciclovir, is now under investigation.

3.3 Herpes simplex viruses

In the past, neonatal infections were almost always caused by HSV-2, but the increasing proportion of HSV-1—now about 40 per cent—reflects its greater prevalence in genital infections. Infants usually acquire the virus during passage through the birth canal, although there are reports of a few infants born with severe defects who must have become infected *in utero*. Signs of intrapartum infection become apparent within a few days of birth; they range from a few trivial skin vesicles to massive and mostly fatal infections involving the brain, liver (Fig. 31.7), and other viscera. In these infants, the clinical picture is similar to those of rubella and CMV (Table 31.3), but is characterized by

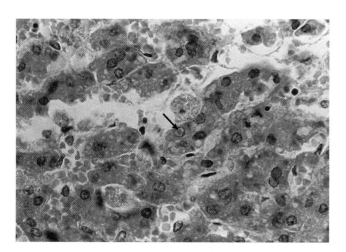

Fig. 31.7 Generalized congenital herpes simplex. Section of liver showing damaged hepatocytes, some of which contain intranuclear herpes inclusions. The clear halo (arrowed) surrounding the inclusion is characteristic.

vesicles in which herpes virions can readily be detected. The reported incidence of such massive infections varies from country to country; and is significantly higher in the USA than elsewhere. However, the small number of cases diagnosed overall bears no relation to the number of women who must be infected. This may well be because mothers who have been infected for some time possess IgG antibody that crosses the placenta and protects the infant at birth. One would thus anticipate danger if a mother acquires a **primary** genital infection (Chapter 18) too late in pregnancy to have formed antibody by the time of delivery. Recognition of this situation demands Caesarean section.

Diagnosis and management

Pregnant women who undergo a **primary** infection with genital herpes near the time of delivery should be offered Caesarean section. Those with a past history should be swabbed every week from the 36th week until term to detect a **recurrence**: Caesarean section should be performed in the case of a positive result near the time of delivery, or if herpetic lesions are visible in the maternal genital tract. **Infants** born to mothers with known HSV infection should be checked carefully during the first week, and swabbed from the nose, mouth, and skin. The appearance of herpetic vesicles dictates immediate treatment with ACV (Chapters 18 and 38).

Although ACV is not licensed for use in pregnancy, treatment of the mother should certainly be considered if she develops a primary infection in the later months.

The TORCH screen

This is a group of laboratory tests sometimes requested for neonates in whom there is any suspicion of a congenital infection with the viruses discussed so far. TORCH is an acronym for *TO*xoplasmosis, *R*ubella, *C*MV, and *H*erpes simplex. A glance at Table 31.3 shows how many features these infections have in common; but such blanket requests are not very popular with laboratory staff, as a careful history and clinical examination often rules out one or more of these infections, making some or all of the tests redundant.

3.4 Varicella-zoster

Of the herpesviruses that infect the fetus, VZV is fortunately the most rare; fortunately, because chickenpox in the mother during the first half of pregnancy may result in the birth of an infant with **severe scarring of the skin**—a particularly characteristic feature—often associated with limb malformations and lesions of the eye and CNS. Infections of this type probably result from maternal viraemia. More often, a mother who acquires varicella around the time of delivery transmits it to her infant *in utero*; if birth takes place less than 5 days after the maternal rash, the infant is liable to have a severe infection, with a fatality rate of up to 30 per cent. If the interval is 5 days or more, the infection is milder, probably because the mother has developed antibody and passed it to the fetus. Occasionally, latent infection of the infant may be established, resulting in shingles a year or two later.

By contrast with chickenpox, mothers suffering from an attack of herpes zoster around the time of delivery do not appear to transmit VZV to their infants.

Diagnosis and management

Diagnosis is based on the distinctive vesicles, in which herpesvirus virions can be found by EM, and by the appearance in the maternal and neonatal blood of specific antibody. Although ACV is not as yet licensed for use in pregnant women, there is no evidence that it harms the fetus, and its use should be considered if the mother develops severe varicella or zoster at any stage of pregnancy. Neonates born within the perinatal period who have not yet developed a rash may be given prophylactic ZIG (Chapters 18 and 37), or ACV if a rash does appear.

In hospitals, appropriate precautions must be taken to prevent cross-infection to susceptible patients and staff.

3.5 Parvovirus

Although parvovirus B19 (Chapter 13) can cross the placenta, the evidence to date does not suggest that it is teratogenic in the same way as rubella or CMV. As in postnatal infections, the target cells are erythroid precursor cells. The consequent depletion of red cells, coupled with a shortened life span, may lead to **fetal loss** or **hydrops fetalis**. Prospective studies in the UK and Germany suggest an excess rate of fetal loss of ≈10 per cent. There are a few reports of fatal hydrops fetalis following infection later in gestation, but this condition is not usually fatal for the fetus. If severe, as diagnosed by ultrasonic examination, **transfusion of the fetus with concentrated erythrocytes** may be beneficial. As fetuses that survive the infection are not damaged there is no indication for advising termination. Needless to say, however, women with signs of parvovirus infection who know or suspect that they are pregnant must be rigorously tested to exclude rubella, which may be circulating in the community at the same time and has a similar incubation period; two such outbreaks in the UK were due to echovirus 11.

3.6 Human immunodeficiency virus

The decades since the start of the AIDS pandemic in 1981 have seen an accumulation of reports of unfortunate infants infected before, during, or shortly after birth by seropositive mothers, not all of whom had overt infection. We still lack detailed knowledge of modes of transmission and pathogenesis; so far, it seems that roughly 20 per cent of infected mothers transmit HIV to their infants at birth, the outcome varying from a silent infection to full-blown AIDS within the next 2 years.

The Public Health Laboratory Health Service stated that to the end of January 1997 there were reports of more than 700 HIV-infected children in the UK, of whom over 30 per cent had AIDS. Of the 700, 55 per cent had acquired the infection from their mothers, compared with 40 per cent contracting it from blood products. HIV can cross the placenta in early pregnancy, but the main mode of transmission seems to be during labour, or by breast-feeding. The great majority of congenital infections are due to HIV-1 rather than HIV-2.

Management

The risk of congenital infection can be reduced by:

- Caesarean section or delivery not later than 4 hours after rupture of the membranes;
- chemotherapy of mother and infant with antiviral agents such as HIV protease inhibitors;
- avoidance of breast-feeding.

3.7 Enteroviruses

Polioviruses, coxsackieviruses, and echoviruses are able to cross the placenta in late pregnancy, but the more usual mode of infection is during birth.

Poliovirus infection during pregnancy is now very rare in well immunized populations. The virus can cross the placenta and may cause abortion. The results of infection at term range from mild febrile illness to neurological deficits similar to those seen in later life. Although live polio vaccine is not advised in pregnancy, there is no evidence that it actually damages the fetus; termination should not be suggested on the ground of inadvertent vaccination.

Group A coxsackieviruses rarely affect the newborn. **Coxsackie B viruses**, on the other hand, may cause severe myocarditis, encephalitis, or a sepsis-like illness, which must be distinguished from a bacterial infection.

Echoviruses usually give rise to respiratory or gastrointestinal disease. Severe multisystem disease, affecting particularly the CNS and liver, has also been reported;

3.8 Hepatitis E

For some unexplained reason, the attack rate of this predominantly water-borne infection is much higher in pregnant than in non-pregnant women. Furthermore, the mortality rate is about 20 per cent, about 20 times higher than in non-pregnant women and men.. Fulminant hepatitis is most likely to develop during the third trimester, and limited observations in India suggest a high probability of maternal infections contracted at this time being passed to the fetus, with consequent abortion or perinatal death from hepatitis. It remains to be seen whether this pattern is confirmed by study of larger series.

3.9 Hepatitis B

HBV infection is not acquired *in utero*, but its perinatal transmission plays a major part in perpetuating the infection in highly endemic areas, and is therefore described in Chapter 22.

Table 31.4 Congenital infections of limited clinical importance

Virus	Possible effects on the fetus or neonate
Human papillomaviruses	HPV-6 and -11 may be transmitted to the neonate during delivery, and in later years give rise to benign laryngeal papillomas
Hepatitis C	Histological and biochemical evidence of hepatitis; long-term effects unknown
Lymphocytic choriomeningitis	The few published studies suggest that infection in early pregnancy may cause hydrocephalus and severe ocular defects
Influenza A	Circumstantial evidence suggests that some clusters of abortions and stillbirths are associated with outbreaks of influenza A

3.10 Other viruses

Table 31.4 lists a few other congenital viral infections concerning which information is scanty, or which occur too seldom to merit detailed descriptions.

4 Reminders

- A number of viruses can seriously damage the fetus or neonate; with some, transmission via the **placenta** is the usual mode of infection, whereas others predominantly infect the baby during or shortly after delivery (**perinatal infection**).

- Some viruses—notably rubella and CMV—infecting the mother during early pregnancy are **teratogenic**, i.e. they interfere with organogenesis; these and others can also damage organs and tissues that are already formed.

- Because the immune system of the fetus and neonate is immature, **maternal IgG antibodies** transported across the placenta and **IgA antibodies** in colostrum and breast milk are important protective factors.

- The adverse effects of most intrauterine viral infections include **fetal death, severe disease in the neonate** affecting a number of body systems, and **persistent postnatal infections**, with or without overt illness. Persistent but silent antigenaemia is an important aspect of perinatal HBV infection transmitted by carrier mothers.

- **Primary** infections of the mother with **rubella, CMV**, and **HSV** are more likely to damage the fetus than are reinfections or reactivations.

- The finding of **specific IgM antibody** is used to diagnose recent rubella in the mother; and, because it does not cross the placenta, **IgM antibody in the cord or peripheral blood** is a good indicator of infection of the neonate by rubella and other viruses.

Chapter 32

Viral infections in patients with defective immunity

1 Introduction

In the preceding chapters there are many examples of the damage that can be wrought in otherwise healthy people by viruses despite the formidable battery of immune responses normally mounted against them. Much worse then is the plight of those unfortunates who lack the ability to respond adequately to microbial invasion. The problem is compounded by the fact that some viruses themselves impair immunity by damaging the cells that mediate immune responses. To put it briefly:

impaired immunity ⟷ some virus infections

There are many types of immune defect, resulting in infection with all sorts of microbes, but here we must concentrate on those relating to viruses.

The immunodeficiencies fall under the following main headings:

1. **primary**, or congenital;

2. **acquired**:
   - secondary to other diseases (including some virus infections);
   - secondary to various treatments for other conditions ('iatrogenic').

Of these, the acquired or secondary forms are much more often encountered than the congenital varieties.

2 Primary immunodeficiencies

Although these syndromes are comparatively rare, more than 20 varieties are listed. For practical purposes, however, we can classify them in two main groups (Table 32.1): **those predominantly involving B cells and hence immunoglobulin and antibody production**; and others **mainly affecting T cells and hence CMI**. However, as we showed in Chapter 5, there is an intimate relationship between these two major arms of the immune system, and in a number of syndromes both are involved to varying degrees. We shall here consider only those in which virus infections play a significant part.

Table 32.1 Primary immunodeficiencies predisposing to virus infections

Predominantly affecting B cells and antibody production	Predominantly affecting T cells and cell-mediated immunity
Agammaglobulinaemia or hypogammaglobulinaemia (X-linked or) rarely, autosomal recessive trait)	Severe combined immunodeficiencies
Common variable immunodeficiencies (late onset)	Thymic aplasia (DiGeorge's syndrome) Purine nucleoside phosphorylase deficiency
Selective immunoglobulin deficiencies	Lymphoproliferative syndrome with unusual response to EB virus Interferon deficiencies (α and γ)

2.1 Deficiencies predominantly affecting B cells and antibody production (Table 32.1)

Agammaglobulinaemia (or more often hypogammaglobulinaemia, as small amounts of immunoglobulin are usually detectable), presents between the ages of 6 and 24 months, at a time when the infant has lost its complement of maternal antibodies; its abnormal susceptibility to infection, usually bacterial but sometimes viral, is often the alarm that triggers investigation of its immune system. One variety is X-linked, affecting only males; a family history of severe infections in male infants is a good diagnostic pointer. More rarely, the trait is autosomal recessive. **The defect is a failure of maturation of B cells**; T-cell function is normal. Replacement therapy with intravenous immunoglobulin is useful.

The **common variable immunodeficiencies** are also characterized by defective production of immunoglobulins but as the name implies, the faults in lymphocyte production are diverse, involving B cells and T-cell subsets in varying degrees. These syndromes are **late in onset**, usually presenting in young adults of both sexes; they are often familial. The patients often suffer from bacterial infections of the respiratory tract, intestinal giardiasis, and pernicious anaemia.

There is also a variety of **selective immunoglobulin deficiencies**, most often affecting production of IgA; people with this defect are usually healthy, although some of them get frequent respiratory infections. Defects in IgM and IgG production have also been reported.

2.2 Deficiencies predominantly affecting T cells and cell-mediated immunity (Table 32.1)

Severe combined immunodeficiency syndromes occur in young children and may be X-linked, or autosomal recessive, affecting both sexes. They carry a high mortality, death being frequently due to fulminating bacterial or virus infections. They

are associated with abnormalities of the thymus and thus of T-cell development, but antibody production is also defective.

Thymic aplasia due to a developmental failure of the third and fourth pouches (**DiGeorge's syndrome**) is not so serious; these children too may be predisposed to virus infections, particularly with CMV, but in many instances there is spontaneous recovery of T-cell production. They often respond well to fetal thymus and bone marrow grafting.

Purine nucleosidase phosphorylase deficiency is a rare condition resulting from a structural defect in chromosome 14; the end result of absence of the enzyme is impairment of T-cell function and these children often die from overwhelming herpesvirus infections.

At least in the Western world, infection with **EBV** is not normally dangerous. There is, however, a rare T-cell defect, usually but not invariably X-linked, which impairs the immune response to this virus; such patients develop a range of potentially fatal syndromes including severe mononucleosis, B-cell lymphomas, bone marrow aplasia, and agammaglobulinaemia.

In some people, possibly several per cent of the population, there are **defects in production of IFN-α or IFN-γ**, i.e. the varieties produced in T cells. There is some evidence that such persons are unusually prone to respiratory and herpesvirus infections; a more serious situation arises if they are unlucky enough to contract hepatitis B, as they are then liable to become chronic carriers (see Chapter 22).

2.3 Virus infections associated with primary immunodeficiencies (Table 32.2)

In Chapter 4, Section 3.2, we mentioned briefly that the sort of cytopathogenic effect induced by a virus gives a clue to its behaviour in relation to the immune responses: lytic viruses (the 'bursters'), e.g. the enteroviruses, are influenced more by antibody, whereas the 'creepers', notably the enveloped agents such as herpes-, myxo-, and paramyxoviruses, are controlled more by CMI. Table 32.2 shows that the immune deficiency syndromes illustrate this point rather well.

B-cell defects are associated particularly with **enterovirus** and occasionally **rotavirus** infections. Poliomyelitis is especi-

Table 32.2 Virus infections associated with primary immunodeficiencies

Defect	Infections
B cells	Polioviruses (natural infection and live vaccine): paralysis Enteroviruses: encephalomyelitis, myositis Rotaviruses
T cells	Myxo- and paramyxoviruses Herpesviruses Papillomaviruses
Interferon	Respiratory viruses Herpesviruses

ally dangerous, with a high rate of paralysis; inadvertent immunization with the live vaccine is also liable to cause paralysis. According to the serotype, echoviruses may cause severe meningoencepalitis or myositis and rotavirus infection may persist for long periods, with chronic diarrhoea and shedding of virus.

That impairment of T-cell activity and CMI opens the way for the 'creeper' viruses. was dramatically illustrated when smallpox vaccine was widely used; children with agammaglobulinaemia but with intact CMI responded normally, whereas those who also had defective T-cell function developed generalized vaccinia, which often proved fatal. In **measles**, impaired CMI may result in a life-threatening infection characterized by absence of rash and giant cell pneumonitis. Nowadays, the main danger to such patients in Western countries is from chronic and occasionally generalized infections with **parainfluenza and influenza; herpesviruses**, particularly CMV and varicellazoster (Fig. 32.1) are also a threat.

A rare condition in which CMI is greatly depressed, epidermodysplasia verruciformis, is particularly associated with papillomavirus infections causing warts, which in these patients may become malignant (see Chapter 15).

3 Acquired immunodeficiencies secondary to other diseases and their treatment (Table 32.3)

Some **malignancies**, notably those of the blood and lymphoreticular system, are notorious for impairing the immune response and increasing susceptibility to virus infections. Paradoxically, this problem has in recent years been enhanced by the successful use of drug and radiation therapy given both for their direct cytotoxic effects on the tumour cells and as a preliminary to bone marrow transplant (BMT) for leukaemia; such treatments are profoundly immunosuppressive, a property that is also exploited to prevent rejection of transplanted solid organs such as the kidney.

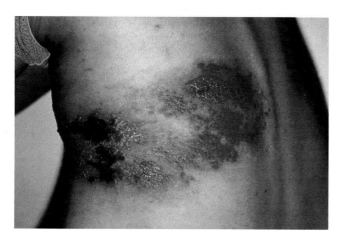

Fig. 32.1 Herpes zoster in an immunosuppressed child. In addition to the characteristic dermatomal distribution, there are vesicular lesions elsewhere on the chest and abdomen.

Table 32.3 Acquired immunodeficiencies

Immunodeficiency secondary to	
Other illnessess	Treatment
Malignancies, especially of blood and lymphoreticular system	Cytotoxic and immunosuppressive drugs and irradiation for tumour therapy or to prevent transplant rejection
Renal failure/dialysis AIDS Measles/malnutrition	

Certain **virus infections** are themselves immunosuppressive. The prime example, and the one best understood, is that of the **human immunodeficiency viruses**, which destroy T-helper cells and thus open the door to so-called opportunistic infections by a variety of microbes. As well as being a hazard to the immunocompromised patient, **CMV** is itself immunosuppressive and may facilitate reactivation of other herpesviruses. That infection with **measles virus** impairs CMI is well known and is neatly demonstrated by the failure of tuberculin to induce a delayed hypersensitivity skin reaction in positive subjects tested within 3 weeks of being given live measles vaccine. The opposite side of this coin is the observation in African children that malnutrition depresses CMI and thus delays recovery from measles.

Table 32.4 gives an idea of the relative frequency and severity of various virus infections in the main categories of immunodeficiency; but remember that although such infections figure most prominently in the column headed 'Primary defects', these conditions are much more rare than those resulting from disease or therapy.

Types of infection

First and foremost it is the **T lymphocytes** that are suppressed, immediately suggesting that infections with herpes and other 'creeper' viruses will dominate the scene. That this is so is apparent from Tables 32.4 and 32.5. Other viruses often infecting immunosuppressed patients include **adenoviruses**, which often cause respiratory and enteric infections, and **papillomaviruses**, which may give rise to persistent warts. **Progressive multifocal leucencephalopathy** is a demyelinating disease occasionally seen in older patients whose immunity is impaired by malignant disease or cytotoxic treatment. It is caused by the JC strain of **polyomavirus** and is uniformly fatal (Chapter 15).

4 Some special problems (Table 32.5)

Many severe virus infections are associated with immunodeficiencies due to malignant disease and cytotoxic therapy and are thus particularly likely to be encountered in hospital practice.

Table 32.4 Relative frequency and severity of virus infections in different immunodeficiency states

Virus infection	Immunodeficiency due to				
	Primary defects	Solid tumours	Haematological malignances	Cytotoxic treatment	AIDS
Herpes simplex	+ +	+	+ +	+ +	+ +
Varicella	+ + +	+ +	+ + +	+ +	
Herpes zoster		+	+ +	+ +	+ +
Cytomegalovirus	+ +	+	+	+ + +	+ + +
Epstein–Barr virus	+ + +			+ +	
Myxo- and paramyxoviruses	+ +		+ +		
Adenoviruses				+ +	+ +
Enteroviruses	+ + +	r	r	r	
Rotaviruses	+ +				
Papovaviruses	+ +			+ +	+

Based in part on data from Wong, D.T. and Ogra, P.L. (1983). *Medical Clinics of North America*, **67**, 1075–93.

+ + +, very common and often severe; + +, common, moderately severe; +, infrequent or mild; r, rare.

Table 32.5 Virus infections associated with malignancies, transplants, and related cytotoxic treatment

Virus	Remarks
Herpesviruses	
Herpes simplex	Severe local infection Encephalitis Occasional generalization
Chickenpox	In children ⎫ **Pneumonitis**
Herpes zoster	In adults ⎭
Cytomegalovirus	Primary infection (from transplant); more often reactivation. **Pneumonitis**
Epstein–Barr virus	Occasional B-cell lymphoma, especially after renal allograft
Other viruses	
Adenoviruses	Gastrointestinal and respiratory infections
Myxo- and paramyxoviruses	Persistent influenza, parainfluenza, and respiratory syncytial virus infections
Papillomaviruses	Persistent warts
Polyomavirus (JC)	Progressive multifocal leucoencephalopathy in older immunosuppressed patients

4.1 Renal failure and long-term dialysis

The antibody responses of these patients are intact but CMI is depressed. The main danger used to be hepatitis B, acquired from blood transfusions: the initial infection was often mild, but often developed into the carrier state, so that hepatitis B was endemic in dialysis units. Screening of blood donors for hepatitis B and C and the institution of rigorous safety procedures has for practical purposes eliminated this problem in the UK, but it still exists in some countries. Circumstances occasionally make it necessary for a patient normally resident in the UK to be dialysed abroad; caution is needed when making such arrangements, first to protect the individual, who must be given hepatitis B vaccine, and second to protect the home dialysis unit against the possibility of importation of infection when the patient is readmitted.

4.2 Renal transplant patients

In addition to the immunosuppression resulting from chronic renal failure, renal transplant patients are subject to other hazards.

1. **Immunosuppressive drugs** such as azathioprine and cyclosporin. A designed to prevent graft rejection enhance both susceptibility to new infections and reactivation of latent herpesviruses.

2. **CMV infection** presents special problems. From 50 to 80 per cent of adults are infected with this agent and the risks to transplant patients are twofold:
   - reactivation of a latent infection;
   - acquisition of the virus by a seronegative (i.e. non-immune) recipient from a seropositive (i.e. infected) donor either of transfused blood or of the kidney itself; in the case of blood, the virus appears to be transferred in the granulocytes.

Active CMV infection can be demonstrated in the great majority of these patients within the first 6 months after transplant. It may not cause overt illness and is then recognized only by laboratory tests. On the other hand it may give rise to an episode of fever, glomerulonephritis with graft rejection, hepatitis, or worst of all pneumonitis, which carries a mortality of over 80 per cent and is the main cause of death in renal transplant recipients. Fortunately, this complication occurs only in a small minority of cases.

Prevention of cytomegalovirus infection

Ideally, seronegative recipients of renal and other allografts should receive organs from seronegative donors, but this is not always feasible. Another approach now being tried is prior immunization of seronegative recipients with an experimental CMV vaccine; the evidence so far suggests that this procedure may not prevent subsequent CMV infections but diminishes their severity.

A substantial proportion of renal transplant patients start to excrete polyomavirus (usually the BK strain but sometimes JC) in their urine a few weeks after operation. These infections are usually reactivations; they are nearly always subclinical, but occasionally cause temporary depression of kidney function.

4.3 Malignancies of the blood and lymphoreticular systems

The immune responses of patients with malignant diseases of the blood and lymphoreticular systems are impaired even in the absence of treatment. Their susceptibility to infection is increased even more by the intense chemotherapy and irradiation preceding allogeneic **BMT**, during which the cells of the immune system—B and T lymphocytes, macrophages and other APCs—are virtually destroyed, to be replaced eventually by donor cells. This situation is obviously fraught with danger; and particularly in view of the successes now being obtained in the

treatment of children with acute lymphoblastic leukaemia, it is a tragedy to lose such a patient as a result of infection. Infections with herpesviruses, mostly due to reactivation, are a particular problem.

Herpes simplex virus

HSV is usually the first to reactivate with a peak at about 2 weeks. Dissemination is unusual, but in bone marrow recipients the local lesions may be very extensive. If HSV infection threatens, it can be prevented or modified with ACV.

Epstein–Barr virus

EBV reactivates in about 50 per cent of patients but does not usually cause significant illness, although EBV-associated lymphomas have been reported.

Primary infection with varicella-zoster virus

VZV is a serious hazard in leukaemic children, whether or not they have had BMTs. Reactivations cause herpes zoster in about 50 per cent of BMT recipients and may disseminate like chickenpox. **Pneumonitis** is a serious complication but can be treated with ACV.

Cytomegalovirus

CMV infections pose the major threat to BMT patients, who are at greater risk than recipients of solid organs: **interstitial pneumonitis**, with a mortality rate of 80–90 per cent, occurs in about a third of them. As the treatment of these infections with antiviral drugs is relatively ineffective, other measures must be employed.

- **Frequent monitoring for CMV reactivation by tests giving rapid results** is important, as timely modification of the immunosuppressive regimen may help to reduce the severity of infection.

- Administration of **anti-CMV immunoglobulin** to seronegative patients before and after BMT has been claimed to reduce the infection rate.

- A different approach has shown promising results. Workers in the UK found that immunization of donor marrow cells *in vitro* with tetanus toxoid or hepatitis B vaccine results in adoptive transfer to the recipient of B-cell responses to these antigens. They then showed that the incidence of CMV pneumonitis was significantly reduced in seropositive recipients receiving marrow from seropositive donors. A possible explanation is that B stem cells from the donor, which are already primed to produce CMV antibody, are stimulated to do so when exposed to CMV antigen in the recipient.

Asymptomatic infections with polyomaviruses

Asymptomatic infections with polyomaviruses also occur, and are similar to those in renal transplant patients (Section 4.2).

Contact with cases of measles or chickenpox

Contact with cases of measles or chickenpox is a particular hazard for leukaemic children who are not already immune as both viruses can give rise to giant cell pneumonitis with high mortal-

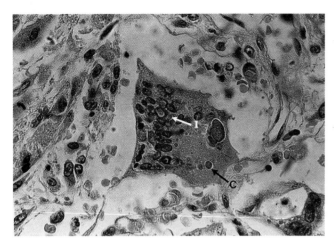

Fig. 32.2 Section of lung from measles pneumonitis. Note giant cell containing intranuclear (I) and cytoplasmic (C) inclusions (arrowed).

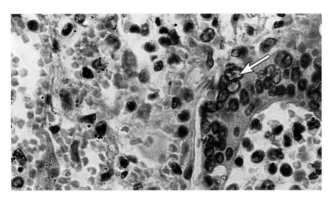

Fig. 32.3 Section of lung from varicella-zoster pneumonitis. By contrast with the measles giant cells (Fig. 32.2), the inclusions (arrowed) are all intranuclear.

ity rates (Figs 32.2 and 32.3). VZV may also cause hepatitis or encephalitis. Immunization of such children with live vaccines is normally contraindicated; but in case of exposure to **measles**, prompt administration of HNIG will abort infection or diminish its severity. A live vaccine against **chickenpox** has been developed in Japan and used successfully to prevent leukaemic children in hospital acquiring this infection. In view of the danger of using live virus vaccines in immunodeficient patients, it must have taken some courage to mount the first clinical trials, but fortunately the vaccine seems to have no side-effects other than causing a very mild attack of varicella in a minority of patients. This vaccine is not as yet licensed in the UK for general use, but is available for immunodeficient individuals on a named patient basis.

4.4 Solid tumours

Table 32.4 shows that these patients, who tend to be older than the leukaemics, suffer mostly from **herpesvirus infections**, VZV often being particularly troublesome in the elderly.

4.5 AIDS

This is the prime example of immunosuppression by a virus; HIV destroys the T-helper cells and thus opens the way to so-called opportunistic infections by a wide variety of pathogens and to various tumours.

As far as other viruses are concerned, **HSV eruptions** in the orofacial, perianal, and genital areas are common; **herpetic oesophagitis** also occurs. **CMV** is so constantly present in these patients that before the isolation of HIV it was suggested as a possible cause of the syndrome. It may cause **febrile illness**, **pneumonitis**, or **chorioretinitis**. Adenovirus and papovavirus infections also occur.

The liability of AIDS patients to develop various malignancies—invasive cervical carcinoma, Kaposi's sarcoma, and lymphomas—is also a sign of a damaged immune system.

5 Diagnosis and treatment

Presentation with a variety of infections is a tell-tale sign that a patient is suffering from a dysfunction of the immune response. It is important to take a careful family history as defects of immunity may have a **genetic component**. Investigations should include tests for **T-cell-mediated immunity** (primarily lymphocyte numbers and functions; cytokine functions); **antibody-mediated immunity** (primarily B cells and the quantity and quality of the various classes of antibody they produce); and functionality of the **complement system**.

Much of the management of immunodeficiencies is directed at the prevention and treatment of infections by antibiotics. Therapy of this nature is necessarily a second best alternative to treatment of the underlying disease, and here progress is being made with replacement therapy, using transplants of fetal thymus and liver. Other promising techniques include the use of stem cells, and, in suitable patients, gene replacement therapy.

6 Reminders

- Patients with defects of immunity are **abnormally susceptible to infections with microbes, including viruses; and some viruses** (e.g. HIV, measles, CMV) can themselves impair immunity by damaging the cells that mediate immune responses.

- The **primary** (congenital) immunodeficiencies are comparatively rare. Those predominantly affecting **B-cell** function are mostly associated with infections by **cytolytic viruses**, e.g. enteroviruses, whereas patients with defects mainly of **T-cell** functions are at most risk from **enveloped cell-associated viruses**, e.g. herpes and paramyxoviruses.

- **Acquired immunodeficiencies** are secondary to infection by HIV, to **malignant disease** and to **cytotoxic drugs** and **irradiation** given therapeutically or to prevent transplant rejection. They are met much more often than the primary immunodeficiencies.

- In these patients **T-cell function is impaired** so that the main risks are **reactivations of herpesviruses**, particularly CMV. Graft recipients who are not immune to CMV may acquire a primary infection from a seropositive donor.

- Cytotoxic treatment apart, children with **leukaemia** are at particular risk of primary infection with **measles** or **chickenpox**, both of which may cause serious **giant-cell** pneumonitis. They should receive passive protection with normal immunoglobulin if exposed to measles; varicella-zoster vaccine is licensed in some countries, but is available only on a named patient basis in the UK.

- Treatment of immunodeficiencies includes:
  - antibiotics to control infections
  - transplants of bone marrow and other tissues.

Chapter 33

Respiratory infections

Just as several syndromes may be caused by one virus, infections of some body systems may be due to a number of viruses. These can sometimes be dealt with by allotting individual chapters to them, as in the case of hepatitis and herpesviruses. Sometimes, however, so many viruses are involved that it is useful to summarize them in short 'minichapters'. This section of the book, on special syndromes, starts with two such chapters, on respiratory infections and sexually transmitted diseases respectively.

Virus infections of the upper and lower respiratory tract cause immense clinical problems worldwide, both in the primary

Table 33.1 Viruses causing common respiratory infections

Diseases	Virus
Common cold	Rhinoviruses
	Coronaviruses
	Parainfluenza viruses
Pharyngitis	Parainfluenza viruses
	Cytomegalovirus
	Influenza A and B
	Rhinoviruses
Bronchitis	Parainfluenza viruses
	Respiratory syncytial virus
	Influenza A and B
	Metapneumovirus
Bronchiolitis	Parainfluenza viruses
	Respiratory syncytial virus
	Metapneumovirus
Croup	Parainfluenza viruses
	Respiratory syncytial virus
	Metapneumovirus
Influenza	Influenza A and B
Bronchopneumonia	Influenza A and B
	Respiratory syncytial virus
	Parainfluenza viruses
Pneumonia	Influenza, SARS

healthcare setting, and in hospitals. Of all acute viral infections, those of the respiratory tract are among the most frequent, with yearly rates as high as 85 illnesses per 100 persons. As over one-third of these episodes need medical attention and result in at least 2 days lost from school or 1 day from work the impact is obvious, in terms both of morbidity and mortality.

The viruses

Table 33.1 summarizes the viruses that may infect the respiratory tract. The vast area of its epithelial lining, over which

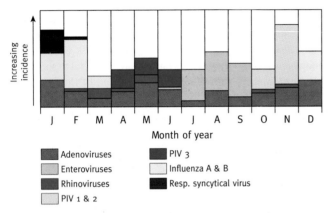

Fig. 33.1 The seasonal incidence of various respiratory viruses.

Legend:
- Adenoviruses
- Enteroviruses
- Rhinoviruses
- PIV 1 & 2
- PIV 3
- Influenza A & B
- Resp. syncytical virus

pass large volumes of air, makes it an ideal portal of entry for a range of viruses, both those that infect the respiratory tract itself, and others that simply pass through to cause disease elsewhere.

There are over 200 recognized respiratory viruses belonging to five families, including orthomyxoviruses (influenza), paramyxoviruses (RSV, parainfluenza), coronaviruses, picornaviruses (common cold), herpesviruses, and adenoviruses.

Seasonality

Most of these viruses are predominant during a particular season (Fig. 33.1), especially in the more northerly and southerly parts of the hemispheres, although nearer the equator these virus 'seasons' are not so apparent and infections occur all the year round. Good examples of seasonality are acute infections by influenza and RSV, which tend to cause outbreaks in midwinter in both hemispheres. Parainfluenza type 3 viruses predominate in the spring, whereas types 1 and 2 cause outbreaks in the autumn months. Both adenoviruses and common cold viruses are prevalent throughout the year.

The precise conditions that result in seasonal spread are not known with certainty but may be attributed more to changes in social behaviour with the seasons, e.g. overcrowding in cold weather, than with variations in humidity and temperature.

Chapter 34

Sexually transmitted viral infections

As references to sexually transmitted infections occur throughout this volume, we thought it would be useful to provide a mini-chapter summarizing them. They can be considered under the headings of **localized** and **generalized** infections (Table 34.1). The first group are those that bring their victims to the STD clinic, and are usually thought of under the label of 'sexually transmitted diseases'. The second group present more dangers, as they cause no local lesions that might indicate acquisition of a potentially serious illness.

How does the frequency of the localized infections compare with their bacteriological counterparts? In the UK, the incidence of syphilis is too low to affect the equation; the most valid comparison is with gonococcal and chlamydial infections. Figure 34.1 shows the incidences of these infections in people aged from 16 to 24 years in England and Wales during 1995; for simplicity, the figures for males and females are pooled. The viral infections outweigh those due to bacteria, mainly because of the very high incidence of papillomavirus infections, which is now six times higher than the figure for gonorrhoea. Furthermore, their treatment presents greater problems.

Table 34.1 Sexually transmitted viral diseases

(a) Predominantly localized infections

Virus	Relevant chapter	Main clinical features
Herpes simplex	17	HSV-2 more severe than HSV-1. Painful, itchy vesicular lesions on genitalia, anal, perineal areas, possibly mouth. Urethritis, proctitis, cervicitis. Tendency to recurrence.
Papillomaviruses	15	Warts, intraepithelial dysplasias, epidermodysplasia verruciformis, carcinomas on skin, anogenital mucosa, cervix, possibly larynx
Adenoviruses	8	Types 19 and 37 cause ulcers on external genitalia, urethritis
Molluscum contagiosum	14	Characteristic molluscum lesions on genitalia

Table 34.1 Sexually transmitted viral diseases—*cont'd.*

(b) Generalized infections

Virus	Relevant chapter	Remarks
Hepatitis A	23	May be transmitted between male homosexuals, especially if promiscuous
Hepatitis E	23	Risk difficult to quantify: probably not high
Hepatitis B	22	The most commonly transmitted hepatitis virus; very high risk of acquisition from HBeAg-positive carriers if intercourse is unprotected
Hepatitis D (delta)	22	Sexual transmission rare
Hepatitis C	24	Risk difficult to quantify: probably not high
Human immuno-deficiency viruses HTLV-I/II, HIV-1/2	25	Unprotected intercourse carries high risk, especially in early stage of infection. Male to female transmission more efficient than female to male. Spread favoured by presence of genital lesions due to, e.g. herpes, syphilis, chancroid
Human cytomegalovirus	19	Usually acquired in childhood, but may be sexually transmitted to seronegative adults

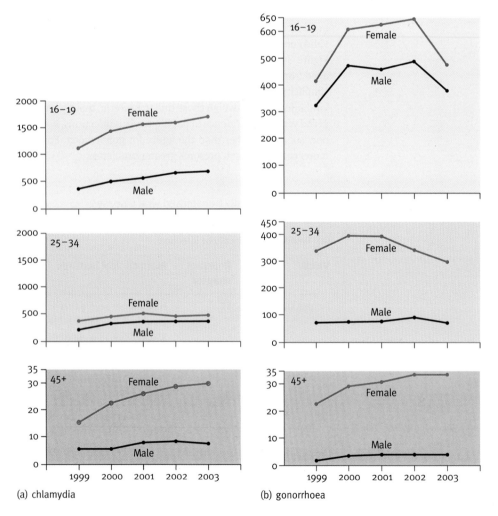

(a) chlamydia (b) gonorrhoea

Fig. 34.1 STDs in England and Wales during 1995 in people aged 16–24 years. Ordinates = rates per 100 000 (Data from CDR Review (1997). *CDR Review*, **7**, p. R174, table 1.)

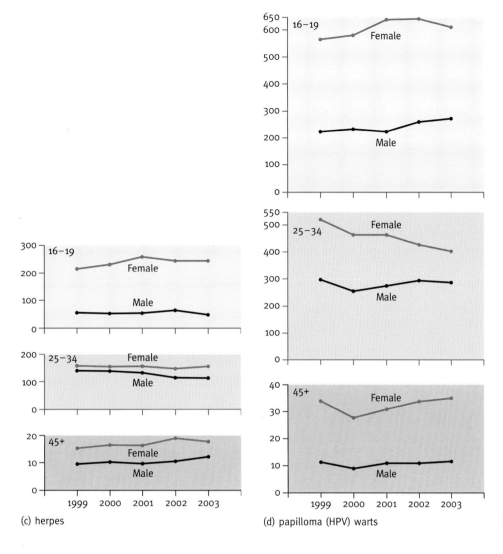

(c) herpes

(d) papilloma (HPV) warts

Fig. 34.1 *cont'd.*

Chapter 35

Resurgent and emergent viral infections

1 Introduction

The last half of the twentieth century saw both victories and defeats in the constant battle against viruses. One major infection, smallpox, was completely eradicated and in some countries the incidence of childhood diseases such as polio, measles, and rubella was drastically reduced. However, other infections have arisen to take their place, so that the overall picture is not as happy as appears at first sight. Such infections can be considered under two headings.

- Known infections that have, in the last three decades, increased significantly; we refer to these as **resurgent** (or re-emergent) **infections**.

- Infections caused by viruses discovered during the last three decades or so, designated as **emergent infections**.

Although this grouping (Table 35.1) is somewhat arbitrary, and there is some overlap between the two categories, there is a real distinction to be made between them.

Table 35.1 Differences between resurgent and emergent infections

Resurgent infection	Emergent infections
Laboratory test available for many years; widespread, often severe, may cause epidemics	Viruses identified relatively recently; some infections may be silent or mild
Usually diagnosed by conventional isolation or serological methods	Usually diagnosed by molecular techniques
Examples:	Examples:
Influenza, viral haemorrhagic fevers, dengue, HIV-1, HIV-2, rabies, West Nile	Human herpesviruses 6, 7, 8; hepatitis viruses D (delta agent), G, GBV-A,–B, and -C; papillomaviruses, hantaviruses, SARS, Hendra, Nipah

Table 35.2 Factors influencing the resurgence of viral infections

Factor	Example
Viral factors	
Breakdown of species barriers	Probable transfer of HIV from a simian reservoir to humans. Spread of influenza viruses from animals or birds to humans, transfer of BSE to humans.
Genetic	RNA viruses, particularly HIV and influenza, have extremely high mutation rates, which favour the spread of strains resistant to immune barriers or chemotherapy.
Host factors	
Ecology and modern agriculture	New farming practices encourage human contact with rodents carrying Hantaan and other exotic RNA viruses. BSE has spread to humans, from beef, as a new form of CJD as a result of feeding animal protein to ruminants.
Medical or surgical interventions	Organ transplants and the use of immunosuppressive drugs have encouraged latent herpesviruses to emerge, such as CMV.
Human behaviour	Changes in sexual habits have enhanced the spread of sexually transmitted viruses, e.g. HIV, HBV, herpes, and papillomaviruses
Intermediate hosts	Hantaviruses, carried harmlessly in rodents infect humans when rodent populations expand because of increased availability of food. Recently, fruit eating bats have been recognized as a source of novel viruses such as Hendra and Nipah, and possibly Ebola. Migrating birds carry potential pandemic influenza viruses.
Population increase	Increasing population densities and urban poverty encourage the spread of waterborne and airborne viruses.
Defects in public health infrastructure	Poor control of mosquitoes either because of worries about DTT or poor public health structure, or both, has allowed the re-emergence of dengue, West Nile, and other classic arboviruses.

2 Factors favouring the resurgence of old enemies

Table 35.2 lists the main factors in the resurgence of viral infection.

2.1 Viral genetic factors

Microbes are highly adaptive and because of their extremely short reproductive cycle, usually measured in hours, can react quickly to alterations in the environment. RNA viruses in particular can mutate readily. There are strong species barriers that often prevent transfer of viruses from animals or birds to humans. Nevertheless, mutations in animal or avian influenza A viruses have allowed them to infect humans, and the emergence of drug-resistant viruses is also due to genetic changes.

In 1998, 2003 and 2006 influenza A (H5N1) viruses jumped from chickens to humans as a result of mutations in the HA gene of the virus. So far a pandemic has been avoided by killing hundreds of millions of affected chickens and thereby removing the epicentre of virus replication. The virus reservoir is migrating birds.

2.2 Changes in agricultural methods

Unnatural methods of **animal management** can give rise to emerging infections. An example is the transfer of sheep prions to cattle in protein animal feed and hence to humans. More than 147 persons have contracted a new form of CJD (Chapter 29), and others who ate contaminated beef in the 1980s may now be incubating the disease.

Removal of forests and development of new farmlands expose farmers to disease-carrying arthropods and with increased urbanization there are new opportunities for mosquitoes to breed in static water, e.g. discarded cans and old car tyres. New irrigation systems perturb vectors or may provide new breeding grounds for virus-infected mosquitoes or attract virus-carrying birds.

Breeding of exotic mammals for the restaurant sector has allowed SARS-CoV to emerge from a civet cat to spread to many countries of the world, to infect 8400 persons and to kill 812 by the end of 2003.

2.3 Human migrations and travel

Microorganisms may simply follow humans as they migrate. Measles and smallpox viruses accompanied the first European explorers in the Americas and devastated the local population. Similarly the Black Death bacillus, *Pasteurella pestis*, travelled with explorers, soldiers, and traders from China to Europe in the fourteenth century. Viruses such as HTLV-1 (Chapter 25) may have been carried by Portuguese explorers from Africa to Japan and later by the slave trade to the Caribbean.

With modern tourism, and with millions of persons travelling the globe daily, microbes are liable to emerge and spread with increasing frequency. Aircraft can also carry virus-infected mosquitoes from country to country

2.4 Increase in human or vector populations

With a current population of 5 billion and a doubling predicted over the next few decades, few places in the world remain unvisited. Virus reservoirs can be disturbed. Ebola virus (Chapter 28)

was first discovered in 1976 and has resurged every few years since that time. It appears to have an animal reservoir, so far unidentified, in West Africa. The ecology of Ebola can be disturbed by extension of villages into virgin forest, tree felling, or hunting, with resultant epidemics in the indigenous population.

Zoonotic viruses spread by vectors such as mosquitoes or ticks but residing in an animal reservoir are often encountered by humans moving into jungle areas. A good example is the massive outbreak of YF among workers constructing the Panama Canal (Chapter 27) or, more recently, SARS.

Hantaviruses (Chapter 28) are an interesting example of an emerged virus that normally occupies a quiet niche as a silent infection of small rodents. It is transmitted from animal to animal by contact with excreta, such as urine in the form of dried dust. Should rodent numbers increase significantly, more opportunities arise for the virus to be transmitted to humans. In 1993, a year when mouse infestation was exceptionally severe in New Mexico, a new hantavirus, termed Sin Nombre, spread into humans (and later even from person to person) by aerosolized dried mouse urine on dust particles.

2.5 Defects in public health infrastructure

With the discovery of antibiotics and antimalarial drugs came a more complacent attitude towards pathogenic microbes. In particular there was a relaxation of mosquito control programmes in some countries. **Dengue** (Chapter 27) also depends upon mosquitoes for spread to humans and has now spread to South America; half a million cases were notified in Brazil in 1997. An even more recent example is West Nile virus, transported in wild birds and then spread to humans by mosquitoes sharing blood from both species.

Table 35.3 Recently emerged viruses

Virus	Disease in humans	Location	Reservoir
Monkey pox	Pox lesions	USA	Gambian giant rats and prairie dogs
Nipah	Respiratory disease	Malaysia	Bats
SARS	Respiratory disease	South-east Asia	Civet cat or rat
HIV	Generalized immuno-suppression	Africa	Chimpanzee
West Nile	Encephalitis	USA	Wild birds
Hendra	Respiratory disease	Australia	Horses
Chicken influenza H5N1	Respiratory disease	South-east Asia	Migrating ducks and geese

3 The emergence of new enemies

3.1 Human immunodeficiency virus

The original host of the most notorious human retrovirus (Chapter 25) was a chimpanzee in Africa: these animals can be infected with **HIV-1**, remaining virus-positive for life and rarely showing symptoms. It is possible that the virus spread from a chimpanzee to a human, probably a hunter, followed by limited spread in humans. This quiet ecology of HIV in Africa could have existed for an extended period. Excursions into the area by travellers and holidaymakers for the first time in the 1970s allowed the virus to emerge. In this particular virus a disturbance of the typical ecology and a change in human dynamics, attitude to sexual activity, and access to air travel provided a pivotal set of circumstances resulting in the current pandemic.

3.2 Herpesviruses

HHV-6 was first isolated in 1986 from lymphocytes deriving from patients with lymphoproliferative illnesses. **HHV-7** was first isolated in 1990 from the CD4+ cells of a normal subject. They are both betaherpesviruses (Chapter 19). Their discovery depended on improved methods for culturing and manipulating lymphocytes in the laboratory.

HHV-8 (see Chapter 20) was discovered by demonstrating DNA sequences in tissues from AIDS patients, including Kaposi's sarcoma, closely resembling those of gammaherpesviruses.

3.3 Hepatitis viruses

During the last decade several new hepatitis viruses have been detected by molecular techniques, including sequence analysis and molecular amplification. They include **hepatitis C** and the related flavi-like viruses **GBV-A, B, and C** (Chapter 24); **HEV** (Chapter 23); and hepatitis G (**HGV**). Like HIV, hepatitis B probably emerged from a chimpanzee reservoir, but much earlier in our evolution, possibly 100 000 years ago.

3.4 Orphan syndromes

Along with discussion of whether viruses could spread into new countries or susceptible populations, an equally important topic is whether known viruses can give rise to new clinical syndromes.

Chronic fatigue syndrome

Fatigue is an important component of many virus diseases and may persist long after the acute infection. It is likely to be caused, at least in the acute phase, by the release of cytokines such as TNF-α, IL-2, and IL-6. However, a more complex illness has become recognized called **chronic fatigue syndrome**, known earlier as myalgic encephalitis or Royal Free Disease. The clinical characteristics include recurring fatigue with constitutional symptoms such as myalgia, arthralgia, sore throat, headache, and tender lymph nodes. There may also be short-term memory problems with difficulty in concentrating. Young adults are mainly affected. A sceptic would assert that many suffer from fatigue and concentration loss, and so dismiss the cause as psychosomatic. However, there are viruses that could initiate such a collection of symptoms, which are particularly debilitating and unpleasant in young people.

Not unexpectedly, particular attention has been directed toward viruses known to establish persistent infections, such as the herpesviruses, and at least one prospective study suggested that infectious mononucleosis (EBV) can precipitate chronic fatigue syndrome. It seems sensible to continue investigations with the herpes family and the newly discovered herpes virus types 6 and 7.

Enterovirus RNA has been detected in muscle biopsy samples of cases of chronic fatigue syndrome but muscle strength *per se* is not particularly reduced in these patients.

Insulin-dependent diabetes mellitus

Most strains of Coxsackie B viruses (Chapter 16) destroy pancreatic β cells in mice, and some have been isolated from humans with diabetes. Nevertheless, the association of these viruses with IDDM is rather loose, and the picture is further complicated by the possibility of an autoimmune response.

Attempts to implicate specific viruses in the causation of these syndromes thus remain inconclusive. Indeed, by analogy with the enteric human orphan (ECHO) viruses, some of which are viruses in search of a disease, chronic fatigue syndrome and IDDM so far remain orphan illnesses in search of causal viruses.

4 Reminders

- Some established viral infections have increased significantly during the past three decades. These are resurgent infections. Contributory factors include mutations in the viruses, and changes in patterns of demography and agriculture, prevalence of insect and animal vectors, human sexual behaviour, and travel.

- Several new viruses, not detectable by traditional methods, have been identified by the exploitation of molecular techniques but caused by overpopulation, mishandling of traditional agriculture; they include several herpes and hepatitis agents, SARS, and BSE. These are referred to as emergent viruses.

- Some illnesses, notably chronic fatigue syndrome and IDDM, are possibly caused **by emergent viruses, but the associations are not yet fully established**.

Part 4

Practical aspects

Chapter 36

The laboratory diagnosis of viral infections

1 Introduction

The role of the virology laboratory has changed dramatically. In the year of our first edition the clinical diagnostic laboratory mainly isolated viruses using classical cell culture techniques, whereby viruses were grown in the laboratory over a period of 4–15 days and identified by cytopathic changes in the cells. Retrospective serological diagnosis was also commonly used and in this manner a huge database was established and clinical syndromes were linked to viruses. There was a glimmering of so-called rapid diagnosis, taking 24–48 hours and using immunofluorescence and cell cultures. None of this work was of immediate use to the patient, but by the late 1990s molecular techniques were developed to the point at which some specialized laboratories could amplify viral genomes using PCR for DNA viruses or RT–PCR for RNA viruses. The RT enzyme first transcribed the viral RNA genome into a DNA copy, which was then amplified. Molecular techniques for virus diagnosis have now taken over and are highly commercialized in the form of kits, giving sensitive and reproducible results.

The results of these tests are now clinically useful. Probably the best example is the monitoring of patients suffering from HIV, hepatitis B, or hepatitis C for responses to antiviral drugs. The laboratory provides answers to the questions of whether an antiviral reduces the number of copies of viral genome, whether the virus develops specific mutations to make it drug resistant, or whether the drug 'cocktail' for the patient should be changed to prevent drug resistance.

There are also some bedside tests for diagnosing influenza or RSV, which take 15 minutes and resemble the use of a dipstick for diabetes. Nevertheless, the identification of SARS by the older techniques of EM and cell cultures showed that it would be imprudent to discard them for the time being.

On the other hand, hepatitis C was first identified only by molecular analysis of its genome, so a balance is required: It may be that the smaller virology laboratories will become totally dependent on molecular diagnostic kits, whereas the larger establishments will retain a variety of methods at their disposal.

2 Collecting and sending clinical specimens to the laboratory

From the point of view of the new doctor this is probably one of the most important sections in the textbook, and careful thought must be given—based, one hopes, on a knowledge of viral pathology—as to which clinical samples should be collected. Whichever techniques are used in the laboratory no results will be forthcoming without good quality samples from the patient.

To perform its task properly the laboratory must be provided with:

- the right specimens;
- taken at the right time;
- stored and transported in the right way (for example, some viruses can be completely destroyed by freezing).

Table 36.1 summarizes the types of specimen to be collected when viral infections of various body systems are suspected.

2.1 Clinical sampling

Swabs

The amount of material collected must be adequate. In particular, throat or skin swabs must be taken fairly vigorously. Swabs are broken off into a vial of transport medium, usually tissue culture medium containing antibacterial and antifungal antibiotics to inhibit contaminants, a protein stabiliser (such as bovine serum albumin) to protect sensitive viruses and a buffering solution at pH 7.0. For molecular diagnosis, the clinical material can be placed in a speical transport medium.

Nasopharyngeal aspirates

These are very useful in the diagnosis of upper respiratory tract infections, of young children, e.g. RSV, but obtaining a satisfactory specimen with minimum distress to the child requires skill and practice.

Table 36.1 Specimens required for isolation of virus or detection of antigen

Disease	Specimen
Respiratory infection	Nasal or throat swabs; postnasal washing
Gastrointestinal infection	Faeces (rectal swab not so satisfactory)
Vesicular rash	Vesicle fluid, throat swab, faeces
Hepatitis	Serum, faeces
Central nervous system	Cerebrospinal fluid, throat swab, faeces
AIDS	Unclotted blood

NB. In addition to the above, 5–10 ml of clotted blood for serological tests is always required.

Vesicle fluid

Vesicle fluid for EM, for example for a poxvirus or herpes, is collected on the tip of a scalpel blade, spread over an area about 3–4 mm in diameter on an ordinary microscope slide, and allowed to dry.

Faeces, to identify enteroviruses or rotaviruses

These should be placed in a dry sterile container; they are preferable to rectal swabs for virus isolation.

Clotted blood

As a general rule 5–10 ml blood is taken. A syringe rather than a vacuum tube is used to take blood; the needle should be removed before expelling the blood to avoid haemolysis. EDTA blood is used for detecting various viral genomes.

2.2 Storage and transport

Specimens should be placed in secure plastic bags and labelled in accordance with local practice. They should go to the laboratory as soon as possible after collection; if kept overnight, they should be held at 4°C rather than being frozen, which tends to destroy viruses with a lipid envelope.

Much time will be saved if request forms are properly completed. Brief indications of the **date of onset** of illness, **clinical signs**, and **suspected diagnosis** are much more important than a specification of the tests required.

3 Rapid diagnostic methods

3.1 Immunofluorescence

Principle

Direct fluorescent antibody method

Virus or viral antigen is detected in a specimen from a patient, or alternatively, the clinical sample is cultivated overnight in a susceptible cell line to amplify the amount of virus present. The tissue or cells are reacted with a specific antiserum, which is coupled with a fluorescent dye (fluorescein isothiocyanate, FITC). After thorough washing to remove unattached serum and dye the specimen is viewed in an ultraviolet microscope. The FITC on serum specifically attached to virus or viral antigen becomes visible as a green fluorescence (Fig. 36.1).

The great disadvantage of this method, now little used, is that many specific sera must be labelled in order to test for a range of viruses.

Indirect fluorescent antibody method

The technical details are identical to the direct method, except that the specific serum is unlabelled; instead, the dye is attached to a second serum prepared against globulins from the species in which the specific serum was made For example, antibodies to human immunoglobulins are often made in rabbits or goats.

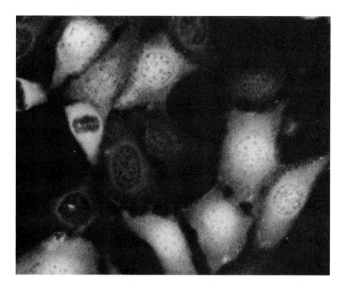

Fig. 36.1 Influenza antigen in VERO cells stained by the indirect immunofluorescence method.

This is called a 'sandwich' method, because there are three layers:

1. The specimen being tested for a specific virus.
2. The specific antiviral serum, prepared in (say) rabbits.
3. FITC-labelled antirabbit antibody.

The principle is the same as that illustrated for an ELISA test in Fig. 36.2(a). The method has the great advantage that only one labelled (anti-species) serum is needed to test for many viruses.

Rather than FITC, the label may be **immunoperoxidase**, which is then reacted with a substrate to give a precipitate visible by ordinary light microscopy.

Applications

The method may be used to identify viral antigen in a clinical specimen, e.g. RSV or influenza virus in cells in throat washings, or in a cell culture previously inoculated with the specimen and incubated for 12–18 hours to allow virus replication and infection of other nearby cells. The latter method has been used with much success to detect early CMV antigens induced in cell cultures within 48 hours of inoculation—a much faster method than waiting many days for a virus-induced CPE in a cell line.

3.2 Enzyme-linked immunosorbent assay and radioimmunoassay

ELISA (Fig. 36.2) has become, alongside PCR, the workhorse of most diagnostic virology laboratories as it is automated, kits are commercially available, and it can be adapted to the identification of many viral antigens, e.g. the p24 antigen of HIV-1, hepatitis B, rotavirus, etc. and the corresponding antibodies.

Principle

This is very similar to that of indirect fluorescent antibody (test). The main differences are:

- Instead of a fluorescent dye, the label is either an **enzyme (ELISA)** or **radioactive iodine (RIA).**
- Specific binding of the labelled antibody (or antigen) is detected by reacting the enzyme with a substrate which then produces a visible colour in the reaction mixture (ELISA) or by counting radioactive emissions (RIA).
- The reaction takes place in a multiwell plastic plate or tube, read by photometry (ELISA) or by a gamma counter (RIA) and printed out automatically. A very commonly used kit contains the 'capture antibody' on a bead.

For various technical reasons, including safety, ELISA has virtually replaced RIA in the routine laboratory. As with indirect fluorescent antibody tests, thorough washing between the various stages to get rid of unbound reagents and the use of positive and negative controls is essential.

Applications

Both ELISA and RIA can provide automated quantitative estimations of the amounts of viral antigen or antibody present.

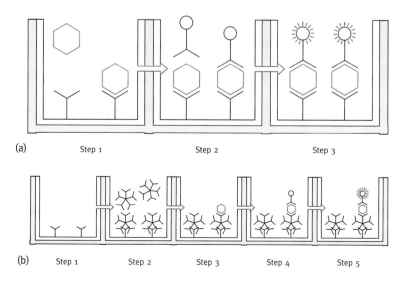

(a) Step 1   Step 2   Step 3

(b) Step 1   Step 2   Step 3   Step 4   Step 5

Fig. 36.2 **(a)** Direct identification of antigen by captures and ELISA. **Step 1**: Addition of specimen containing antigen that combines with the specific 'capture' antibody on a plastic surface. **Step 2**: Addition of enzyme-labelled specific antibody. **Step 3**: Substrate is added, reacts with bound enzyme, and undergoes colour change. **(b)** Identification of specific IgM antibody by capture and ELISA. **Step 1**: Plastic surface coated with antibody to IgM. **Step 2**: Patient's serum added; IgM molecules are captured by the anti-IgM. **Step 3**: After washing to remove unattached IgM, test antigen is added and combines with any captured IgM of the same specificity. **Steps 4 and 5**: as steps 2 and 3 in (a). Note that the captured IgM molecule on the left, having no specificity for the test antigen, does not react.

3.3 Latex agglutination tests

Latex particles are coated with viral antigen and agglutinate when mixed on a slide with specific antiserum. The test is rapid, easy to read, and does not require complicated equipment. It is, however, liable to prozone effects, giving false negative results at low dilutions of serum.

3.4 Electron microscopy and immunoelectron microscopy

Principle

'Samples are negatively 'stained' with phosphotungstic acid, so that the virions, which are not penetrated by the stain, stand out as white particles on a dark background. However, virus particles must be present at a concentration of at least 10^6/ml to stand a chance of being identified; it is therefore sometimes necessary to use simple virus concentration methods. Needless to say an experienced microscopist is needed if the results are to be reliable. The method is used less and less nowadays, but was used to identify the SARS coronavirus.

Applications

EM is used for rapid identification of morphologically distinctive virions, usually directly in clinical specimens, but sometimes in cell culture fluid. HSV and VZV can be readily identified in vesicle fluid, although, being identical in appearance, they cannot be distinguished from each other by EM. The technique is useful where virus cannot be cultivated and yet is present in large quantities, e.g. certain gastroenteritis viruses (Chapter 11) or hepatitis B (Chapter 22).

The value of the test may on occasion be increased by using **IEM**, which is the addition to the specimen of specific immune serum that agglutinates a particular virus, thus making the virions easier to find and adding serological specificity to their identification.

3.5 Detection of viral genome by nucleic acid hybridization

Highly sensitive methods have been devised to detect viral genetic information in infected cells, and are now in routine and extensive use. The first is nucleic acid hybridization; amplification methods are described in Section 3.6.

Principle of hybridization methods

Dot-blot hybridization involves extracting the nucleic acid—usually DNA—from the specimen and denaturing it into single strands. Spots of the extracted DNA solution are placed on a nitrocellulose filter, and treated with a probe consisting of a labelled stretch of DNA or RNA complementary in sequence to the specific region being sought in the specimen. The label may be a fluorescent dye or a radioisotope. The principle of hybridization *in situ* is similar, except that the specific nucleic acid sequences are labelled directly in tissue sections.

Applications

Viral nucleic acid hybridization techniques are very sensitive and can be used, for example, to detect the genomes of papillomaviruses and herpesviruses in tissues and enteric viruses in faeces.

3.6 Detection of viral genomes by nucleic acid amplification methods

These molecular methods are now used in most clinical laboratories to detect and quantify the genomes of HIV provirus, CMV, hepatitis B, and HPV in clinical samples. The methods are exquisitely sensitive: the most important technical problem is the danger of **false positives**. For example, if a different laboratory in the same building has handled plasmid DNA of the same viral origin, contamination of buffers or equipment with a few molecules of plasmid DNA is difficult to avoid. This contaminating DNA could be amplified and, unless rigorous controls are incorporated, give a false positive result. RNA viruses such as HIV, hepatitis C, and influenza can be detected and also quantified by incorporating an initial step of RT to transcribe the viral RNA to a piece of DNA. Viral genome quantification in patients' samples is now a major activity in clinical laboratories, particularly for patients treated with the newer antiviral drugs to measure the reduction in viral load following chemotherapy of HIV, and hepatitis B and C viruses

Polymerase chain reaction

Two distinct oligonucleotide primer sequences, one on each strand of the target viral DNA (solid block, Fig. 36.3) are added to a clinical sample that has been treated with heat (94°C) and detergent to denature and, therefore, physically separate the strands of viral DNA (step 1). The primers specifically hybridize with the homologous nucleotide stretches on the viral DNA genome. A DNA polymerase (open square) termed *Taq* polymerase (from *Thermophilus aquaticus*), which acts at high temperature, is added. After 1 min the temperature is reduced to 52°C for 20 s to allow annealing of primers (step 2) and the temperature is then raised to 72°C for 5 min to allow DNA polymerization to occur (step 3). Under these conditions, and only if the oligonucleotide primers have hybridized, the Taq enzyme generates multiple copies of the nucleotide stretch between the two primers. Multiple cycles of DNA denaturation, annealing of primers, and polymerization can be programmed in the microprocessor-driven heating block. In this manner, a portion of a single molecule of viral DNA can be amplified a million-fold in a few hours to give a quantity of DNA that can be separated in a polyacrylamide gel, and then visualized by addition to the gel of ethidium bromide and exposure to UV light. 'Nested PCR' is even more sensitive. Following initial amplification of a unique stretch of viral DNA, a further set of 'internal' primers is added that anneal to DNA within the original fragment, allowing a smaller stretch to be amplified.

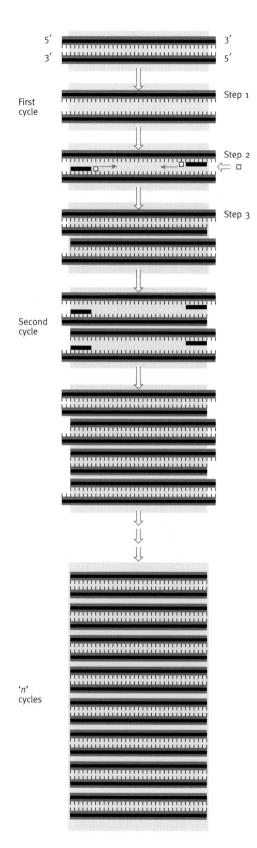

Fig. 36.3 Detection and amplification of viral genome by the polymerase chain reaction. **Step 1**: denaturation (separation) of viral dsDNA. **Step 2**: addition of oligonucleotide primer ■ and *Taq* polymerase □. Annealing of primer. **Step 3**: DNA transcription and amplification.

Branched chain techniques

A technique has been devised for using highly sensitive branched DNA (bDNA) probes to detect and quantify viral RNA sequences. The sensitivity derives from signal amplification rather than the target amplification that provides the basis for PCR.

For example, to measure HIV RNA copy number in plasma, the sample is first centrifuged to pellet the virus particles. The lysed virus containing RNA is added to microtitre plate wells coated with oligonucleotide probes, which match conserved sequences in the HIV genome. The viral RNA forms double-stranded duplexes with the probe sequences and is thereby captured. After the well is washed, bDNA amplifier molecules are hybridized to the bound HIV RNA, and then alkaline phosphatase probes that bind to the bDNA amplifier molecules are added. The HIV-specific bDNA probes are thus linked to an enzyme that catalyses the release of a chemiluminescent molecule from its substrate, and the amount of light produced is proportional to the quantity of viral genome. The method is faster, less laborious and expensive, and requires less technical ability than PCR.

The NASBA amplification technique

This method targets RNA viruses or mRNA transcripts of DNA viruses and uses three enzyme systems at the same time to amplify a particular viral genome sequence. It can be quantitative. The three enzymes are RT, DNA-dependent RNA polymerase, and RNase H.

A viral genome specific primer also incorporates the T7 promoter and hybridizes to the viral genome. This is extended by the RT enzyme. The RNase degrades the RNA strand and the RT, ulitizing a second primer, produces dDNA. Multiple copies of RNA are produced from this DNA template by the T7 DNA-dependent RNA polymerase.

Quantification of viral genomes by real time polymerase chain reaction

Undoubtedly this technique will now become a laboratory workhorse. The best known system is TaqMan. Essentially, this PCR method does not wait for an end quantitation but detects genome amplification as it goes along. A specific probe binds to the viral amplicon under investigation, and is hydrolysed to produce fluorescent molecules, which are immediately detected and quantified. Alternatively a dye is encouraged to intercalate into the dsDNA being produced in the first reaction, and as more dye is trapped fluorescence increases. Often PCR reactions finish within minutes, giving an instant diagnosis.

Monitoring the effects of antivirals

Laboratory help is essential for clinical care of AIDS patients being treated with drug combinations; HAART (Chapter 25). Patients need to be monitored every 2–3 months and expectations are to detect fewer than 50 HIV genome copies per ml of plasma after antiviral drug treatment, compared with a typical figure of 10 000 RNA genome copies at the start of antiviral therapy, say 3–4 months previously.

The laboratory is also essential for the continuing care of patients chronically infected with hepatitis B and treated with a combination of lamivudine, famciclovir, and adefovir. One hundred- to 1000-fold reduction of viral DNA load would be typical following antiviral therapy.

Similarly a rapid and sustained reduction in RNA genome copies of HCV following therapy with IFN and ribavirin would predict successful treatment. With hepatitis C the laboratory can also help by identifying which of the five types has infected the patient, because these respond differently to antiviral therapy.

Analysis of hepatitis B and C and HIV genomes for drug-resistant mutations

The quantitative PCR methods described above give the first warning of a resurgence of viraemia in a patient following long-term therapy. The first possibility to be investigated is point mutations in the RT or protease genes of HIV, for example indicating emergence of a drug-resistant virus. Obviously patients are treated with drug combinations to minimize this possibility. However, rapid clinical action may have to be taken to replace one of the drugs in the combination.

Usually viruses avoid the action of antiviral drugs by a point mutation in the target gene and these mutations are well known. Therefore, a number of molecular tests can be used to search for these particular mutations. In particular a so-called point mutation assay utilizes PCR primers synthesized so as to hybridize to the drug-sensitive or drug-resistant virus only. However, direct nucleotide sequencing is now so automated that this is the method of choice, sometimes used in conjunction with so-called chip technology whereby literally thousands of pre-synthesized oligonucleotides arranged on a microchip are allowed to interact with a PCR-amplified DNA from the virus in question. Computer analysis of these interactions can pinpoint a dominant drug-resistant mutant in a viral population.

The design of the molecular polymerase chain laboratory

To avoid false positive results, the utmost care must be taken to avoid contamination of specimens with foreign nucleic acid molecules. This requires an independently ventilated suite of rooms, each with its own gowns, pipettes, and other equipment, which should be colour coded to avoid cross-contamination. In the case of adjoining rooms, the direction of flow of activities must always be from entrance to exit.

4 Virus isolation in cell cultures

4.1 General principle

This original technology of the virology laboratory is being used less and less but still represents a 'gold standard' for some tests that are superseding it. It was used with great success, to identify the novel coronavirus causing SARS. Most larger laboratories will use three cell lines for screening for viruses mainly from the respiratory tract, CSF, or faeces. Suitable mammalian cells are grown in a single layer (**monolayer**) on the surface of a plastic container and inoculated with the test specimen. They are then observed daily for virus-induced changes (**CPEs**), which are sometimes sufficiently characteristic to be reported without further investigation. Confirmatory tests, e.g. by immunofluorescence, may, however, be necessary.

4.2 Propagation of cell substrates

The **growth medium** used to cultivate cells contains a solution of salts at physiological concentrations, glucose, amino acids, essential vitamins, and antibiotics to inhibit bacterial and fungal contaminants; it is buffered at pH 7.2–7.4. Fetal calf serum is added to a concentration of 10–20 per cent to provide supplements essential for cell growth. When the cells have formed a confluent monolayer the growth medium is replaced by a **maintenance medium** containing only 2–5 per cent serum, which permits little or no further cell multiplication.

When test cells are needed, a stock monolayer is treated with trypsin or versene to disperse it into a suspension of individual cells, which are then diluted in growth medium to a concentration of 10^5–10^6/ml and distributed into other vessels for use. Multiwell plastic dishes are now widely used, but some viruses replicate best in stoppered tubes continuously rotated at a slight angle to the horizontal.

4.3 Types of cell culture

Semicontinuous cell lines

Such cells are derived from human or animal fetal tissue. They have the normal diploid karyotype and hence can be used for vaccine production. Some lines are also used for diagnostic work. Classic cells are called WI-38 and MRC-9.

These cells are termed 'semicontinuous' because they have a limited lifespan and can be subcultured through only 50 or so generations. Even so, millions of cultures can be obtained from a single fetal organ. In practice, several thousand vials of cells suspended in dimethyl sulphoxide are frozen in liquid nitrogen after only a few passages in the laboratory. Each of these can be used to generate further cultures (the 'seed lot' system). For measles, mumps, or rubella vaccine production, only cells at a given low passage level, e.g. the fourth, are used and each batch of cells is carefully tested for karyotype and other properties to exclude the possibility of malignant change. Such strict criteria are not necessary in the diagnostic laboratory, where cells from several successive subcultures may be used for virus isolation.

Continuous cell lines

These are the most widely used for diagnostic work. They are derived either from a tumour or from normal cells, which after repeated culture, have become transformed so that they behave like tumour-derived cells, i.e. they have an abnormal number of chromosomes. They can be propagated indefinitely. Some cell lines such as Vero (monkey kidney) or MDCK (dog kidney) are now used to cultivate viruses for vaccines such as polio and influenza respectively.

Lymphocyte cultures

B lymphocytes will divide and continue to do so indefinitely if infected with EBV. This characteristic, known as '**immortalization**'; is an example of cell transformation by a virus (Chapter 6) and can be used as a marker of isolation of EBV.

T lymphocytes will grow in the presence of a lymphokine, IL-2, formerly known as T-cell growth factor. This finding proved essential to the study of the human retroviruses (HIV

and HTLV, Chapter 25), which can be propagated in such cultures with the formation of syncytial giant cells.

4.4 Test procedure

Suitable cell cultures are inoculated with a small quantity of the clinical specimen contained in transport medium (section 1, above). The cultures are then observed for CPEs (see Fig. 36.4), which may appear within 48 hours (e.g. enteroviruses, herpes simplex), or be delayed for as long as 14 days (e.g. CMV). CPE fall into the following categories according to whether they are

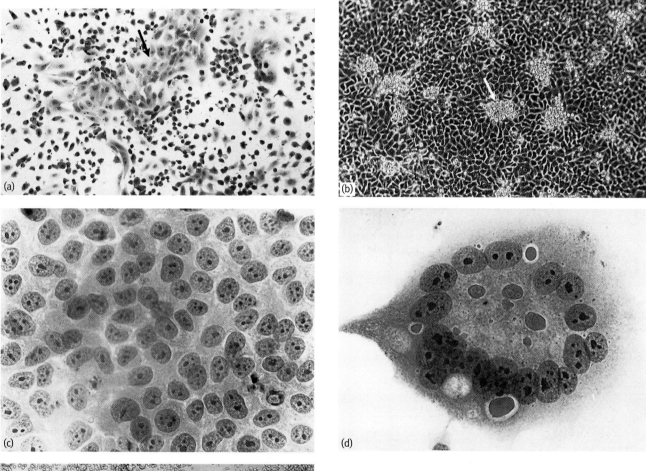

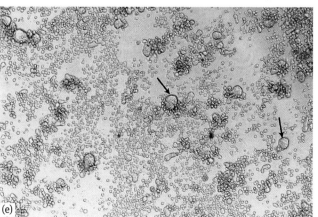

Fig. 36.4 CPEs of viral infection. **(a)** Enterovirus infection of a continuous line of human embryo lung cells (HEL). Areas of rounded, dead, or dying cells lie between islands of normal cells (arrowed). **(b)** HSV type 2 infection of baboon kidney cells (phase contrast). The affected cells (arrowed) are swollen and refractile. **(c)** High-power view of a continuous line of human epithelial cells (c) and a multinucleate giant cell **(d)** resulting from infection with respiratory syncytial virus. **(e)** Infection of a line of human lymphocytes with human immunodeficiency virus (HIV-1). Multinucleate giant cells are arrowed. (Parts (a) and (c) are reproduced with permission from Robinson, T.W.E. and Heath, R.B. (1983). *Virus Diseases and the Skin*. Churchill Livingstone, London.)

caused by viruses of the 'burster' (lytic) or 'creeper' types (Chapter 4).

- 'Burster' viruses (e.g. enteroviruses): rounding up and lysis (Fig. 36.4(a)).
- 'Creeper' viruses (e.g. herpesviruses, paramyxoviruses): formation of multinucleate giant cells (syncytia), with or without 'ballooning' of clumps of cells (Fig. 36.4(b–d)).

A few viruses, although replicating in the cell culture, cause no visible CPE and are detected only by their ability to make the cells resistant to superinfection with a second virus. Other viruses not causing CPE can be detected by immunofluorescence (Fig. 36.1) or by their capacity to bind red blood cells (haemadsorption). Some viruses, e.g. certain enteric and hepatitis viruses cannot be grown in cell culture systems.

For isolating HIV-1 from AIDS patients a special technique had to be developed, since this agent grows only in replicating human lymphocytes, which cannot normally be maintained in culture. This difficulty was overcome by stimulating the cells with a plant lectin, phytohaemagglutinin, and IL-2. The CPE of HIV-1 in such a culture is shown in Fig. 36.4(d).

5 Detection of antiviral antibodies

It must be emphasized that isolation of a particular virus, although suggestive of a diagnosis, does not always prove a

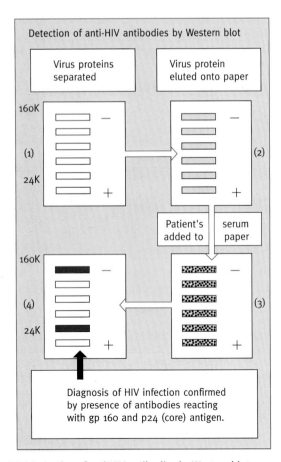

Fig. 36.5 Detection of anti-HIV antibodies by Western blot.

casual association between it and the patient's illness. As we saw in Chapter 4, some viruses are shed from clinically normal people. This uncertainty factor can be greatly diminished by the use of serological tests, in which (1) a rising titre of antibody to a particular virus is sought, or (2) serum is tested for the presence of specific IgM antibody. Method (1) depends on testing paired samples of serum, the first being taken as soon as possible after onset and the second, 10–14 days later. A fourfold or greater rise in titre of the relevant antibody is considered significant. Method (2), more widely used, has the advantage of rapidity in that specific IgM antibody is detectable a few days after the onset of illness. Some modern techniques detect newly secreted antibodies from B cells and so deviate from the paired sera approach.

5.1 Class-specific (IgM) antibody tests

We have already described some of the newer, rapid methods used for detecting viral antigens or antibodies. Among them, ELISA-type 'capture' methods (Fig. 36.2) are readily adaptable to the detection of specific antibodies, of which IgM is the most useful diagnostically. It is detectable within days of infection and remains so for 3–9 months, so that its finding is good evidence of a current or recent infection. In brief, the following steps are involved in testing for IgM antibody to a virus such as rubella (Fig. 36.2(b)).

1. IgM antibody to human IgM (anti-IgM) is adsorbed to a solid surface, e.g. a well in a microtitre plate.
2. The test serum is then added; IgM molecules are 'captured' by the anti-IgM.
3. Rubella antigen is added, and attaches only to rubella-specific IgM.
4. & 5. Enzyme-labelled antibody to rubella is added and detected as described in Section 3.2.

Such tests are very reliable, provided that adequate controls are included and each step is followed by thorough washing to remove unbound, non-specific reagents. IgM antibody rises following secondary infections (e.g. reactivation of herpesviruses) or booster doses of polio or rubella vaccines are possible sources of error.

5.2 Immunoblotting methods

The Southern blot method has no geographical connotation, but was named after the worker who invented a widely used method for DNA hybridization. A similar method used for RNA hybridization inevitably became known as Northern blotting, and Western blotting refers to its application for identifying proteins. It is a well-used method for diagnosis of HIV infection.

As the correct diagnosis of HIV-1 infection has such important personal and social implications, it is necessary to confirm a positive result (see Chapter 25) by a different technique, usually Western blotting (or immunoblotting) (Fig. 36.5; numbers in the description which follows refer to this figure). Virus proteins are separated as bands according to their molecular weights by electrophoresis through a polyacrylamide gel (1). The bands are eluted ('blotted') on to chemically treated paper, to which they bind tightly (2). The test human serum from the patient is added to the paper strip and any specific antibody attaches to the viral proteins (3). As in some other sandwich-type tests, an antihuman antibody labelled with an enzyme is added, followed by the enzyme substrate; the paper is then inspected for the presence of stained bands (4), which indicate the presence of complexes of specific antibody with antigen.

5.3 'Traditional' serological tests

These comprise complement fixation (many virus infections), radial haemolysis (screening test for rubella antibody), and occasionally haemagglutination inhibition to detect postimmunization antibodies to influenza.

Complement fixation is a reliable and versatile test has for many years served as the main diagnostic serological test. It is, however, relatively insensitive and requires large amounts of antigen, which are not available for all viruses. Many antibodies, when reacted with their specific antigen and complement, form a complex. Clearly, such a complex cannot be formed in the absence of the antibody, and any complement present will not be bound (or 'fixed'). The test thus depends on determining whether, at the end of the reaction period, free complement is still detectable (antibody absent, complement not fixed: negative result) or undetectable (antibody present, complement fixed: positive result). The test is used in hospital practice for detecting increases in antibody titre in paired sera: it does not discriminate between IgM and IgG antibodies.

The radial haemolysis test is a variant of the complement fixation test in which the virus is linked to sheep or human red blood cells by chromium chloride. The treated cells are mixed with molten agarose, which is poured into a Petri dish or other suitable plate.

When cool, small wells are punched in the agarose, each then being filled with a serum sample. After overnight incubation to allow diffusion of antibody into the agarose and combination with the antigen on the red cells, a solution of complement is poured over the plate, and lyses those red cells in which both antigen and antibody are present. A well containing antibody is thus surrounded by a clear zone of lysis, the diameter of which gives an indication of the amount of antibody in the sample. A variant of the complement fixation test can be used to test for influenza antibody, but is much more widely employed as a test for rubella antibodies in females. It is not accurate enough for assessing the antibody status of individual patients, but can be used to screen large numbers of sera, e.g. from antenatal clinics.

6 Reminders

- Molecular techniques (PCR, branched chain, NASBA) for quantifying viral genomes by **PCR** or **bDNA assay** and analysing genomes for drug-resistant mutations and reduction in viral genome load following chemotherapy are now making a very significant contribution to the management of patients. TaqMan is a real-time PCR technique able to give instant data.

- Provision of **appropriate specimens** and clinical information is essential.

- **Immunofluorescence, ELISA, latex agglutination**, and **EM** tests are still used. The latter has had a resurgence of interest for identification of pox viruses and was also essential for diagnosing SARS infections. The specificity of many of these tests is enhanced by the use of monoclonal antibodies.

- **Virus isolation in cell cultures** is still useful on occasion, but is slow and becoming superseded by more rapid methods. Viruses cause particular cytopathic changes in cells, which may give a good indication of the virus concerned.

- **EM** is useful for diagnosing infections with **herpes** and **poxviruses** (vesicle fluid) **and gastrointestinal infections** (faeces).

Control of viral diseases by immunization

Not until the germ theory of disease was accepted in the late nineteenth century and concepts of immunity were developed was it possible to develop the scientific framework for the practice of immunization against microbial diseases. We now know that vaccines contain what in modern terminology are virus proteins with antigenic areas called **epitopes**. Viral epitopes induce both B-cell and T-cell immunity; they may be contained in a continuous length of protein, or may have a discontinuous structure whereby two separate pieces fortuitously come together because of the tertiary folding of the polypeptide or protein. Vaccine-induced immunity may last several years or a lifetime, the ability to make these long-term responses being mediated by 'memory cells' (Chapter 5, section 4.2).

The first vaccines to be prepared in the laboratory were those against smallpox and rabies; other milestones of virus vaccine development include attenuated YF vaccine, manufactured from infected chick embryos; poliomyelitis and other viruses propagated in cell cultures, and, most recently, vaccines made from viral proteins and even DNA.

In this chapter, we aim only to cover the general principles of immunization. More detailed information on individual vaccines will be found in the relevant chapters in Part 2.

1 The technology and practicalities of virus vaccine production and development

1.1 Virus vaccine production and standardization

Table 37.1 lists most of the virus vaccines currently licensed around the world, most of which are prepared from live virus strains that have been attenuated in the laboratory by various methods. These vaccine viruses are selected on the basis of their good **immunogenicity** and **lack of pathogenicity**. They must also be **highly stable genetically**, i.e. with a minimal chance of reversion to the pathogenicity of the original 'wild-type' strain.

The preparation of all microbial vaccines demands the highest standards of laboratory practice, and vigorous efforts are made by international organizations such as WHO to ensure that virus vaccine seed material and production facilities in

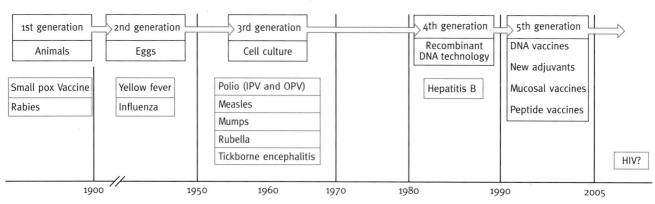

Fig. 37.1 Five generations of virus vaccines.

Table 37.1 Some virus vaccines currently licensed

Vaccine	Source of virus	Inactivated or attenuated vaccine	Route of administration	Comments
Vaccinia	Lymph from scarified animal skin	Attenuated	Scarification of arm	Stocked for emergency use only; US and Russian armies immunized
Yellow fever	Eggs	Attenuated	i.m.	Long immunity induced.
Influenza	Eggs	Inactivated (subunit)	i.m.	Antigenic variation of virus outdates vaccine yearly; 70 per cent effective
Polio	Monkey kidney or human diploid cells	Inactivated Attenuated	i.m. Oral	Both vaccines are highly efficacious
Measles	Chick embryo cells	Attenuated	i.m.	Components of the successful triple vaccine (MMR)
Rubella	Human diploid cells	Attenuated	i.m.	with at least 90 per cent efficacy;
Mumps	Chick embryo cells	Attenuated	i.m.	long-lasting immunity
Rabies	Animal brain	Inactivated	i.m.	Postexposure prophylaxis now superseded in many countries
	Human diploid cells	Inactivated	i.m.	Pre- and postexposure prophylaxis
Hepatitis A	Human diploid cells	Inactivated	i.m.	
Hepatitis B	Human serum	Inactivated (subunit)	i.m.	Superseded in many countries
	Yeast (recombinant)	Subunit	i.m.	Recombinant DNA vaccine

i.m., intramuscular

different countries conform to given standards. Thus, vaccine manufacturers use well characterized stock vaccine viruses and cell cultures for preparing vaccines. A seed virus technique is used whereby a large batch of vaccine virus is frozen at −70ºC. From this, the actual vaccine is produced by infecting cells with virus that is only two passages removed from the seed. This procedure reduces the opportunity for unwanted mutations to occur in the vaccine virus, which might alter its virulence or antigenic characteristics.

The amount of infective virus in a live vaccine is quantified in cell cultures to ensure an adequate infectivity titre. For inactiv-

ated or subunit vaccines such as influenza or hepatitis B, the amount of viral antigen is adjusted to about 10 µg protein per dose. Needless to say, rigorous quality assurance checks, including of course tests for microbial contamination, are carried out from start to finish of the production process.

1.2 Choice of cell substrates

Although we live in an age of biotechnology almost all the current virus vaccines, with the notable exception of hepatitis B, are produced using the traditional technology of cell culture developed half a century ago. However, cloning techniques and expression of viral proteins in yeast or mammalian cells will be key techniques of the near future.

John Enders and his colleagues achieved a major scientific breakthrough in the 1940s when they reported that a strain of polio virus could be cultivated in monkey kidney cells, which, unlike neural tissue, can readily be grown in the laboratory. They were awarded the Nobel Prize for their work. The result of this observation (together with the discovery of antibiotics, which prevented bacterial contamination of cell cultures) was the development of effective vaccines, first against polio and then other viral infections.

In general, the criteria for selection of cells for vaccines are ready availability, the lack of potential oncogenicity, genetic stability, and freedom from demonstrable contamination with extraneous viruses. For most of the earlier vaccines, such as polio and rubella, cells from a variety of mammals were used but, with the growing appreciation of the presence of retroviruses in animal cells and perhaps other, as yet undetected, viruses, together with growing concern about the use of primates, for reasons of conservation, more vaccine viruses are now cultivated in human cells. These are diploid, with a limited lifespan in culture, as in nature. Commonly used cells such as WI-38 or MRC-5 were derived from aborted fetuses and this may raise ethical problems for some people. The cells can be passaged only 40–50 times *in vitro* before dying out so that, in practice, large batches of cells are frozen in liquid nitrogen at an early passage level and are made available for manufacturers to produce virus vaccines.

1.3 The virological basis of killed or attenuated virus vaccines

Chemically killed vaccines

Chemical agents such as **formalin** or **β-propiolactone** inactivate viruses by chemically cross-linking base pairs in virion RNA or DNA. Classic killed vaccines are rabies, influenza, and polio.

Live attenuated vaccines

Most attenuated or 'weakened' virus vaccines are made from RNA viruses such as polio, measles, mumps, and rubella. This is probably no coincidence because the RNA replicase has a low fidelity of transcription (Chapter 3). This means that in every cycle of infection, lasting say 8 hours, an RNA virus might throw off 500 different mutants compared with the 10 000 or so viruses identical to the parent strain. However, advantage can be taken of the observations, dating back even to Pasteur, that some of these mutants may be less virulent than the parent virus. They may be selected or enriched in the laboratory by rapid passage; namely, transfer of virus from cell culture to cell culture; this is the so-called 'attenuation by passage'. Another method, used alone or in combination, is to perform the passages at a low temperature (28–30°C). This allows the emergence of temperature-sensitive (ts) or cold-adapted mutants that replicate preferentially at these temperatures, at the same time losing their pathogenicity. Such strains, with many mutations in the genome, are termed **attenuated**; Dr A. Sabin used such techniques to produce the attenuated live viruses used in the OPV.

The genetic basis of attenuation

When such attenuated viruses are analysed a surprisingly limited number of specific mutations are noted in key genes. Comparison with the genome of wild-type virulent polio type I genome shows that the attenuated strain has undergone 55 substitutions out of 7441 bases; 21 of these substitutions result in actual amino acid changes. With the important type 3 polio vaccine strain, which is known to revert to virulence more easily than type 1, only 10 nucleotides are mutated, of which only three result in amino acid changes in the structural protein. New live attenuated influenza vaccines have about 10 mutations with at least one in each of the eight genes.

For the first time a new technology of **reverse genetics** is being applied to negative-strand RNA viruses. A negative-stranded genome can be excised, transcribed to DNA, mutated, and reinserted into a cell with a reconstituted RNA transcriptase that allows infection of the cell and incorporation of the genetically modified gene. We can anticipate a new generation of GM vaccines.

1.4 Problems with viral vaccines

Although the development of effective virus vaccines is one of the major successes of biomedical research, some serious—but fortunately rare—problems of safety have come to light.

As an example of a totally unexpected problem, an inactivated vaccine against RSV (see Chapter 9) resulted in some immunized children developing a more serious infection than their non-immunized classmates, when they were in contact with virulent virus. It has been reasoned that chemical inactivation distorted the immune response allowing excessive production of IgE against one of the viral spike proteins, but this was 40 years ago. Another problem encountered with some attenuated vaccines such as those for polio and influenza is reversion to parental-type virulence. The incidence of post-vaccination polio is about 1 in 300 000 doses of attenuated vaccine. Such events provide a warning that we still do not fully understand the underlying genetic mechanisms determining virulence or attenuation of most viruses.

All at once or one at a time? The measles, mumps, and rubella (MMR) vaccine controversy

In 1988 a combined MMR prepared from attenuated strains of these viruses was introduced on a large scale. Although even a single dose conferred immunity in about 90% of those receiving it, it was recommended that the vaccine should be normally be given in two doses at 12–15 months of age, but could be given at any age thereafter.

The widespread use of the MMR vaccine use was followed by dramatic reductions in the incidence of all three infections.

However, it was contended by some that the vaccine was responsible for various complications, ranging from febrile reactions soon after its administration to more serious illnesses, in particular autism and Crohn's disease of the lower bowel.

The heated arguments surrounding the validity of these allegations have generated an enormous literature, reminiscent of the earlier debates about the complications of pertussis vaccine, and there is certainly not enough space here to discuss the issues in depth. The main contention of the anti-MMR lobby is that administration of triple vaccine, added to the others recommended in early childhood, is in danger of 'overloading the

immune system'. The vaccine should therefore be given as three spaced single vaccines. This extended schedule is not, however, approved officially because it leaves vulnerable children unprotected for too long against one or other of the three infections; and indeed there is evidence that use of the single vaccines has been followed by increases in their incidences.

It has to be said that there is much misleading information about this topic on the internet, which is often the first port of call for parents who are mistrustful of advice from official sources. This is a pity, because the strong conclusion from many well conducted observations in the field is that there is no evidence for an association between triple vaccine on the one hand, and autism and bowel disease on the other. Furthermore, it is now widely accepted that the early researches on which this conclusion was based were flawed.

Some contraindications and possible side-effects of viral vaccines are listed in Table 37.2.

Table 37.2 Main side-effects and contraindications for licensed viral vaccines

Vaccine	Potential side-effects	Main contra-indications for vaccination
Inactivated vaccines		
Influenza	Local reactions, including redness at inoculation side. Guillain–Barré syndrome is exceedingly rare	Serious egg allergy
Rabies	Mild local reactions with modern human diploid cell vaccine. Local and systemic reactions, including encephalo-myelitis with older animal brain vaccines	None
Polio	None	None
Hepatitis B	None	None
Live attenuated vaccines		
Measles	Mild. Malaise, rash, fever, headache in a low proportion	Pregnancy; the immunocompromised; serious egg allergy (except rubella and polio)
Rubella	Mild. Lymphadenopathy and joint pain in a low proportion	
Mumps	Mild. Fever and parotitis. Post-vaccination meningitis with Urabe strain	
Yellow fever	Mild. Malaise, headache in a low proportion	
Polio	Vaccine-associated paralysis; exceedingly rare. Production of live vaccine will now cease for routine use and killed vaccine will be stockpiled	

2 Virus vaccines and public health

As a result of mass immunization campaigns during the last two decades, childhood infections such as polio, measles, and rubella are well controlled in many of the more wealthy countries, so well in fact that some parents now withdraw their children from vaccination schemes, not wishing to accept a very small risk of side-effects when they perceive that the incidences of the illnesses in question, e.g. measles, mumps, rubella, polio, are now extremely low. However, it should also be remembered that in a global context infectious diseases still take a heavy toll both in mortality and general suffering. Paralytic polio is still present in South America, Asia, and Africa (although the WHO plan will see the virus eradicated by 2006), and measles causes very serious problems in children in these countries. These viruses can be, and are, imported into the USA and Europe. Nevertheless, the scientific problems faced in the development and production of safe and efficacious vaccines for these diseases have been overcome: only the political will and economic resources to use them in developing countries are now needed. As long as reservoirs of any of the viruses remain, importations into apparently 'virus-free' countries will be a constant problem.

Smallpox eradication is the best example of a vigorous international approach to the elimination of an important infectious disease. It was initiated by the USSR (Russia) at a WHO meeting in Alma Ata in the late 1960s and supported fully by the USA; with the necessary funds and scientific expertise the world vaccination campaign was pushed forward by WHO in some of the poorest nations on earth with dramatic success. Similar international co-operation could now result in the vanquishing of polio and even hepatitis B (by 2040).

Cost-effectiveness of vaccines

The increasing availability of effective vaccines inevitably imposes heavy costs on the budgets of national and international health authorities, but there are few more splendid examples of cost-effectiveness than immunization, which produces massive savings on hospitalization and medical treatment. This is particularly the case with polio, measles, and rubella, which sometimes give rise to serious long-term sequelae.

Apart from the vital global strategy of the international WHO programme most national health authorities organize their own childhood immunization schedules. The details vary from country to country; the UK schedule is summarized in Table 37.3. It is most important that these national campaigns are conducted in a vigorous manner to achieve immunization rates greater than 90 per cent in childhood. Sometimes it is impossible to predict at the outset whether a vaccination campaign will produce enough herd immunity to prevent spread of the natural virus. Figure 12.3 shows the results of two successive strategies to prevent rubella epidemics, by immunizing either adolescent girls or babies of both sexes. The latter approach proved by far the more successful (see Chapter 12).

In the UK and Europe, influenza vaccine is administered to individuals at special risk, e.g. the **elderly** and those with **cardiac or respiratory disease**, and, when an epidemic is threatened, to certain groups such as **healthcare staff** and people in public services. Immunization of all medical, paramedical, and dental staff against hepatitis B is now obligatory. In some European countries universal immunization of babies with hepatitis B vaccine is the rule. It is quite likely that the UK and USA will also adopt this approach.

Overseas travel

Before going abroad, especially to the less developed countries, travellers should seek advice on immunization, which may change from time to time according to local circumstances. Visitors from more developed countries often forget that they may be at risk of influenza in the winter period. Decisions as to which inoculations should be given may depend on the type of travel and accommodation: the requirements of backpackers in the interior may differ from those staying in luxury hotels on the coast.

YF may be contracted during visits to endemic areas and immunization is obligatory for entry to these regions and subsequent travel to uninfected countries. Prophylactic **rabies vaccine** is not recommended unless the traveller is visiting an endemic area for an extended period. Travellers to Third World countries may opt for hepatitis A vaccine or the combined **hepatitis A and B** vaccine.

Table 37.3 Schedule of routine immunizations in the UK

Vaccine	Age	Notes
DTP and Hib Polio	1st dose 2 months) 2nd dose 3 months) 3rd dose 4 months)	Primary course
Measles/mumps/rubella (MMR)	12–15 months	Can be given at any age over 12 months
Booster DT and polio, MMR second dose	3–5 years	Three years after completion of primary course
BCG	10–14 years or infancy	
Booster tetanus, diphtheria, and polio	13–18 years	

Children should therefore have received the following vaccines:

By 6 months:	3 doses of DTP, Hib and polio.
By 15 months:	Measles/mumps/rubella
By school entry:	4th DT and polio; second dose measles/mumps/rubella
Between 10 and 14 years:	BCG
Before leaving school:	5th polio and tetanus diphtheria (TD)

Adults should receive the following vaccines:

Women seronegative for rubella:	rubella
Previously unimmunized individuals:	polio, tetanus, diphtheria
Individuals in high-risk groups:	hepatitis B,
	hepatitis A, influenza,
	pneumococcal vaccine

Reproduced with permission from Department of Health (1996). *Immunization against infectious disease*, pp. 46–7. HMSO, London.
D, Diphtheria; T, Tetanus; P, Pertussis; Hib, *Haemophilus influenzae* Type B.

Vaccine storage and usage

All vaccines must be kept at ≈4°C and not allowed to freeze. Live vaccines are particularly susceptible to heat-inactivation and some are provided as freeze-dried powder to be reconstituted with sterile water at the time of use. Vaccines that cannot be freeze-dried, e.g. oral polio, must be transported in special cold boxes containing sensors that give a warning if the internal temperature rises beyond the safety limit.

Live polio vaccines are administered as oral drops, usually on a sugar lump; all the other current viral vaccines, whether live or inactivated, are administered by intramuscular injection.

3 Passive immunization

Injection of **human immunoglobulin** preparations containing appropriate antibodies give immediate partial or complete protection against infection by certain viruses. Table 37.4 summarizes the preparations currently available. Such protection is immediate upon injection of the antibodies but is not sustained beyond about 4 months because of decay of antibodies and the production in the recipient of antibodies against the preparation. This is by no means a universal protective method because administration of antiviral antibodies to persons already infected with certain viruses could actually make the infection worse; with dengue, for example, antibodies may form complexes and provoke an untoward reaction (Chapter 27), but for certain infections, it may be a useful adjunct to active immunization.

Table 37.4 Examples of human immunoglobulins used for passive prophylaxis

Preparation	Comments
Normal human immunoglobulin (HNIG)	For prevention or modification of measles in persons at special risk after contact with an infection, e.g. immuno-compromised children or adults
	For prevention or modification of hèpatitis a in travellers to endemic countries excluding Europe, USA, and Australasia
Hepatitis B Immunoglobulin (HBIG)	Can be co-administered with vaccine to provide rapid protection. Administered to persons with needlestick injuries. Not available for travellers
Human rabies immunoglobulin (HRIG)	To provide rapid protection after exposure to virus until vaccine immunity develops
Zoster immunoglobulin (ZIG)	For immunosuppressed or leukaemia patients; neonates or pregnant contacts of cases
Lassa convalescent plasma	Used therapeutically
SARS convalescent plasma	Used therapeutically in a few patients
TBE convalescent plasma	Used therapeutically in affected areas

4 New approaches to vaccine development

4.1 Genetically engineered virus vaccines

Strong new ideas and the techniques of molecular biology have been introduced in the last two decades into vaccine technology. Thus genes or portions thereof can now be **cloned in plasmid vectors** and transferred to yeast cells, as is already done in the manufacture of hepatitis B vaccine. In the example of cloning illustrated in Fig. 37.2, a viral gene coding for an immunogenic protein is excised from the virus and cloned into a plasmid vector, which is then inserted into a bacterial cell. The plasmid replicates alongside the bacterium and provides the necessary genetic information for synthesis of the viral protein. This protein may be produced in large quantities in a bacterial

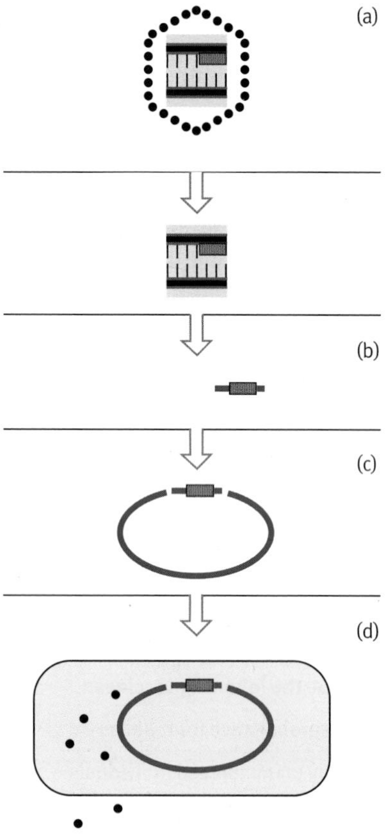

Fig. 37.2 The cloning and expression of a viral gene in a caterium. **(a)** A viral gene ▬, coding for an externally situated viral protein (•), is excised **(b)** and inserted into a plasmid vector **(c)**. The vector is used to transfect a bacterium **(d)**, in which the gene is translated to produce large amounts of viral protein. Such 'genetically engineered' proteins may be used for vaccine production.

fermentation apparatus and purified from the bacterial culture. Of course, the vector may be cloned into eukaryotic cells, insect cells or larvae, or even into plants and plant viruses for efficient expression of the viral protein.

Perhaps the most exciting molecular technique is the cloning of viral genetic information into the genome of other large DNA viruses, such as vaccinia, canarypox, or adenovirus, which are thus used as 'Trojan horses' to carry the genes of the new vaccine virus into the recipient. Thus immunogenic proteins of rabies, influenza, HIV, and hepatitis have been cloned into the TK locus of the genome of vaccinia poxvirus. Moreover, insertion of new genetic information at this point in the vaccinia genome is expected to attenuate this virus further. The vaccinia virus genome is so large (≈150 kbp) that viral functions are not compromised by excision of a portion and reintroduction of a new gene. After inoculation into the skin, vaccinia virus replicates and at the same time as producing its own proteins codes for the new antigens specified by the cloned viral gene.. Other viruses such as adenovirus can be used as vectors and, perhaps surprisingly, some RNA virus such as VEE where a replicon system is designed whereby a vaccine virus only replicates when the additional RNA replicase is co-administered.

4.2 Short peptides as vaccines

Our understanding of the nature of the B- and T-cell epitopes (antigenic determinants) on virus proteins is progressing rapidly. Some viral epitopes consist of only eight amino acids. Cattle can be protected against foot and mouth disease virus by immunization with short synthetic peptides of the correct amino-acid sequence. In theory, many such epitopes for different viruses could be synthesized and linked together as a single immunogenic protein able to induce B- or T-cell immunity to a wide range of infective agents.

4.3 DNA vaccines

Unexpectedly, researchers discovered that injected **viral DNA** would penetrate mammalian epithelial cells and be transcribed and copied into viral proteins by the cellular protein translating system. More important, these newly synthesized viral proteins, would be processed into viral peptides and presented on MHC class I molecules exactly as if the cell had been infected with the virus itself. Viral DNA could thus act like an attenuated virus vaccine. Even the RNA genome of viruses such as influenza or HIV may be transcribed into DNA by RT and the DNA utilized to infect cells. DNA vaccines have an important future and experimentation is particularly critical with HIV.

4.4 Adjuvants

Adjuvants of various compositions can prolong and enhance the immune response to inactivated or subunit vaccines. Aluminium hydroxide is the only one so far licensed for use in humans. It must be acknowledged that the scientific basis of these molecules is still obscure. New research is focused on stimulating the innate immune system via Toll-like receptors, which are present on the outer membrane of macrophages and dendritic cells and can sense viral RNA and some viruses themselves.

Methods of presentation of viral antigens to the immune cells are important and immunogenicity can be enhanced if viral proteins are aggregated in novel ways with or without adjuvants. For example, aggregation of viral proteins by saponin molecules results in formation of **immune-stimulatzing complexes**; and viral proteins have been incorporated into lipid spheres **(liposomes)** containing muramyl dipeptides, which increase the immunological response and memory of the host.

5 Reminders

- Viral vaccines prevent infection by antigenic stimulation of the host and induction of memory T cells, resulting in the generation of neutralizing antibody and cytotoxic T cells. Immunity starts to develop some days after vaccination and memory cells may persist for decades.

- **Inactivated** (killed) vaccines consist of chemically inactivated whole virions (e.g. rabies, formalin-killed polio vaccine). Non-living vaccines are also prepared from fractionated virus containing immunogenic proteins, (e.g. 'split' influenza vaccine), or by recombinant DNA techniques (e.g. HBsAg vaccine).

- **Live vaccines** are prepared from viruses, which, by manipulation in the laboratory are no longer pathogenic but retain their immunogenicity (e.g. YF, oral polio, mumps, measles, rubella).

- Vaccines are not without serious side-effects but these are extremely rare. **Pregnancy and immunocompromised states are contraindications to live attenuated vaccines in case the virus crosses the placenta.**

- Smallpox has been completely eradicated and some other viral infections such as polio have been virtually eliminated. Humanitarian considerations apart, **immunization is one of the most cost-effective public health measures available.**

- **Passive prophylaxis with human immunoglobulin preparations** gives a measure of immediate protection against infection of measles, hepatitis A and B, rabies, VZV, and Lassa. Immunoglobulin may be co-administered with inactivated vaccines such as rabies and hepatitis B.

- Certain viruses remain uncontrolled by immunization because of multiplicity of serotypes, i.e. rhinoviruses and arboviruses, or major antigenic change, i.e. HIV.

- New approaches to vaccine development include recombinant DNA techniques, the use of DNA itself as the immunogen and the improvement of adjuvants and new adjuvants targeting the innate immune system. Replication-deficient VEE or adenoviruses are forming the basis of a new class of GM vaccines.

Antiviral chemotherapy

Certain important virus diseases such as measles and rubella can be kept under very good control with live virus vaccines, and some (e.g. smallpox and polio) even eradicated. But, as we saw in Chapter 37, it is difficult to imagine the development of successful vaccines for many other viruses, because of a multiplicity of serotypes, or variability or complexity of their antigenic structure. These are the target viruses for antiviral chemotherapy. There are currently 30 or so antiviral compounds licensed for use against herpes, HIV-1, RSV, and influenza A virus. A negative feature of all the known antivirals, with the exception of ribavirin, is their very narrow spectra of activity; thus antiherpes compounds have no effect against influenza and vice versa. All the drugs so far have been discovered by random biological screening in the laboratory but chemists are now using three-dimensional structures of virus proteins, accurately determined by X-ray crystallography, to design inhibitory molecules that fit into sites of important activities on viral proteins. Examples are the new influenza NA inhibitors that have been designed to bind tightly to the active site of the viral enzyme without binding to host cell or bacterial NAs.

However, would it not be possible to devise a universal antiviral against all viruses, or does such a compound exist already as IFN? The answer is unfortunately, no. The great hopes raised over 40 years ago when IFN was discovered by Isaacs and Lindenmann have not been realized, and its applications in viral chemotherapy are still limited to certain hepatitis B and C infections. However, the work of these pioneers has given rise to a wide range of molecules—the cytokines—which have important effects in the immune system.

1 Points of action of antivirals in the virus life cycle

Scientists have searched for the last 40 years for molecules that would inhibit virus-directed events without interfering with normal cellular activities. The potential points of inhibitory action of antiviral drugs include:

- **Binding to the free virus particle.** This represents a rather unusual target in the sense that drugs may stabilize the virus by cross-linking its structural proteins so that release of nucleic acid from its interior is impeded. This could stop virus infection at a very early stage. There is also considerable interest in **virucidal compounds**, which could destroy enveloped viruses such as HIV or influenza H5N1 on

Table 38.1 Examples of antiviral drugs affecting different steps in virus multiplication (the list is not complete)

Target	Drug	Virus inhibited
Viral adsorption or fusion	Enfuvirtide	HIV-1
Penetration and uncoating	Amantadine	Influenza A
	Rimantadine	
Viral nucleic acid synthesis	Aciclovir	Herpes simplex and varicella
	Penciclovir	Zoster
	Ganciclovir	CMV
	Ribavirin	Influenza A and B, hepatitis C
	Lamivudine (3TC) NRTI	HIV-1
	Zidovudine (AZT) NRTI	HIV-1
	Didanosine (ddi) NRTI	HIV-1
	Stavudine (d4t) NRTI	HIV-1
	Zalcitabine NRTI	HIV-1
	Abacavir NRTI	HIV-1
	Nevirapine NNRTI	HIV-1
	Efavirenz NNRTI	HIV-1
	Delavirdine NNRTI	HIV-1
	Emtricitabine NNRTI	HIV-1
	Tenofovir (nucleotide analogue)	HIV-1
	Interferon	Range of viruses
	Foscarnet	HIV-1 and herpes simplex
Binding to intact virus particle	Disoxaril	Rhinoviruses
Virus release	Zanamavir	Influenza A and B NA
	Oseltamivir	Influenza A and B NA
	Saquinavir	HIV protease
	Indinavir	HIV protease
	Ritonavir	HIV protease
	Lopinavir	HIV protease
	Nelfinavir	HIV protease
	Amprenavir	HIV protease

contact. These 'disinfectants' are being explored with caution: in the case of HIV, toxicity for cells lining the vagina could actually enhance the infection.

- **Interference with virus adsorption** or attachment to the receptor-binding site on the cell. Synthetic cell receptors could act as 'decoys' and hence prevent infection of cells. An example is the attempted use of soluble CD4 and other molecules to prevent HIV infection. Most successful has been the use of drugs to prevent fusion of HIV with the cell membrane to allow virus entry.

- **Inhibition of virus uncoating** or release of nucleic acid from the virus interior. The most investigated inhibitor in this group is amantadine, an antiviral against influenza A targeting the viral M2 protein.

- **Inhibition of viral nucleic acid transcription and replication.** Certain viruses code for specific enzymes of their own, such as influenza RNA transcriptase, herpes TK and DNA polymerase, and HIV RT, integrase, and protease. These viral enzymes form the most important targets for inhibition.

- **Interference with cellular processing of viral polypeptides**, by preventing addition of sugar or acyl groups. This may be the least successful approach because cellular and viral proteins are processed in similar ways.

- **Prevention of virus budding or interference with virus maturation.** The newest antivirals under investigation inhibit influenza virus NA, which normally acts at the virus release stage. Some anti-HIV proteases block events catalysed by viral proteases immediately after release of virus and during its maturation.

The current licensed antivirals are very effective inhibitors and, although few in number compared with antibacterials, are now widely used in hospital and in general practice. Their chemical structures are illustrated in Fig. 38.1.

2 The use of antivirals: general considerations

A list of antivirals according to their clinical usefulness and effectiveness would be headed by ACV, the L-valyl ester prodrug valaciclovir, and the chemically related penciclovir against alpha-herpesviruses. ACV cream is now licensed as an 'over the counter' drug for use against herpes cold sores; as the development of antivirals expands, this could be a portent of things to come. AZT and other dideoxynucleoside analogues such as ddi, ddC, and 3TC, non-nucleoside analogues inhibitors, and protease inhibitors are widely used for treating HIV-1 infections. The NA inhibitors such as oseltamivir are being increasingly used to treat influenza in the elderly and will have an important role in future pandemics and are being stockpiled. Less used are ribavirin against RSV infection in children and amantadine against influenza A. Pegylated IFNs are used to treat SARS patients and also hepatitis B and C patients, often alongside ribavirin.

Anti-influenza

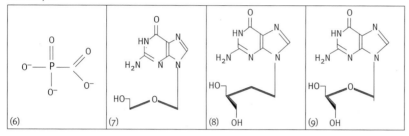

Anti-herpes

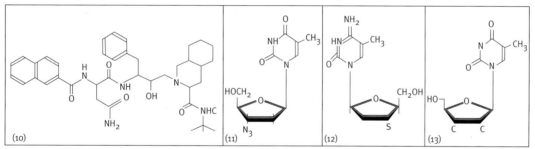

Anti-HIV

Fig. 38.1 The chemical structures of some antiviral compounds. (1) zanamivr; (2) Oseltamivir; (3) amantadine; (4) rimantadine; (5) ribavirin; (6) foscarnet; (7) ACV; (8) penciclovir; (9) ganciclovir; (10) saquinavir; (11) zidovudine; (12) lamivudine; (13) stavudine.

2.1 Therapy and prophylaxis

Antivirals are mostly used therapeutically and are administered as soon as possible after the first signs of infection. For example, ACV should be taken as soon as possible after the onset of herpetic lesions (i.e. at the early itching stage), and amantadine, when the patient first begins to feel ill with influenza. Speed of use is essential, and if there is a delay even of 24 hours, the drugs are much less effective.

To a lesser extent antivirals are used to prevent a virus infection, (e.g. amantadine and oseltomivis in the prophylaxis of influenza A; Sections 4.1 and 4.2).

Compared with vaccines, prophylaxis with a chemical antiviral has the advantage of speed of action, as some protection would be anticipated within an hour or so of administration.

The converse is also true: when prophylaxis is discontinued the patient again becomes susceptible to infection.

A good example of antiviral prophylaxis is the long-term administration of ACV by mouth to prevent recurrent attacks of genital herpes, a condition that causes much discomfort and sexual disability. The NIs or M2 blockers are used to prevent infection with influenza in the family or workplace.

Following oral or intravenous administration, effective tissue concentrations of the drug may be achieved in minutes. The half-life of an antiviral drug is only a few hours and therefore frequent dosing is required to maintain optimal levels in plasma and tissues. Penciclovir has the same antiviral spectrum as ACV against herpes type I, but sufferers need only take three tablets a day rather than five because the former drug is more tightly bound inside the cell and its half-life is prolonged.

2.2 Pharmacology and side-effects

All drugs have side-effects and antiviral compounds are no exception. Even the very safe antiherpes drug **ACV,** which has been used for two decades in millions of patients, can cause gastrointestinal symptoms such as nausea and vomiting. Particular care must be exercised in patients with renal failure, as even with normal kidney function about 70 per cent of the drug is excreted unchanged in the urine. Severe renal malfunction can result in undesirably high concentrations of drug in the blood. The structurally related anti-CMV drug, **ganciclovir,** induces more serious side-effects: for example, neutropenia occurs in one-third of patients and thrombocytopenia, rash, and nausea may also occur.

Zidovudine at the original dosage prescribed for AIDS patients induced anaemia, neutropenia and leucopenia in approximately one-third of patients. These side-effects are now avoided by using lower doses of drug which are, however, still effective. **Amantadine** causes the slight neurological effect of 'jitteriness' in a few patients, which ceases immediately the drug is discontinued. Again, with careful adjustment and lowering of dosage, particularly for the elderly or for patients with renal problems, these side-effects can be avoided.

IFNs are not free of side-effects such as depression and other psychiatric changes, fatigue, and even severe somnolence.

Pregnancy is usually an important contraindication for the use of all these drugs because of potential damage to the fetus. Unexpectedly, however, AZT and 3TC administered to an HIV-positive mother during pregnancy can have a beneficial effect by reducing the chance of spread of the virus from mother to fetus.

2.3 The use of prodrugs

The most recent pharmaceutical innovation is antiviral prodrugs with chemical side groups attached to the active antiviral molecule that enhance adsorption and tissue penetration. Host enzymes then cleave off the side chain from the prodrug to release concentrations of the active drug that are often higher than could otherwise be achieved. For example valaciclovir, the prodrug of ACV, is absorbed from the gastrointestinal tract and converted to ACV in the intestine and liver. Approximately 60 per cent of the prodrug given by mouth is absorbed, compared with 20 per cent absorption of ACV. Similarly, famciclovir is a diacetyl prodrug of penciclovir. Hydrolysis in the intestinal wall and metabolism in the liver remove both acetyl groups, and oxidation of this deacylated form converts famciclovir to penciclovir.

3 Herpes infections

3.1 Aciclovir and related compounds

Mode of action

ACV and **penciclovir** possess an excellent combination of biochemical and pharmaceutical properties, which explains their unique anti-herpesvirus specificity. Indeed, they approach the ideal specification for an antiviral drug. First, the compounds are phosphorylated to the monophosphate only in herpes-infected cells, as this biochemical step requires a **herpesvirus TK** and cannot be achieved by normal cellular TK. The viral TK is less 'precise' than the corresponding cellular TK and so, unlike the latter, will accept 'fraudulent' substrates such as ACV. Once ACV is phosphorylated in the cell it cannot emerge because of the charged phosphate group that has been added by the TK enzyme. Moreover as the pool of 'normal' unphosphorylated ACV in the cell is depleted, more ACV molecules move across the plasma membrane and these are in turn phosphorylated. In this manner the drug accumulates only in virus-infected cells. Phosphorylation to the di- and triphosphate is then achieved by cellular enzymes.

Thus the drug is likely to be of low toxicity as its tissue distribution is limited to virus-infected cells. The second specific feature of the drug is that the triphosphate, the active moiety, binds to and specifically **inhibits the herpesvirus DNA polymerase**. It has little effect on cellular DNA polymerase and hence is not toxic. These drugs can terminate DNA chain formation and so, at least in theory, might inhibit DNA replication in uninfected cells. However, if this happens at all, the effect must be very slight and the compounds are considered to be safe in clinical use: for example, patients with recurrent herpes simplex have been effectively treated with daily doses for many years without side-effects. However, a latently infected cell cannot be cleared of herpesvirus by ACV, which is thus unable to eradicate the infection.

The related antiviral, penciclovir, has a similar mode of action to that of ACV but is retained more tightly within the cell as the mono-, di-, or triphosphate and therefore needs to be given less often. Penciclovir has approximately one-hundredth the potency of ACV in inhibiting herpesvirus DNA polymerase, but as it accumulates in very high concentrations and has an extended half-life, its clinical effect is similar.

Clinical application

The nucleoside analogue predecessors of ACV, such as idoxuridine and trifluorothymidine, were useful for treating herpetic eye infections, particularly keratitis, and adenine arabinoside previously had a role in the treatment of herpes simplex encephalitis and serious paediatric infections. However, ACV and now penciclovir are so much more effective and so free from problems of toxicity that their use has transformed the often difficult clinical management of herpes simplex and varicella-zoster.

ACV or penciclovir are used in the prophylaxis of herpes simplex and zoster infections in bone marrow and heart transplant patients, and to prevent the spread of virus in those already infected. The drugs are also very effective in treating herpes simplex encephalitis, if administered early. Continuous treatment prevents recurrent HSV-1 and -2 infections, particularly those of the genital tract, and some patients have taken ACV orally for many years. Treatment of severe VZV infections in the elderly and in immunocompromised patients requires higher dosage than herpes simplex infections and more effective anti-VZV drugs are required.

A derivative, **ganciclovir**, has mild antiviral activity against CMV and is used to treat life-threatening CMV pneumonia after BMTs and eye infections in AIDS patients with serious CMV infection.

Nucleotide analogues such as **cidavir** have recently proved effective in CMV eye infections.

3.2 Foscarnet

Mode of action

This drug inhibits herpes DNA polymerase by blocking the pyrophosphate binding site on the enzyme. It can, however, accumulate in bone and is toxic for the kidneys, and hence is mainly used in life-threatening situations.

Clinical application

Foscarnet (Foscavir®) is sometimes useful in treating severe ACV-resistant alphaherpesvirus infections.

4 Influenza

4.1 Amantadine and rimantadine

Mode of action

One of the structural proteins of the influenza virus, M2, normally acts as an ion channel across the viral membrane, allowing passage of hydrogen ions to the interior of the virus, particularly when it is within cellular lysosomes during early infection. Under these conditions two virus core proteins, NP and M, which bind closely with the viral RNA, dissociate and thus allow the viral RNA to enter the nucleus to replicate. Blockage of the ion channel by amantadine stops the induction of low pH and therefore inhibits all subsequent events that would normally lead to infection.

Clinical application

Prophylactic administration of antiflu drugs—the neuraminidase inhibitors (NIs)—or **amantadine** will prevent influenza A in 80 per cent of individuals. The antiflu drugs may be used prophylactically when the presence of influenza A virus in the community is confirmed. Prophylactic use can continue for 5 weeks or until the end of the epidemic is in sight. As with influenza vaccines, chemoprophylaxis is recommended only for the 'special risk groups', such as the over-75s, diabetics, and persons with chronic heart or chest diseases who have not been immunized or who wish to receive extra protection. The NIs (see below) can be used but must be given quickly, within 24 hours of onset. The NIs are very much under-used as antivirals. The situation may change dramatically with the advent of a new pandemic influenza A virus, when no vaccines would be available for the first waves of infection and the NIs and amantadine would be expected to have some clinical benefit.

4.2 Inhibitors of influenza neuraminidase (NIs)

Two drugs that bind tightly to the influenza mushroom-shaped NA have been discovered and refined, using X-ray crystallography of drug–protein interactions (oseltomivis and zanamivir). These antivirals are effective against influenza A and B viruses, preventing infection and reducing symptoms in persons already infected.

NA normally acts at the stage of virus release from the cell and inhibition of the enzyme by the new drug causes virus particles to aggregate at the cell surface rather than releasing themselves to infect adjacent cells. The NIs are already overtaking M2 blockers as the drugs of choice against influenza.

4.3 Ribavirin

Mode of action

The nucleoside analogue ribavirin possesses antiviral effects in cell culture. However, selectivity may be poor because it inhibits cellular inosine-5′-monophosphate dehydrogenase rather than any important viral enzyme.

Clinical application

Ribavirin has been used to treat a wide range of viruses including influenza. It is licensed in several countries for use as an aerosolized drug in children seriously ill with RSV. It has also been used, with variable success, to treat Lassa fever, hantavirus infections, and, in combination with IFN, hepatitis C.

5 HIV infections

5.1 Nucleoside RT inhibitors (NRTIs)

Mode of action

AZT was the first RT inhibitor to be used for treating HIV infection. Like ACV, it must be phosphorylated intracellularly to produce the active antiviral drug, which is the triphosphate. The latter is a very potent inhibitor of viral RT and prevents nucleotide chain elongation much in the same manner as ACV.

The 3′ positioning of the azido group of AZT blocks the essential phosphodiester linkage, which would normally enable the next nucleotide to be added to the growing DNA chain. Furthermore, AZT triphosphate binds to the viral RT rather than to the cellular DNA polymerase, giving some specificity of action. By contrast with ACV, cell enzymes rather then viral enzymes phosphorylate the molecule and hence intracellular concentrations of the drug increase in normal cells as well as in virus infected cells; this partly explains its toxic effects. The other dideoxynucleosides have a similar mode of action to that of AZT.

Clinical application

Remarkably, within 2 years of the isolation of HIV-1 a series of compounds that inhibit this virus had been discovered and one of them, AZT, was shown quite quickly to be effective in prolonging the lives of AIDS patients by about 18 months. It was noted recently that in patients given a drug holiday the immune system rebounded and could be expected to suppress virus. This new, and as yet to be fully explained clinical approach, is called interrupted therapy.

HIV-1 strains quite quickly mutated in the RT gene, the point of action of the drug, to become AZT drug-resistant. The patterns of resistance are quite complex. Four mutations in the RT are dominant in AZT-resistant viruses. But it was rather surprising to find that resistance to AZT could be reversed by other mutations induced in the RT by, for example, the dideoxynucleoside analogue ddi. Entirely new drugs can act synergistically with AZT to avoid drug resistance problems and can be used in lower dosages to avoid side-effects. Molecules such as ddi, ddC, and 3TC are used in **combination chemotherapy** with AZT, often with the addition of a viral protease inhibitor. This use of a combination of drugs is called HAART (highly active antiretroviral therapy).

5.2 Non-nucleoside RT inhibitors (NNRTIs)

The non-nucleoside RT inhibitors comprise several hundred antiviral compounds of very varied chemical structure but only a handful have been tested in the clinic. They are powerful inhibitors of HIV in the laboratory but drug-resistant HIV mutants appear almost immediately a patient is treated. Many of these compounds are highly selective for HIV-1 and bind tightly to the viral RT close to the polymerase active site, where they distort this region of the viral enzyme. They are used in combination with nucleoside and protease inhibitors.

5.3 Protease inhibitors

The virus-coded protease has the important function of cleaving certain HIV structural proteins at the **maturation** stage of viral replication (see Chapter 3). Without such cleavages the newly released virus does not mature and is not infective. At least six new drugs have been found that inhibit HIV protease but not mammalian cell proteases. These are powerful anti-HIV-1 drugs in the laboratory and the clinical data suggest that they are effective in AIDS patients. They are well tolerated but are difficult to manufacture and patients require large doses, up to 2 or 3 g/day. Drug-resistant mutants are easily selected and the cross-resistance patterns are complex.

5.4 Nucleotide inhibitors

This class of drug represented by tenofovir also targets the viral reverse transcriptase enzyme and can be used in place of a NRTI drug in the HAART scheme.

Fusion inhibitors

These drugs stop the virus from binding to and entering the cell and the most well tested molecule at present is enfuvirtide (Fuzeon).

5.5 Combination chemotherapy (HAART)

The most recent clinical strategy is to use a **combination** or 'cocktail' of drugs, e.g. AZT, 3TC, a non-nucleoside analogue, and a protease inhibitor.

It is now possible to quantify effects of drug treatment by assaying the amount of viral genome in the plasma of the patient—the **viral genome load**. Drug combinations can reduce the load to undetectable levels and therefore there is some optimism that HIV, like certain leukaemias for example, may be held in check by such complex drug treatments. Patients are monitored carefully for viral load. Cocktail antiviral chemotherapy is expensive and complicated to monitor and patients have to take perhaps 15 tablets at specific times each day. Default can allow a very rapid rebound of drug-resistant virus, which is thus not totally eradicated. Nevertheless, many AIDS patients have benefited from the effects of these new combinations of drugs and can even return to work.

Hepatitis C virus

This important and widespread virus causes both acute and chronic infection of the liver. Persistent infection can lead to chronic liver disease and the virus is the leading cause for liver transplantation in developed nations.

Approved treatments for patients are restricted to IFN-α (either in the native or pegylated forms) alone or in combination with the nucleoside analogue ribavirin. However, treatment failure is relatively high at about 60%. The three recombinant IFNs used are IFN-α2a, IFN-α2b (which is similar to 2a with a substitution of a single amino acid), and alfacon-1, a bioengineered consensus IFN-α, that has activity similar to natural IFN. Pegylated IFN used in combination with ribavirin is probably the most favoured treatment at present.

Hepatitis B virus

Despite the availability of vaccine, hepatitis B remains a major public health problem with up to 400 million carriers. Antiviral chemotherapy is the only option to control chronic HBV infection, which is unresponsive to vaccination. Most attempts to eradicate HBV infection using chemotherapy have only had a modest success to date. A subgroup of patients with active liver disease and low-level viraemia do respond to treatment with IFN-α given subcutaneously. This treatment gives rise to side-effects of the IFN. Surprisingly nucleoside analogues originally developed to treat HIV or HSV, such as lamivudine (3TC), can be potent and well tolerated inhibitors of HBV. The drug acts by inhibiting reverse transcription during the replicative cycle of hepatitis B. It is effective in patients who fail to respond to IFN and can be given orally. Relapses can occur, however, in most patients when they discontinue therapy. It is also used as prophylactic treatment in liver transplants. Nevertheless, drug-resistant mutants emerge using monotherapy. A second nucleoside analogue, adefovir, an acyclic analogue of deoxyadenosine monophosphate has also been licensed for chronic hepatitis B patients.

Clinical trials are in progress with famciclovir (dGTP competitor), adefovir (dATP), and enlecavir (dGTP). Meanwhile treatment of choice uses IFN-α, which is effective in 20–30% of patients, followed by 3TC. More drugs are being synthesized and undoubtedly drug combinations will be favoured to reduce the emergence of drug-resistant viruses.

Cellular proteins as targets for antiviral drugs

The existing antivirals described above have been found or even designed to target viral proteins and thereby ensure specificity and safety. However, the biggest problem is that the viruses can often mutate and thereby become resistant to the drug. A second problem is that drugs that target viral proteins have a narrow spectrum. In contrast many cellular proteins are being identified as essential for viral replication. Most of the drugs used in the wide pharmacopoeia target cellular proteins. Thus cellular toposomerases, nuclear transport proteins, protein kinases are all required for viral replication and experimental inhibition of these proteins has already been shown to repress viral replication. These may be the antivirals of the future.

RNA interference

Mammalian cells have evolved many systems to resist viral infection. dsRNAs, a sign of viral infection in a cell, can activate RNA-dependent protein kinase-mediated responses that include inhibition of translation and even induction of cell death. As a counterbalance, viruses may express dsRNA binding proteins that prevent PCR activation by sequestering dsRNA binding proteins. Short interfering RNAs or micro RNAs downregulate gene expression by binding to complementary mRNAs and either triggering mRNA climation or arresting mRNA translation into protein. There are now the first indications that interference RNAs can be synthesized specifically to a viral mRNA sequence to block viral mRNA but not host mRNA.

6 Interferons

IFNs and their mode of action are described in Chapter 5.

6.1 Clinical application

The possibility of using IFN in the clinic was limited for a long time by the small quantities available. With the development of cDNA cloning technology the situation changed and controlled trials of genetically engineered IFNs have now been conducted. Five IFN preparations are licensed: alpha 2a (Roferon A); alpha 2b (Intron A®); and alpha N3 (Alferon N®), Beta 1B (Betaseron®), and gamma 1B (Actimmune®). Pegylated IFNs have a polyethylene glycol molecule attached to slow absorption and extend serum half life. Thus the standard 3 MIU three times weekly can be reduced to one weekly injection.

Successful trials of recombinant IFNs have been carried out in volunteers infected with rhinoviruses and also in patients with hepatitis B and C, but clinical and laboratory responses are not uniform. Approximately one-third of patients with chronic HBV respond to treatment with 5 million units daily of IFN and remissions may be sustained. The most common side-effects are those of fever, chills, headache, and myalgia, which has led to the supposition that in many acute viral infections these symptoms may in fact be caused by IFNs stimulated by the virus itself.

7 The future

Although chance and virological screening will continue to play a part in the discovery of new antivirals, knowledge of viral gene structure and functioning is leading to a new generation of drugs. To give an example, the interaction between an antiviral compound (disoxaril) and a rhinovirus protein has been visualized at the atomic level by X-ray crystallography. This low molecular weight inhibitor of the common cold virus has been identified as binding in a 'cave' at the bottom of the receptor-binding pocket of the virus. The drug–virus interaction blocks pores in the virion through which ions would normally pass to its interior to aid uncoating. Infection of cells is aborted. Such computer-aided studies at the atomic level can assist the design of new inhibitors. The most exciting example is modification of a drug first discovered 30 years ago and known to block the NA function of influenza. The original drug was not active in animals but computer-guided modification led to synthesis of a related molecule, which can prevent influenza infection in animals and in humans.

In parallel with the search for new drugs, more intensive study of existing ones could give clues to the synthesis of molecular varieties with broader spectra of antiviral activity or prolonged intracellular retention. The antiherpes drug penciclovir is an example.

The emergence of **drug resistance**, a major consideration in antibacterial chemotherapy, is being closely monitored. Strains of HIV, resistant to zidovudine and other dideoxynucleoside analogues, non-nucleoside RT inhibitors, and protease inhibitors have been recovered from AIDS patients. Herpesviruses resistant to ACV have been isolated and may be a problem in immunosuppressed patients, although not yet in normal patients. These drug-resistant herpes variants either have no TK enzyme, or have a genetic change in the viral TK gene. The altered TK does not phosphorylate ACV and so the active antiviral triphosphate molecule is not produced in the virus-infected cell. Similarly, after a few days of treatment with amantadine, drug-resistant strains of influenza A with specific nucleotide changes in the M2 gene may be detectable.

New viruses such as SARS, Nipah, West Nile, and Hendra have emerged recently and have become a focus for drug discovery. The worry about bioterrorism has renewed work on drugs against smallpox and polio. The future will tell whether, as with tuberculosis, combinations of drugs can overcome the high propensity of the dominant variants (quasi-species) of RNA viruses such as influenza and HIV to develop drug resistance; already, mixtures of four drugs are used to treat AIDS patients.

8 Reminders

- Vulnerable points for attack in the virus life cycle are **adsorption** to cells, **penetration, replication of viral genome**, and viral **budding and maturation**. Viral enzymes such as RNA transcriptase, DNA polymerase, protease, and RT are excellent targets for antiviral drugs.

- Antiviral compounds are usually used **therapeutically** to treat infections but **prophylactic** use to prevent infection is sometimes possible. Unlike immunization, administration of an antiviral can give rapid protection against infection, whereas its premature discontinuation may allow the infection to recur.

- At least 30 antiviral drugs acting at various stages of viral replication are licensed for clinical use. They are mostly active against **herpesviruses, influenza A**, and **HIV**, and more recently **hepatitis B**.

- The active form of ACV is the **nucleoside triphosphate**. ACV requires a herpes-coded TK enzyme to add the first phosphate. The triphosphate inhibits herpes DNA polymerase.

- **Prodrugs** namely Famciclovir, the diacetyl version of penciclovir, and valaciclovir, the L-valyl ester of ACV have good bioavailability when given by mouth and are used clinically. The dideoxynucleoside analogue inhibitors of HIV such as AZT are prodrugs and are phosphorylated in both normal and virus-infected cells. Such compounds have a less specific virus inhibitory activity than ACV, which is phosphorylated only in herpes-infected cells.

- Most antiviral drugs have a very narrow spectrum of activity: amantadine or NA inhibitors, such as oseltamivir, inhibit only influenza, ACV inhibits only herpesviruses, and many dideoxynucleoside analogues inhibit only HIV.

- IFN has unexpectedly opened up a new field of cytokine research and is also used in the clinic against hepatitis B and C infection.

- Antivirals have so far been discovered by random biological screening, but viral nucleotide sequence data and X-ray crystallography of virus proteins may lead to a generation of 'designer' drugs. An example is the new class of **inhibitors of influenza NA (oseltamivir and relenza)**.

- **Combination chemotherapy** employing four antiviral drugs each with a different molecular target is now used to treat AIDS patients and reduces the emergence of drug-resistant viruses (HAART).

- Emerging viruses such as **SARS** or **West Nile** or biothreat viruses such as **smallpox** are new target viruses for chemotherapists.

Appendices

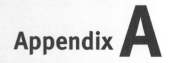

Safety precautions: codes of practice, disinfection, and sterilization

1 Introduction

The question of microbiological hazards of course applies not only to viruses but to all infective agents. It is a large subject, on which much has been written, but its history is littered with disasters befalling those who have ignored the good advice available in abundance. Nowadays, such incidents are comparatively rare, because of greater awareness of the dangers, and the rigorous implementation of safety precautions.

On no account should the following notes be regarded as a guide to safety precautions. They are intended only to give you a general idea of the sort of considerations that apply when dealing with potentially hazardous materials or situations. Since they are extensive, and in any event vary somewhat from place to place, they cannot readily be summarized; at the end of this Appendix we have listed some publications that provide detailed guidance.

The subject falls under two main headings:

(1) Safety in the ward or outpatient department and during transport to the laboratory, which we shall call for convenience the clinical phase.

(2) Safety during processing in the laboratory, the laboratory phase.

Most readers will be mainly concerned with (1).

2 The clinical phase

2.1 Wards and outpatient clinics

In the UK, the handling of clinical specimens must conform with the relevant provisions of the Health and Safety at Work Act and other statutory requirements, which are supplemented by rules that apply to local circumstances. These codes of practice must be readily available to all staff coming into contact with infectious or potentially infectious patients or specimens.

Every hospital must have a Control of Infection Officer, who is often a microbiologist, and a written Control of Infection Policy covering such matters as isolation of infectious and immunocompromised patients; disinfection methods; and procedures for dealing with hazardous microbial diseases, including those due to viruses, AIDS, hepatitis B, and haemorrhagic fevers. There should also be contingency plans for dealing with outbreaks of infection within the hospital; this information must be available to all staff coming into contact with patients.

Another point of particular importance to medical and nursing staff is the safe handling of clinical specimens during collection, storage and transport to the laboratory, and the procedures for dealing with spills or leakages of potentially infective material. The safe disposal of 'sharps' needles, scalpel blades and the like is an essential feature of daily life in the wards and clinics.

All microbiology specimens—including blood samples—must be regarded as potentially infective and handled accordingly.

2.2 Dental departments

Microbiological safety within dental units presents special problems: students are advised to read the appropriate chapters in the book by Samaramayake (1996), Appendix C. Here, we shall mention only the following general points.

Infection of dental staff by patients

It is usually possible to identify potentially infective medical patients, but this is not so with dental patients, any of whom is liable to be shedding one or another virus from the mouth, often without symptoms. Viral infections associated with an enanthem in the mouth are listed in Table 4.4; in all these infections, virus is likely to be present in the saliva. Herpes simplex virus is often shed intermittently in the absence of symptoms and presents a risk of herpetic whitlow to the operator. Cytomegalovirus is also shed in the absence of symptoms, but does not present a hazard. As far as viral infections are concerned, hepatitis B and HIV infections give the greatest cause for concern.

Hepatitis B (Chapter 22)

The blood and oral secretion of HbeAg-positive but symptomless carriers may be infective. Recorded cases of dentists acquiring this infection from patients are rare, but the risk is significant and the appropriate precautions must be taken. It is advisable for all dental care staff having direct contact with patients to receive hepatitis B vaccine.

HIV (Chapter 25)

Patients with full-blown AIDS often have fungal infections of the mouth and the characteristic purplish lesions of Kaposi's sarcoma. Viral infections include chronic herpetic stomatitis, hairy leucoplakia of the tongue (possibly due to EBV infection) and oral condylomata caused by papillomaviruses. Any of these appearances should arose strong suspicion of AIDS, if it has not already been diagnosed. The transmissibility of HIV is

substantially less than that of HBV, but the precautions to be taken are the same.

The golden rule for dentists and oral hygienists is: Always wear rubber gloves when operating in the mouth.

Infection of patients by dentists

There have been several transmissions of hepatitis B to patients from HbeAg-positive dentists. HIV has been transmitted to patients in a dental practice in the USA, and in Romania, patient-to-patient transfer via inadequately sterilized syringes has been reported. Dentists suffering from either of these infections are not necessarily debarred from contact with patients, provided adequate precautions are taken, but obviously, any dental worker suffering from either infection must follow the advice given by an appropriate expert.

Disinfection and sterilization of instruments, prostheses etc

The main considerations here are prevention of cross-infection from patient to patient and from patient to dental laboratory staff. Prostheses and some delicate dental instruments cannot be treated by heat, the most effective method, and recourse must be made to glutaraldehyde (see below). Disposable items are of course preferred whenever possible.

3 The laboratory phase

Microbiology laboratories have their own codes of practice which include an absolute ban on smoking, eating and drinking, and applying cosmetics. Instructions in these rules is given to all new staff, who must sign an undertaking that they have read and understood them. Again, this is not the place for an extended description of these specialized regulations, but you should be aware that laboratories handling microbes, whether for research or diagnostic purposes, are classified in terms of the level of containment they provide, usually on a scale of 1 to 4. Thus routine clinical or teaching laboratories are classified as containment level 1, and those dealing with the most hazardous pathogens, e.g. the haemorrhagic fever viruses, as containment level 4.

3.1 Disinfection and sterilization: routine procedures

Disinfection is the microbiological decontamination of infective material; preliminary cleansing of re-usable items, such as instruments, is an essential part of the process.

Sterilization is the destruction of all infective microbes on a clean article so that it may safely be used for clinical purposes.

Except for the prions (see below) viruses are inactivated by the same procedures as those used for other microbes. Heat is by far the most effective method; typical treatments are autoclaving at 121 °C for 20 min. or hot air oven at 160 °C for 60 min.

Disinfectant solutions are used only when heating is not possible, e.g. for treating contaminated surfaces, pipettes, delicate instruments etc.

The phenolic disinfectants used to kill bacteria are less active against viruses, which are however, readily activated by hypochlorite solutions and, rather less effectively, by glutaraldehyde.

Hypochlorite solutions

These are highly corrosive; gloves and aprons should be worn when making up or using them and they should not be employed on metal equipment. The following working concentrations should be used.

Decontamination of spills of blood or body fluids	10000 parts per million (ppm)
Decontamination of potentially (i.e. not visibly) contaminated surfaces	1000 ppm

Glutaraldehyde solution

Objects to be treated should be first cleansed in detergent and hot water, since glutaraldehyde does not penetrate coagulated protein. They are then immersed in a freshly prepared (same day) 2 per cent solution for at least an hour but preferably overnight. Glutaraldehyde fumes are toxic so that good ventilation is essential when preparing or using it and all containers must be closed. Rubber gloves must be used when handling it.

Prions (Chapter 29)

The agent of Creutzfeld-Jacob disease (CJD), is, like others in this group, unusually resistant to all forms of disinfection. In the UK, the Department of Health and Social Security have issued guidelines for dealing with potentially contaminted instruments and tissues. They include a recommendation that such material should be autoclaved with one cycle at 134 °C for 18 min. holding time, or six cycles each at 134 °C for 3 min. holding time.

4 Further reading

Essential microbiology for dentistry Samaramayake, L.P. (1996), Churchill Livingstone, London.

Guide to blood-borne viruses and the control of cross-infection in dentistry. British Dental Association, 1987

Lloyd, G. and Kiley, M.P. Safety in the virology laboratory (1998) In Topley and Wilson's microbes and microbial infections, 9th edn, pp. 933–46. Arnold, London.

Viral infections notifiable in the UK

Under the Public Health (Infectious Diseases) Regulations 1988, the following are notifiable.

Viral infections	Infections possibly caused by a virus
Haemorrhagic fevers, viral	Encephalitis (acute)
Yellow fever	Meningitis
Hepatitis, viral	Food poisoning
Hepatitis, A, B, and C	
Measles	
Mumps	
Rubella	
Poliomyelitis (acute)	
Rabies	

Suggestions for further reading

This book supplies all the information needed both for passing final undergraduate examinations in virology and for general clinical practice; however, we recognize that in view of the increasing importance of the subject, some of our readers will want to explore various aspects in greater depth. The following list of reference works should prove useful in this respect. In compiling it we have not quoted edition numbers that might become out of date during the life of this book.

General virology

Topley & Wilson's Principles of Bacteriology, Virology and Immunity.
Virology, Volumes 1 and 2.
Mahy, B.W.J. and Volker ter Meulen (eds). Hodder Arnold, London.

A comprehensive account (70 chapters) of general virology, individual viruses and their diseases.

Field's Virology.
Knipe, D.M. and Howly, P.M. (eds). Lippincott Williams & Wilkins, Philadelphia.

A very large reference work (2560 pages) in two volumes. Comes with a CD-ROM.

Viral Infections of Humans: Epidemiology and Control.
Evans, A.S. (ed.). Plenum Publishing Corporation, New York.

This is a first-rate book on the epidemiology of viral infections; it also contains much general information about viruses themselves. Comes with a CD-ROM.

Dictionary of Microbiology and Molecular Biology.
Singleton, P. and Salisbury, D. John Wiley & Sons, Chichester.

Concise and authoritative monographs on the topics covered by the title. Expensive, but a mine of information.

Immunology

Immunology: Instant Notes.
Lydyard, P.M., Whelan, A., and Fanger, M.W. BIOS Scientific Publishers, Oxford.

The importance of immunology to our understanding of the pathogenesis and control of viral infections cannot be overstated. This book is a useful presentation of basic immunology, illustrated with black and white line drawings.

Index